Alfaro's
CLINICAL
JUDGMENT in
NURSING

A How-To Practice Approach

Alfaro's
CLINICAL
JUDGMENT in
NURSING

8th EDITION

A How-To Practice Approach

Donna D. Ignatavicius, MS, RN, CNE, CNEcl, ANEF, FAADN
President,
DI Associates, Inc., Littleton, Colorado

Susan Andersen, MS, RN, CNE
Director of Assessment Evaluation and Quality Improvement,
University of Kansas School of Nursing,
Kansas City, Kansas

ELSEVIER

ELSEVIER
3251 Riverport Lane
St. Louis, Missouri 63043

Notice

Practitioners and researchers must always rely on their own experience and knowledge in evaluating and
using any information, methods, compounds or experiments described herein. Because of rapid advances
in the medical sciences, in particular, independent verification of diagnoses and drug dosages should
be made. To the fullest extent of the law, no responsibility is assumed by Elsevier, authors, editors or
contributors for any injury and/or damage to persons or property as a matter of products liability, negligence
or otherwise, or from any use or operation of any methods, products, instructions, or ideas contained in
the material herein.

Senior Content Strategist: Sonya Seigafuse
Senior Content Development Manager: Lisa Newton
Content Development Specialist: Andrew Schubert
Publishing Services Manager: Deepthi Unni
Project Manager: Kamatchi Madhavan
Design Direction: Patrick Ferguson

Printed in India

Last digit is the print number: 9   8   7   6   5   4   3   2   1

Working together
to grow libraries in
developing countries

www.elsevier.com • www.bookaid.org

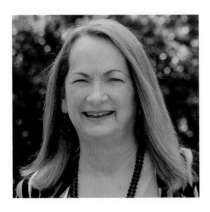

Donna D. Ignatavicius received her diploma in nursing from the Peninsula General School of Nursing in Salisbury, Maryland. After working as a charge nurse in medical-surgical nursing, she became an instructor in staff development at the University of Maryland Medical Center. She then received her BSN from the University of Maryland School of Nursing. For 5 years she taught in several schools of nursing while working toward her MS in Nursing, which she received in 1981. Donna then taught in the BSN program at the University of Maryland, after which she continued to pursue her interest in gerontology and accepted the position of Director of Nursing of a major skilled-nursing facility in her home state of Maryland. Since that time, she has served as an instructor in several associate degree nursing programs. Through her consulting activities, faculty development workshops, and international nursing education conferences (such as Boot Camp for Nurse Educators®), Donna is nationally recognized as an expert in nursing education. She is currently the President of DI Associates, Inc. (http://www.diassociates.com/), a company dedicated to improving health care through education and consultation for faculty. In recognition of her contributions to the field, she was inducted as a charter Fellow of the prestigious Academy of Nursing Education in 2007, received her Certified Nurse Educator credential in 2016, and obtained her Academic Clinical Nurse Educator certification in 2020. Additionally, Donna was inducted as a fellow into the Academy of Associate Degree Nursing in 2021.

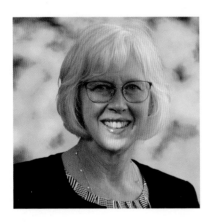

Susan Andersen is the Director of Assessment, Evaluation, and Quality Improvement at the University of Kansas School of Nursing in Kansas City, Kansas. She is an experienced nurse administrator and has served as the Director of Nursing for both an associate degree registered nursing program and a licensed practical nursing program. Sue has taught in the didactic, clinical, and simulation areas at the baccalaureate and associate degree levels, and is experienced in curriculum development, concept-based curriculum, curricular revision, program assessment, and evaluation. She obtained her Certified Nurse Educator® (CNE) credential in 2020 and is a contributor for the Certified Nurse Educator® (CNE) and Certified Nurse Educator Novice® (CNE®n) Exam Prep textbook (2023) edited by Donna Ignatavicius.

Donna:
To my husband Charles for his continued support of my writing; to nursing faculty for their dedication in preparing students to think like nurses to ensure safe entry into practice.

Susan:
To my husband Brian for his continued support, encouragement of my writing, and journey through nursing; to my parents for their encouragement and for providing me the opportunity to become a registered nurse; to my fellow nurses and faculty colleagues as we work together to prepare the next generation of nurses.

PREFACE

The concept of critical thinking has been explored for the past 40 years in nursing practice and education. However, researchers have found that critical thinking is only one type of thinking nurses use when making clinical judgments for diverse clients. As the author of the previous seven editions of this book, Rosalinda Alfaro helped students learn how to become better thinkers as the concepts of critical thinking, clinical reasoning, and clinical judgment (CJ) were evolving.

For this updated eighth book edition, we focus on how to use multiple types of thinking to clinically reason and make safe, appropriate clinical judgments. To facilitate this focus, we restructured this edition to align with the six National Council of State Boards of Nursing (NCSBN) CJ cognitive skills.

ORGANIZATION OF THIS EDITION

According to the NCSBN, about 50% of a nurse's time is spent making clinical judgments for clients who are experiencing or are at risk for experiencing clinical deterioration or medical complications. Therefore, we organized this new edition to help students learn how to make safe, evidence-based clinical judgments for diverse clients in a variety of health care settings.

- **Chapter 1** provides the introduction to the concept of clinical judgment and describes the interrelationships of critical thinking, clinical reasoning, and clinical judgment. Examples of the newest Next-Generation NCLEX® (NGN) test items that measure the ability to apply CJ cognitive skills are also presented.
- **Chapters 2 through 7** focus on each NCSBN cognitive skill needed to make safe clinical judgments. Each chapter provides a practical, evidence-based, how-to approach with multiple Thinking Exercises in which students can practice applying one of the cognitive skills. Thinking Exercises are interspersed throughout each chapter and at the end of each chapter. These exercises provide diverse client situations from multiple clinical specialties and health care settings. Answers and rationales for all exercises are included at the end of their respective chapters.
- **Chapter 8** provides a brief summary on how to make safe clinical judgments followed by multiple unfolding case studies and stand-alone test items for student practice in applying all six cognitive skills. Answers and rationales for all test questions are included at the end of the chapter.

CHAPTER FEATURES IN THIS EDITION

Each chapter of the new eighth edition provides special features, as appropriate, to make content accessible and reader-friendly. These features include:

- **This Chapter at a Glance:** A list of major headings within the chapter is presented to help students easily access information.
- **Chapter Learning Outcomes:** A list of learning outcomes that students can achieve by reading the chapter and completing the thinking exercises is provided.
- **Key Terms:** A list of important terms found within the chapter are listed with definitions for quick reference; each key term is bolded within the chapter.

- **Bulleted Content:** Some content is listed in an accessible, easy-to-read format rather than presented in a long, run-on sentence or paragraph.
- **Clinical Judgment Tips:** Boxes highlighting essential information to remember are interspersed throughout each chapter.
- **Tables and Boxes:** Important content within the chapter is highlighted or expanded in easy-to-read tables and boxes. Tables have at least two columns; boxed content does not.
- **Evidence-Based Practice Boxes:** Summaries of recent research that support chapter content are presented.
- **Chapter References:** Citations for chapter references are provided; classic references are specified as such.

HOW TO USE THIS BOOK

The eighth edition of this book is an essential interactive learning resource for all prelicensure nursing students. This completely revised new edition expands the basic description on clinical judgment presented in most other nursing textbooks by providing the evidence, theoretical foundation, and thinking exercises for every CJ cognitive skill.

One suggestion for using this book is to require its introduction in the first nursing semester and integrate its content throughout the program. The focus of the first nursing semester is typically on client assessment and the role of the professional nurse. The first three chapters of the eighth edition include an introduction to clinical judgment, how to recognize cues, and how to analyze cues. These chapters could be assigned for students in the first semester because they align with client assessment and the nurse's role.

For the second semester, Chapters 4 through 7 are appropriate to assign; students can work through the thinking exercises in these chapters and discuss in class. Chapter 8 could be assigned for the third nursing semester where students can practice NGN-style test items to "put it all together" and apply the six CJ cognitive skills. Additional NGN practice items can be found in the primary author's (DI) workbooks entitled *Developing Clinical Judgment* (RN and PN/VN versions) published by Elsevier, Inc.

During each semester, faculty should facilitate and assess student learning regarding how to use CJ cognitive skills. Suggestions for facilitating and assessing this learning include:

- Thinking "out loud" to explain the clinical reasoning process for the book's Thinking and End-of-Chapter Exercises
- Reviewing the Clinical Judgment Tips to reinforce the most vital content for practice readiness
- Discussing how research findings from the Evidence-Based Practice boxes contribute to understanding clinical judgment and clinical reasoning using the six cognitive skills
- Practicing diagraming thinking for each cognitive step of the clinical judgment process using the Thinking and End-of-Chapter Exercises.
- Practicing completing Unfolding Case Studies and Stand-Alone items before or during class; discussing the answers and rationales for correct and incorrect responses
- Adding newer NGN test item types on unit exams and/or quizzes

Another suggestion is to use this book as a guide to accompany a stand-alone course (or courses) focusing on Clinical Judgment. Students could begin using the book in the first semester in foundational courses, especially focusing on the first three chapters to become familiar with the cognitive skills of clinical judgment and focus on Recognize and Analyze Cues. In the Clinical Judgment course, Chapters 4 through 8 would then be appropriate to assign; students can work through the thinking exercises in these chapters and discuss in class. Students could then practice

NGN-style test items to "put it all together" and apply the six CJ cognitive skills towards the end of the Clinical Judgment course. This process will prepare students to apply the cognitive skills when providing care for clients in clinical learning experiences.

We hope you will enjoy using this book and encourage your students to fully engage with the content, thinking exercises, and NGN-style test items.

Donna Ignatavicius and Susan Andersen

ACKNOWLEDGMENTS

The author team is grateful for the Elsevier editorial, production, and design staff. Special thanks to Sonya Seigafuse, Senior Content Strategist; Andrew Schubert, Content Development Specialist; Kamatchi Madhavan, Senior Project Manager; and Patrick Ferguson, Senior Book Designer, who provided ongoing editorial guidance and support and worked to keep the text production on track.

CONTENTS

Introduction to Clinical Reasoning and Clinical Judgment

1

THIS CHAPTER AT A GLANCE...

Nurses' Role in Client Safety
Brief Review of the Nursing Process
- Historical Perspective
- NCSBN Definition

Clinical Reasoning
- Definition
- Phases

Essential Types of Thinking for Clinical Reasoning
- Novice Versus Expert Thinking
- Critical Thinking

Thinking Ahead, Thinking-In-Action, and Thinking Back
Clinical Judgment
- Description
- NCSBN Definition
- Models
- Thinking Skills

Developing Clinical Judgment Skills for Nursing Practice and NGN Readiness
- Nursing Practice Readiness
- NGN Readiness

LEARNING OUTCOMES

1. Identify commonly occurring nursing errors (missed nursing care) that can cause undesirable client outcomes.
2. Describe the six steps of the nursing process as outlined by the most recent ANA *Nursing Scope and Standards of Practice.*
3. Differentiate clinical reasoning and clinical judgment.
4. Distinguish the types of thinking needed for clinical reasoning.

5. List the six cognitive (thinking) skills needed to make sound clinical judgments.
6. Explain why clinical judgment skills are essential for nursing practice and Next-Generation NCLEX® (NGN) readiness.
7. Identify the new test item formats that are part of the NGN.

KEY TERMS

Abductive reasoning: The ability to use reflection on the explanation for a conclusion or observation about a client.

Clinical judgment: The observed outcome of critical thinking and decision-making. It is an iterative process that uses nursing knowledge to observe and assess presenting situations, identify a prioritized client concern, and generate the best possible evidence-based solutions in order to deliver safe client care.

Clinical reasoning: The cognitive (thinking) process of identifying a client's actual or potential problems or needs, collecting and analyzing client assessment data, hypothesizing and performing nursing actions, and evaluating and reflecting on the actions to determine if they were effective.

Critical thinking: The cognitive process in which the nurse examines client assessment data using reflection and reasoning to determine appropriate action.

1

Deductive reasoning (deduction): The ability to determine specific hypotheses or client problems from multiple general possibilities.

Inductive reasoning: The ability to make generalizations when observing, identifying, and organizing important signs and symptoms (cues) into patterns to make a conclusion about what a client is experiencing.

Missed nursing care: Any aspect of required client care that is omitted or delayed; may be deliberately missed.

Nursing process: A systematic method for problem-solving to make safe, client-centered care decisions.

Critical thinking, clinical decision-making, clinical reasoning, and clinical judgment are concepts that are sometimes used interchangeably in the nursing profession. However, although they are interrelated, these terms are not the same. This chapter introduces and differentiates these concepts to help you better understand their importance in preparing for entry into nursing practice and ensuring client safety.

NURSES' ROLE IN CLIENT SAFETY

All nurses, including new graduates, must be able to care for clients competently and safely. According to the latest *Nursing Scope and Standards of Practice*, client safety is the "condition of preventing harm or other undesirable outcomes" (American Nurses Association, 2021, p. 41). Harm to clients can be caused by individual (nurse or other health care team member) or health care system errors. Client errors can be either an act of commission (doing something wrong like administering an incorrect medication) or omission (failing to do the right thing like not frequently turning a client to prevent pressure injury).

Classic research by Benner et al. (2010) identified commonly occurring examples of client errors caused by nurses, which include:

- Lack of attentiveness and client monitoring
- Inadequate actions to prevent health complications
- Failure to carry out interventions in an appropriate and timely manner
- Lack of ability to make safe clinical judgments

These examples could also be described as missed nursing care according to Kalisch et al. (2009) in their classic concept analysis. Missed nursing care includes any aspect of required client care that is omitted or delayed, and may be deliberate. Intentional missed nursing care, also called undone nursing care, occurs when you do not have the time or skill to perform a nursing activity or task. The errors identified by Benner et al. (2010) are *not* intentional and are often caused by lack of critical thinking. The ANA *Standards of Practice* specify expected competencies using the nursing process as the critical thinking model for professional practice (ANA, 2021).

BRIEF REVIEW OF THE NURSING PROCESS

Many American and Canadian nursing programs include the nursing process in their curricula (Doane & Varcoe, 2021). The nursing process is a systematic method for problem-solving to make safe, client-centered care decisions (Ignatavicius, 2024).

Historical Perspective

The nursing process model has been used since the 1960s as the gold standard to guide professional nursing practice and has been measured on the nursing licensure examination (NCLEX®) for many years. The American Nurses Association states that the "common thread uniting different types of nurses who work in varied areas is the nursing process" (https://www.nursingworld.org/practice-policy/workforce/what-is-nursing/the-nursing-process/).

The original four steps of the nursing process in the late 1960s were:
1. Assessment
2. Planning
3. Implementation
4. Evaluation

In the early 1970s, a new organization called the North American Nursing Diagnosis Association (NANDA) was formed in an attempt to develop a common nursing language (nursing diagnoses) based on nurses' interpretation of assessment data. This additional step of Diagnosis modified the nursing process to ADPIE, a five-step approach to problem-solving. You probably learned these steps in your nursing program:
1. Assessment
2. Diagnosis
3. Planning
4. Implementation
5. Evaluation

The most recent ANA *Nursing Scope and Standards of Practice* added Outcomes Identification as an additional step in the nursing process (ANA, 2021). Table 1.1 briefly describes each step of the most current version of this model.

TABLE 1.1   Nursing Process Steps With Descriptions

Steps of the Nursing Process	Descriptions of Nursing Process Steps
Assessment	Collecting pertinent information about the client situation through observation, interview, and health assessment
Diagnosis	Analyzing client information to determine actual or potential diagnoses, problems, and issues
Outcomes identification	Identifying expected outcomes for a plan of care individualized for a client situation
Planning	Developing a collaborative plan of care to prioritize client needs and achieve expected outcomes
Implementation	Performing evidence-based interventions and strategies to meet expected outcomes
Evaluation	Determining progress toward achieving expected outcomes

Adapted from American Nurses Association (ANA). (2021). *Nursing scope and standards of practice.* (4th ed.). Silver Spring, MD: ANA.

Although the nursing process was not intended to be used in a linear manner, students and nurses entering the profession often use this model from the first step through the last step in sequential order.

NCSBN Definition

According to the National Council of State Boards of Nursing (NCSBN) who regulates the nursing profession and administers the nursing licensure exam (NCLEX®), the nursing process is an appropriate model for managing *basic* client problems and remains an Integrated Process in its licensure test plans. The most recent definition of the nursing process in the 2023 NCLEX-RN® test plan is "a scientific, clinical reasoning approach to client care that includes assessment, analysis, planning, implementation and evaluation" (NCSBN, 2023, p. 4). This five-step approach does not include Diagnosis but rather substitutes the term "Analysis." Because Diagnosis suggests the use of NANDA nursing diagnoses, the NCLEX® does not assess your ability to use this specific language to identify client problems or conditions. The 2023 NCLEX-PN® test plan defines the problem-solving process (nursing process) as a scientific approach to client care that includes data collection, planning, implementation, and evaluation.

Many health care settings do not use NANDA nursing diagnoses but rather use common medical terminology like signs and symptoms that can be communicated and clearly understood by all members of the interprofessional health care team, including the client and client's family. In addition, permission to use NANDA terminology is costly and research supporting the diagnoses is weak or outdated. Analysis as a nursing process step is a broader term used to describe the ability to process and interpret appropriate assessment data (clinical cues) to identify actual and potential client problems or conditions.

CLINICAL JUDGMENT TIP

Remember: When communicating with members of the health care team, use common terms like signs and symptoms that can be clearly understood.

CLINICAL REASONING

The NCSBN definition of the nursing process includes "scientific clinical reasoning." Clinical reasoning is an essential skill for all health care professionals today more than ever, especially for nurses who spend more time providing direct care than other professionals for increasingly complex clients in acute, long-term, and home health care settings.

Definition

Many articles on clinical reasoning and clinical judgment have been published over the past 25 years, but definitions of these concepts have been overlapping and confusing. The definitions of "reasoning" in major dictionaries generally include:
- Action of thinking in a logical, sensible manner
- Process of making a conclusion or inference
- Process of thinking to make a decision

While these definitions vary somewhat, all of them refer to reasoning as a deliberate thinking *process*.

To help clarify the role of clinical reasoning for nursing practice, Simmons (2010) performed a major concept analysis. As part of that analysis, the author defined clinical reasoning as a complex process that uses cognition (thinking) and nursing knowledge to collect and analyze client information, interpret its significance, and weigh alternative nursing actions.

Levett-Jones et al. (2010) developed a model outlining the *five rights* of clinical reasoning to help nursing students identify and manage clients who are at high risk for medical complications or clinical deterioration:
1. Right cues
2. Right action
3. Right client
4. Right time
5. Right reason

In other words, effective clinical reasoning depends on your ability to recognize the right cues to take the right action for the right client at the right time for the right reason.

More recently, Joplin-Gonzales and Rounds (2022) applied this updated definition of clinical reasoning for their nursing research: **Clinical reasoning** is the cognitive (thinking) process of identifying a client's actual or potential problems or needs, collecting and analyzing client assessment data, hypothesizing and performing nursing actions, and evaluating and reflecting on the actions to determine if they were effective. Sometimes referred to as *clinical decision-making*, this more current definition includes reflection and analysis, which are integrated throughout the clinical reasoning process.

Phases

All health care professionals need to use the clinical reasoning process when providing client care. Yet despite many studies focusing on clinical reasoning, there has been no consensus on the phases or elements of clinical reasoning. A recent Delphi study by Joplin-Gonzales and Rounds (2022) identified five phases of clinical reasoning that you will use in daily practice (Table 1.2).

TABLE 1.2   Phases of Clinical Reasoning With Descriptions

Phases of Clinical Reasoning	Descriptions of Clinical Reasoning Phases
Client problem presentation	Recognizing and identifying one or more client problems
Client problem assessment	Collecting client data (subjective and objective) and recognizing patterns
Client problem analysis	Analyzing and interpreting data to determine relationships
Client problem hypothesis	Categorizing data to determine client priority problem (hypothesis) and actions
Client problem evaluation	Testing and evaluating the hypothesis to determine client response to actions

Adapted from Joplin-Gonzales, P., & Rounds, L. (2022). The essential elements of clinical reasoning. *Nurse Educator,* *47*(5), E145–E149.

During the clinical reasoning process, nurses use several types of reasoning including:

- Inductive reasoning
- Deductive reasoning
- Abductive reasoning

Inductive reasoning (induction) is the ability to make generalizations when observing, identifying, and organizing important signs and symptoms (cues) into patterns to make a conclusion about what a client is experiencing. Induction is used during the client problem presentation and assessment phases of clinical reasoning (see Table 1.2). For example, let's say you are caring for a hospitalized client who experienced abdominal trauma, and the client suddenly experiences sharp chest pain, dyspnea, tachycardia, and decreased peripheral oxygen saturation. Knowing clients who have trauma or surgery are at risk for venous thromboembolism and having knowledge of pathophysiology, you would conclude that this client's signs and symptoms are consistent with this complication. Or, the client could be experiencing a new problem not associated with previous trauma such as a myocardial infarction.

Deductive reasoning (deduction) is the ability to determine specific hypotheses or client problems from multiple general possibilities. Deduction is used during the client problem analysis and hypothesis phases of clinical reasoning (see Table 1.2). In the example of the client who experienced abdominal trauma, the client is likely developing one of several conditions. You would want to collect additional assessment data, including a full set of vital signs and more specific information about the client's pain, to narrow down the likely health condition.

Abductive reasoning is the ability to reflect on the explanation for a conclusion or observation about a client. This reflective thinking is used during the evaluation phase of clinical reasoning (see Table 1.2). For example, after actions for the client's health condition or medical complication are implemented, you would reassess the client reflecting on the care to determine if the actions were effective or not and if the condition has improved, stayed the same, or worsened.

ESSENTIAL TYPES OF THINKING FOR CLINICAL REASONING

All nurses are novice practitioners at some point in their careers. Novice nurses, including new graduates, demonstrate novice clinical reasoning skills. But experienced nurses can be novices at times, too, such as when they care for clients with conditions with which they are not familiar. For example, when the COVID-19 pandemic emerged, many experienced nurses were novices and used novice thinking when caring for clients with this new type of viral infection. This example demonstrates that nurses must continually acquire knowledge and experiences to enhance and refine their thinking skills and nursing expertise. Don't ever be afraid to say, "I'm unfamiliar with dealing with clients with these conditions and need help."

Nurse thinking also changes depending on context (circumstances); what works in one clinical situation may not work in another. For example, think about the difference between caring for children versus caring for adults. Growth and development issues and differences in anatomy and physiology affect many aspects of care. Realize that you may be an expert nurse, but if the circumstances change and you are unfamiliar with giving care under those circumstances, you will likely use novice thinking.

CLINICAL JUDGMENT TIP

Remember: Nurse thinking changes depending on context (circumstances); what works in one clinical situation may not work in another.

Novice Versus Expert Thinking

Benner (2001) described the five stages nurses go through as they progress from novice to expert during their career, which include:

1. *Novice:* Beginning practitioners who lack experience in specific clinical situations (e.g., a new graduate with no experience in nursing or an experienced acute psychiatric nurse who is beginning to work in long-term care).
2. *Advanced beginner:* Those with marginally acceptable performance based on a foundation of experience with real clinical situations (e.g., a nurse who is in the first year of employment or the first year of a new clinical specialty).
3. *Competent:* Those with 2 or 3 years of experience in similar clinical situations (e.g., a nurse who has practiced critical care nursing for 2 or 3 years).
4. *Proficient:* Those with broad experience that allows meaning to be understood in terms of the "big picture" rather than isolated observations (e.g., a nurse who is in charge of making client assignments).
5. *Expert:* Those with extensive experiences that enable an intuitive grasp of situations and problems (e.g., an experienced nurse who serves as charge nurse, preceptor, or member of a health care committee).

This classic research demonstrated that the novice nurse advances toward becoming an expert nurse through developing thinking skills and gaining nursing experience. These experiences provide the novice the opportunity to use clinical reasoning to improve clinical outcomes. Box 1.1 compares novice to expert thinking.

BOX 1.1 Novice Versus Expert Thinking	
Novice Nurses	**Expert Nurses**
• Often unaware of what they don't know	• Know the limitations of their own knowledge
• Knowledge is organized as separate facts. Rely heavily on resources (e.g., texts, notes, preceptors). Lack knowledge gained from experience (e.g., listening to breath sounds)	• Knowledge is organized and structured, making recall of information easier. Have a lot of experiential knowledge (e.g., what abnormal breath sounds are like, what subtle changes look like)
• Focus so much on actions that they tend to forget to assess before acting	• Assess and think things through before acting
• Need clear-cut rules	• Know when to bend the rules
• Hampered by unawareness of resources	• Aware of resources and how to use them
• Hindered by the brain-drains of anxiety and lack of self-confidence	• Self-confident, less anxious, and more focused
• Have limited knowledge of suspected problems; therefore, they question and collect data more superficially	• Have a better idea of suspected problems, allowing them to question more deeply and collect more relevant and in-depth data
• Rely on step-by-step procedures. Tend to focus more on procedures than on the client response to the procedure	• Know when it's safe to skip steps or do two steps together. Are able to focus on both the parts (the procedures) and the whole (the client response)
• Become uncomfortable if client needs prevent performing procedures exactly as they were learned	• Comfortable with rethinking procedure if client needs necessitate modification of the procedure
• Follow standards and policies by rote	• Analyze standards and policies, looking for ways to improve them
• Learn more readily when matched with a supportive, knowledgeable preceptor or mentor	• Are challenged by novices' questions, clarifying their own thinking when teaching novices

The progression of thinking from novice to expert requires the development of critical thinking skills as the foundation of clinical reasoning.

Critical Thinking

Numerous definitions of critical thinking are cited in the literature and tend to vary based on the discipline in which they are used. Unlike thinking in general, critical thinking is deliberate, important, and purposeful. It is an intellectual process involving your ability to analyze and use logic, and is influenced by habits of the mind, such as open-mindedness, confidence, and reflection (Lunney, 2010). From a nursing perspective, critical thinking is the cognitive process in which the nurse examines client assessment data using reflection and reasoning to determine appropriate action (Connor et al., 2022). Critical thinking requires left-brain thinking (logical and *analytical*—judging the worth of those ideas) and right-brain thinking (*creative* and intuitive—generating new ideas), and is a building block for clinical reasoning and judgment.

Analytical thinking follows a logical process of eliminating ideas to narrow the range of possibilities to one most likely specific solution or condition. Similar to deductive reasoning, it is the mental process of taking complex information and breaking it down into basic parts to arrive at the best or correct option. Part of analysis is the ability to interpret client information (cues) to determine a client's actual or potential condition.

According to a recent concept analysis, creativity in nursing care can be defined as development and acceptance of new ideas for client care such that the new methods are simple, useful, efficient, affordable, and safe. Creative nursing care requires a creative vision and *creative thinking* (Cheraghi et al., 2021).

> ### CLINICAL JUDGMENT TIP
>
> *Remember:* Critical thinking requires left-brain thinking (logical and *analytical*—judging the worth of those ideas) and right-brain thinking (*creative* and intuitive—generating new ideas), and is a building block for clinical reasoning and judgment.

THINKING AHEAD, THINKING-IN-ACTION, AND THINKING BACK

Tanner (2006) coined the term "thinking like a nurse" to emphasize the importance of clinical reasoning and judgment in today's complex clinical settings. In addition to exploring types of thinking needed for making clinical decisions, you need to consider when thinking should occur. Thinking can be divided into three phases based on time:

1. Thinking ahead
2. Thinking-in-action
3. Thinking back

Thinking ahead involves anticipating what might happen and being proactive by identifying what you can do to be prepared. For novices, thinking ahead is difficult and sometimes restricted to reading policies and procedures. An important part of being proactive is asking questions like, "What can I do to help jog my memory and stay focused and organized?"

Thinking-in-action is often called "thinking on your feet." It is rapid, dynamic reasoning that considers several things at once, making it difficult to describe. For example, suppose you find your stove on fire. As you spring into action, your mind races, thinking about many things at once ("How can I put this out?" "Where's the fire extinguisher?" "Should I call the fire department?"). Thinking-in-action is highly influenced by previous knowledge and clinical experience. To keep safety first in all important situations, refer to experts nearby who have extensive experiential knowledge stored in their brains. If you encountered a fire, wouldn't you like to have a fireperson standing at your side? Thinking-in-action is prone to "knee-jerk" responses and decisions. For instance, an untrained person may throw water on a grease fire, which can make it worse.

Thinking back (reflecting on thinking) involves analyzing and deconstructing your reasoning to look for flaws or errors, gain a greater understanding of the situation, and make corrections. Experienced nurses double-check their thinking in dynamic ways during thinking-in-action. However, this process does not replace reflective thinking that happens *after* a situation occurs.

Considering all three of these phases of thinking helps you examine thinking in a holistic way. If you look only at *one phase*, you will likely miss important components of the thinking process.

CLINICAL JUDGMENT

Although the nursing process, critical thinking, clinical reasoning, and clinical decision-making have been discussed in the literature and taught in nursing education for decades, nursing errors remain high in practice, especially among novice nurses. About two-thirds of adverse events among hospitalized clients are a result of poor clinical decision-making; 80% of employers are *not* satisfied with the decision-making abilities of entry-level nurses (Saintsing et al., 2011).

As you are probably aware, nurses are required to provide safe and effective care in multilayered complex health care settings that demand higher level cognitive and clinical skills when compared to previous decades (Clemett & Raleigh, 2021). Making sound clinical judgments is the foundation of professional nursing practice, positively influencing client outcomes and ensuring client safety (Manetti, 2019). Improving the quality of client care is dependent on your ability to develop strong clinical judgment skills. While clinical reasoning is the *process* for nurse thinking, clinical judgment is the result or *outcome* of that thinking (Fig. 1.1).

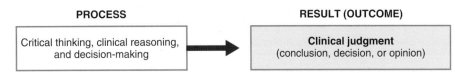

FIG. 1.1 Clinical judgment—the result of critical thinking, clinical reasoning, and decision-making.

A number of definitions reinforcing clinical judgment as an outcome have been published in the nursing literature. Classic research by Tanner (2006) demonstrated the most common thinking process used by nurses is clinical reasoning rather than the nursing process. This researcher made the following conclusions to describe clinical judgment based the analysis of the nursing literature:

1. Clinical judgments are more influenced by *what the nurse brings to the situation* (like knowledge and experience) than the objective data about the situation.
2. Sound clinical judgment rests to some degree on *knowing the client* and the client's pattern of responses.
3. Clinical judgments are influenced by the *context* in which the situation occurs and the culture of the nursing unit.
4. Nurses use a *variety of reasoning patterns* alone or in combination when making clinical judgments.
5. *Reflection on practice* is critical for the development of clinical knowledge and improvement in clinical reasoning.

Since Tanner's study was published, several nursing education organizations have published their definitions of clinical judgment. For example, the National League for Nursing (NLN) states that nurses make judgments in practice, supported by sound evidence (best practices), that integrate nursing science to provide safe, quality care (outcome) (NLN, 2012). Most recently, the American Association of Colleges of Nursing (AACN) *Essentials* document defines clinical judgment as a process in which nurses make decisions (outcomes) based on nursing knowledge, critical thinking, and clinical reasoning (AACN, 2023).

CLINICAL JUDGMENT TIP

Remember. While clinical reasoning is the *process* for nurse thinking, clinical judgment is the result or *outcome* of that thinking.

Description

Although multiple definitions and descriptions of clinical judgment have been published, all of them emphasize that clinical judgment uses the reasoning process to make a decision to achieve positive client outcomes. Several nursing authors have explored the concept of clinical judgment in more detail by conducting concept analyses. The most recent analysis by Connor et al. (2022) defined clinical judgment as a reflective and reasoning process that is informed by a nursing knowledge base to form clinical conclusions (outcomes) (Box 1.2).

> **BOX 1.2   Evidence-Based Practice**
>
> **What Is Clinical Judgment in Nursing?**
> Based on Connor, J., Phil, M., Flenady, T., Massey, D., & Dwyer, T. (2022). Clinical judgement in nursing—An evolutionary concept analysis. *Journal of Clinical Nursing, 32*(13–14), 3328–3340.
>   The authors conducted a concept analysis using Rodgers' evolutionary method to develop a contemporary definition of clinical judgment in nursing. Eighteen peer-reviewed journal articles were analyzed. Three commonly cited elements of clinical judgment were identified in the literature:
> * The ability to clinically reason
> * The ability to use one's own knowledge base and clinical experience within the situation
> * The ability to use reflection to make decisions
>   Decision-making was identified as the major consequence (outcome) of clinical judgment in nursing.

Jacobs et al. (2018) conducted a descriptive survey of practicing nurses to identify their perception of clinical judgment characteristics. Examples of study findings included that nurses perceive clinical judgment:

1. Is essential for safe client care
2. Is context (circumstance) dependent
3. Requires interpretation of client needs
4. Requires knowledge based on experience

These findings validated the results of previous research and the conclusions drawn from other literature sources.

NCSBN Definition

As a result of continued client errors caused by practicing nurses, especially those entering into practice, in 2012 the National Council for State Boards of Nursing (NCSBN) began to examine the need for a potential change in the nursing licensure examinations (NCLEX®) to measure clinical judgment abilities. Based on an in-depth review of multiple studies and related journal articles, the NCSBN determined that nurses use clinical judgment skills to manage *complex* client conditions. An analysis of new graduates found that making sound clinical judgments is one of the most essential skills needed for nursing practice.

The NCSBN's definition of clinical judgment is *"the observed outcome of critical thinking and decision-making. It is an iterative process that uses nursing knowledge to observe and assess presenting situations, identify a prioritized client concern, and generate the best possible evidence-based solutions in order to deliver safe client care"* (NCSBN, 2023, p. 4). Consider the following key points in this definition:

* Clinical judgment is the result or *outcome of thinking* to make decisions about client care when potential or actual health problems occur. The same process of thinking to make clinical decisions occurs repeatedly as you manage client problems (*iterative process*).
* Clinical judgment requires recall of *nursing knowledge* to make appropriate clinical judgments. (However, having knowledge does not guarantee an accurate or appropriate clinical judgment will be made.)
* Clinical judgment requires the nurse to *prioritize* a client's need for care based on the data presented about a clinical situation.
* Clinical judgment requires the use of *best current evidence* regarding a presented client situation so you can come up with possible solutions or approaches for care to keep the client *safe*.

The NCSBN recently added Clinical Judgment with its definition as an additional Integrated Process in the NCLEX-RN® and NCLEX-PN® Test Plans.

Models

One of the first models of clinical judgment was developed by Tanner (2006), who described four phases:

1. *Noticing:* Having a "grasp" on a clinical situation by being proactive regarding client expectations.
2. *Interpreting:* Determining the meaning of the client's clinical situation.
3. *Responding:* Deciding on whether to act on the client's clinical situation; if action is needed, selecting the most appropriate actions.
4. *Reflecting:* Determining how the client is responding to the nurse's actions and if actions need to be adjusted based on that response.

The NCSBN created a clinical judgment model from a blend of several models, including Tanner's work, called the NCSBN Clinical Judgment Measurement Model (NCJMM). As the name implies, this more recent model was created to measure the nursing graduate's ability to make clinical judgments. While it is not important for you to be familiar with the entire model, it is essential that you master the cognitive (thinking) skills associated with clinical judgment. The NCJMM identifies six cognitive (thinking) skills that are needed for effective professional nursing practice and will serve as the basis for the new NGN test item types. These skills are Layer 3 of the NCJMM, also called the Clinical Judgment Practice or Action Model.

The NCJMM also identifies factors that influence the ability of nurses to make appropriate clinical judgments. Examples of these environmental and individual factors, sometimes referred to as Layer 4 of the NCJMM, are listed in Box 1.3. Individual factors are those related to the practicing nurse or candidate taking the nursing licensure examination.

BOX 1.3 Example of Environmental and Individual Factors That Influence Clinical Judgment

Examples of Environmental Factors	Examples of Individual Factors
Environment	Knowledge
Medical records	Skills
Time pressure	Specialty
Task complexity	Prior experience
Resources	Level of experience
Cultural considerations	Nurse or candidate characteristics
Client observation	
Consequences and risks	

Thinking Skills

The Next-Generation NCLEX® (NGN) includes new test item types that measure the six cognitive steps of clinical judgment, often referred to as clinical reasoning or thinking skills. Each of these thinking skills is briefly introduced in this chapter. Chapters 2 through 7 in this book describe these skills in more detail and present examples of NGN test items as Thinking Exercises that are designed to measure each skill. The definitions of the six thinking skills essential for clinical judgment are listed in Box 1.4 with key questions that summarize the focus of each skill.

BOX 1.4   Clinical Judgment Skills with Definitions and Key Questions

Recognize Cues: Identify relevant and important information from different sources (e.g., medical history, vital signs). *What matters most and now?*

Analyze Cues: Organize and connect the recognized cues to the client's clinical presentation. *What could it mean?*

Prioritize Hypotheses: Evaluate and prioritize hypotheses (urgency, likelihood, risk, difficulty, time constraints, etc.). *Where do I start?*

Generate Solutions: Identify expected outcomes and use hypotheses to define a set of interventions for the expected outcomes. *What can I do?*

Take Actions: Implement the solution(s) that address the highest priority. *What will I do?*

Evaluate Outcomes: Compare observed outcomes to expected outcomes. *Did it help?*

From National Council of State Boards of Nursing (NCSBN). (2023). *Next-Generation NCLEX®: NCLEX-RN® Test Plan.* Chicago, IL: NCSBN.

Recognize Cues

For clients in any health care setting, the nurse collects client data from a number of sources. Cues, also called clinical cues, are client findings or assessment data that provide information for nurses as a basis for decision-making to make appropriate clinical judgments, and can be divided into four major types as listed below.

1. Environmental cues; e.g., presence of family member
2. Client observation cues; e.g., signs and symptoms
3. Medical record cues; e.g., lab values and vital signs
4. Time pressure cues; e.g., rate of clinical decline

In actual clinical practice, the nurse reviews all client findings to determine which data are abnormal, relevant, and of immediate concern. To help you *Recognize Cues*, ask yourself, "Which client data are most important in the presented clinical scenario?" Carefully review the client's presenting data, such as developmental age and medical diagnosis, to determine their relevance. Chapter 2 discusses how to recognize cues in detail.

Analyze Cues

After relevant cues are identified in a clinical scenario, the nurse organizes and links them to the client's presenting clinical situation. Ask yourself: "What do the relevant client data mean or indicate at this time?" For example, consider a client who has a history of transient ischemic attacks and begins to experience difficulty speaking, facial drooping, and right-arm weakness. To link these assessment findings with an acute ischemic stroke, you need knowledge of pathophysiology, especially signs and symptoms. In some clinical situations, the client may have *multiple* relevant cues that are associated with several different client conditions. Chapter 3 describes how to analyze cues in detail.

CLINICAL JUDGMENT TIP

Remember: To recognize and analyze cues, you are not required to make a medical diagnosis but rather will be expected to connect or link client findings with selected client conditions or health problems, either actual or potential.

Prioritize Hypotheses

After organizing, grouping, and linking relevant client findings with actual or potential client conditions, the skill *Prioritize Hypotheses* requires you to narrow down what the data mean and prioritize the client's problems or needs. While you may have learned about priority decision-making models such as the ABCs or Maslow's Hierarchy of Needs, these models are not very useful in helping you make clinical judgments in *complex* clinical situations. Clients typically have multiple comorbidities that affect their primary health problems, needs, or concerns, which add to the complexity of their care.

To prioritize hypotheses, review and evaluate each of the client's needs or health problems in the clinical situation. Then rank them to decide what is *most likely* the priority health problem. Evaluate factors in the clinical situation such as urgency, risk, difficulty, and time sensitivity for the client. Chapter 4 discusses how to prioritize hypotheses in detail.

Generate Solutions and Take Actions

After identifying the client's priority problem in a given clinical situation, you want to think about all possible actions that can be used to resolve or manage the problem. To assist in selecting the possible actions or approach to care you might include, first determine what outcomes are desired or expected for the client. The next step in this thinking process is to identify potential nursing actions that could achieve the desired outcomes. Also identify which actions should be avoided or not indicated. Some nursing actions may focus on collecting additional information about the client through frequent monitoring.

After the list of potential actions is identified for each desired outcome, determine which actions should be implemented to meet the priority needs of the client. Deciding which actions to take is the focus of taking actions. After generating a list of possible actions, determine the most appropriate action or combination of actions that will resolve or manage the client's priority health problems or concerns. Also determine how each action will be implemented. Examples of methods to accomplish or implement actions include what to communicate, document, perform, administer, teach, or request from a health care provider or other member of the health care team. Chapters 5 and 6 discuss how to generate solutions and take actions in detail.

Evaluate Outcomes

The last clinical judgment thinking skill is to determine if the actions implemented for the client resolved or effectively managed the health problem(s). The best way to make that determination is to compare what the desired or expected outcomes are with current client findings or observed outcomes. Ask yourself "Which assessment findings/signs and symptoms indicate that the client's condition has improved?" "Which findings indicate that the client's condition has worsened?" Chapter 7 discusses how to evaluate outcomes in detail.

DEVELOPING CLINICAL JUDGMENT SKILLS FOR NURSING PRACTICE AND NGN READINESS

Using clinical judgment skills effectively is essential for professional nursing practice, and based on nurses' knowledge, experience, and thinking ability. In a practice analysis of new RN graduates, the NCSBN (2018) found that nurses use clinical judgment in almost half of daily tasks and activities.

Nursing Practice Readiness

Nursing graduates who take and pass the NCLEX® are expected to be ready for entry into practice and have the knowledge and skills needed to provide safe, effective client care. Currently there is no universally accepted definition of nursing practice readiness or standardized expectations for new graduate competencies in most countries. However, most experts suggest that nursing practice readiness includes the skills, competencies, and confidence to provide safe, effective client care. Some authors also include the need for informed clinical judgment skills (AlMekkawi & El Khalil, 2021; Mirza et al., 2019).

A recent study of 5000 new RN graduates found that only 23% could demonstrate *beginning* clinical judgment competencies when analyzing clinical situation vignettes as part of the Performance-Based Development System (PBDS) (Kavanagh & Szweda, 2017). New graduates were better able to identify problems in clients who were clinically deteriorating when compared to their ability to identify how to manage those problems. Box 1.5 lists the clinical judgment competency areas measured by the PBDS.

BOX 1.5   Clinical Judgment Competency Areas Using the PBDS

- Problem/urgency identification focus
  - Problem/risk identification
  - Relative priority-urgency
  - Justification for actions
- Problem management focus
  - Identification of individual nursing interventions

- Communication of essential information
- Anticipation of orders
- Justification for actions

Data from the Kavanagh and Szweda (2017) study, the nursing practice analysis, and other literature sources motivated the NCSBN to change the nursing licensure examinations (both RN and PN) to include measurement of clinical judgment skills. These changes resulted in new test item formats that measure each of the six cognitive (thinking) skills in the NCJMM as described earlier in this chapter. In April 2023 these test items were added to the existing NCLEX-RN® and NCLEX-PN® as part of the NGN.

NGN Readiness

The NGN includes test item types that were previously included on the licensure examinations plus a number of new item types. The new item types are presented in two ways—unfolding cases and Standalone items. This book includes numerous opportunities for you to practice taking these new items and are labeled as *Thinking Exercises* in Chapters 2 through 8.

Currently all candidates taking the NCLEX-RN® and NCLEX-PN® have three unfolding cases with six new test item types each as part of the licensure examinations. For candidates who do not meet the passing standard after answering the minimum number of licensure exam items, additional Standalone items are included in their adaptive NCLEX®. The combination of older style NCLEX® test items and NGN test items will likely continue to evolve over the next few years.

Most of the NGN test items are scored using a partial credit scoring system. In other words, you will receive credit for the correct responses, even if part of a test item is incorrect.

Unfolding Cases

Unfolding case studies are also called "evolving" cases because the client's clinical situation changes or evolves over time—usually minutes, hours, or days. Unfolding cases as part of NGN present realistic situations in which the client either clinically deteriorates or develops a medical complication during the case.

All of the case presentations are commonly occurring situations that novice nurses encounter in a variety of health care settings. Client information is presented within a variety of tabs to simulate parts of an actual health care (medical) record. These tabs may include:

- Orders
- Nurses Notes
- Progress Notes
- Laboratory Results
- Diagnostic Results
- Vital Signs
- History and Physical
- Nursing Flow Sheet

Presented laboratory results include the normal reference ranges similar to an actual medical record. An example can be found in Box 1.6.

BOX 1.6 Example of Laboratory Results

History and Physical	Laboratory Results	Orders	Nurses Notes

Serum Laboratory Test and Reference Range	Yesterday	2 Weeks Ago	4 Weeks Ago
Uric acid (<6 mg/dL [<0.36 mmol/L])	7.8 mg/dL (0.46 mmol/L)	6.4 mg/dL (0.38 mmol/L)	5.7 mg/dL (0.34 mmol/L)
Creatinine (0.5–1.1 mg/dL [44.2–97.3 µmol/L])	2.3 mg/dL (203.4 µmol/L)	2.1 mg/dL (185.7 µmol/L)	1.3 mg/dL (115 µmol/L)
Hematocrit (>33%)	34%	35%	35%
Platelets (150,000–400,000/mm^3 [150–400 × 10^9/L])	100,000/mm^3 (100 × 10^9/L)	145,000/mm^3 (145 × 10^9/L)	158,000/mm^3 (158 × 10^9/L)
Fasting blood glucose (74–106 mg/dL [4.1–5.9 mmol/L])	110 mg/dL (6.1 mmol/L)	104 mg/dL (5.8 mmol/L)	100 mg/dL (5.6 mmol/L)

Each NGN unfolding case includes six test items to measure each of the six clinical judgment cognitive (thinking) skills in this order:

1. Recognize Cues
2. Analyze Cues
3. Prioritize Hypotheses
4. Generate Solutions

5. Take Actions
6. Evaluate Outcomes

The NCLEX® is a computer-adaptive test that allows you to use a mouse to answer the items. Because this book is a print product, the Thinking Exercises (NGN test items) are sometimes presented in a slightly different format. However, additional Thinking Exercises on the book's Evolve site provide you with the ability to practice computer-based test items that are very similar to the newer item types on the NCLEX®. Box 1.7 lists the newer NGN test item types (divided into five categories) that are used as part of unfolding case studies.

BOX 1.7   Test Item Types Used in NGN Unfolding Case Studies

- Highlight items
  - Highlight In-Text
  - Highlight In-Table
- Drag-and-Drop items
  - Drag-and-Drop Cloze
  - Drag-and-Drop Rationale
- Matrix items
  - Matrix Multiple Response
  - Matrix Multiple Choice
- Drop-Down items
  - Drop-Down Cloze
  - Drop-Down Rationale
- Extended Multiple Response items
  - Extended Multiple Grouping
  - Extended Select-All-That-Apply
  - Extended Select-N

While the list of newer NGN test item types may seem overwhelming, several types have similar features but require different actions with a computer mouse to answer them. Keep these characteristics in mind as you answer test items in the unfolding cases:

- Highlight items require you to "highlight" the answers within the computer mouse. You will want to use a color highlighter for this book's Thinking Exercises.
- Any Cloze item means that there are one to three fill-in-the-blanks for you to complete in one or two sentences.
- Any Rationale item is a Cloze item but the sentence includes a dependent clause connected by terms such as "as evidenced by," "due to," or "because."
- Any Matrix item means that you will need to respond to information in a table.
- Similar to the familiar and older Select-All-That-Apply (SATA) test item types, the correct response for the NGN SATA can be one, some, or all of the provided choices. However, the number of choices in the new SATA items is between 5 and 10.
- Select-N test items specify the number of correct responses you need to select.

CLINICAL JUDGMENT TIP

Remember: Unfolding cases as part of NGN present realistic situations in which the client either clinically deteriorates or develops a medical complication during the case. Each case includes six test items that measure each of the six clinical judgment thinking skills.

Directions for each type of test item are consistent throughout the NCLEX® and this book. The following boxes illustrate examples of NGN test items used in unfolding cases with which you may not be familiar. These items are used as part of unfolding cases in Thinking Exercises in this book. Box 1.8 shows a Highlight-in-Table item using the Laboratory Results described earlier in this section. Note that the answers have been highlighted.

BOX 1.8 Example of Highlight-in-Table NGN Test Item

The nurse is caring for a 39-year-old client who is 32 weeks pregnant. Highlight the findings below that require **immediate** follow-up.

History and Physical	Laboratory Results	Orders	Nurses Notes
Serum Laboratory Test and Reference Range	Yesterday	2 Weeks Ago	4 Weeks Ago
Uric acid (<6 mg/dL [<0.36 mmol/L])	7.8 mg/dL (0.46 mmol/L)	6.4 mg/dL (0.38 mmol/L)	5.7 mg/dL (0.34 mmol/L)
Creatinine (0.5–1.1 mg/dL [44.2–97.3 µmol/L])	2.3 mg/dL (203.4 µmol/L)	2.1 mg/dL (185.7 µmol/L)	1.3 mg/dL (115 µmol/L)
Hematocrit (>33%)	34%	35%	35%
Platelets (150,000–400,000/mm^3 [150–400 × 10^9/L])	100,000/mm^3 (100 × 10^9/L)	145,000/mm^3 (145 × 10^9/L)	158,000/mm^3 (158 × 10^9/L)
Fasting blood glucose (74–106 mg/dL [4.1–5.9 mmol/L])	110 mg/dL (6.1 mmol/L)	104 mg/dL (5.8 mmol/L)	100 mg/dL (5.6 mmol/L)

As you likely noticed, not all abnormal client assessment findings need *immediate* follow-up. Although the blood glucose is slightly elevated, the serum uric acid, creatinine, and platelet count are more important to follow up because the client could be experiencing a potentially life-threatening complication of pregnancy, which could endanger both the client and the fetus. This item measures your ability to *Recognize Cues*.

Drag-and-Drop and Drop-Down items present a sentence or two for you to complete using a list of choices (see Box 1.9).

The Drag-and-Drop Cloze item in Box 1.9 measures the ability to *Analyze Cues*. To answer this item, you need to identify all relevant client findings and determine for which potential complication the client is at high risk. The Drop-Down Rationale measures the ability to *Prioritize Hypotheses*. To answer this item, you need to determine what the client's priority need is and why. Based on changes in the client's condition as documented in the Nurses Notes, the client needs close monitoring of the airway.

BOX 1.9 Examples of Drag-and-Drop and Drop-Down NGN Test Items

Drag-and-Drop Cloze Item
The nurse is caring for a 45-year-old client in the ED.

History and Physical	Nurses Notes	Orders	Laboratory Results

1420: Client admitted to ED with report of burns to both hands and left side of face. Was burning leaves when a gust of wind blew sparks onto the nearby grass. Client used blankets and water from hose to control fire but sustained burns. Second-degree burns on both palms of hands; first- and second-degree burns to left cheek and chin for total of 4% burn to body. Hair near cheek slightly singed. States facial burns much more painful than hand burns; reports pain level is 9/10 on a 0–10 pain scale. Alert and oriented ×4. Lung sounds clear throughout all fields; no adventitious breath sounds. S$_1$ and S$_2$ present. Bowel sounds present ×4. Moves all extremities freely. VS: T 98.8°F (37.1°C); HR 86 BPM; RR 22 bpm; B/P 114/70 mmHg; SpO$_2$ 98% on RA.

Continued

BOX 1.9   Examples of Drag-and-Drop and Drop-Down NGN Test Items—cont'd

Complete the following sentence by selecting from the list of Word Choices below.

Based on analysis of documented assessment findings, the nurse determines that the client is currently at high risk for [**Word Choice**].

Word Choices	
Infection	Airway obstruction
Hand contractures	Scarring

Answer:

Based on analysis of documented assessment findings, the nurse determines that the client is currently at high risk for **airway obstruction**.

Drop-Down Rationale Item

The nurse is caring for a 45-year-old client in the ED.

History and Physical	Nurses Notes	Orders	Laboratory Results

1420:   Client admitted to ED with report of burns to both hands and left side of face. Was burning leaves when a gust of wind blew sparks onto the nearby grass. Client used blankets and water from hose to control fire but sustained burns. Second-degree burns on both palms of hands; first- and second-degree burns to left cheek and chin for total of 4% burn to body. Hair near cheek slightly singed. States facial burns much more painful than hand burns; reports pain level is 9/10 on a 0–10 pain scale. Alert and oriented ×4. Lung sounds clear throughout all fields; no adventitious breath sounds. S_1 and S_2 present. Bowel sounds present ×4. Moves all extremities freely. VS: T 98.8°F (37.1°C); HR 86 BPM; RR 22 bpm; B/P 114/70 mmHg; SpO_2 98% on RA.

1510:   Partner present with client. Client alert and oriented ×4. Has nonproductive cough and states feeling "a little short of breath." VS: T 98.6°F (37°C); HR 90 BPM; RR 26 bpm; B/P 126/78 mmHg; SpO_2 94% on RA.

Complete the sentence by selecting from the lists of options below.

The nurse determines that the client's **_priority_** for care is frequent _____ **1 [Select]** _____ because the client has a(an) _____ **2 [Select]** _____ and _____ **3 [Select]** _____.

Options for 1	Options for 2	Options for 3
Pain assessment	Nonproductive cough	Bilateral hand burns
Skin assessment	Increased blood pressure	Bradypnea
Airway assessment	Pain level of 9/10	Decreasing SpO_2

Answers:

The nurse determines that the client's **_priority_** for care is frequent **airway assessment** because the client has a(an) **nonproductive cough** and **decreasing SpO_2**.

Matrix test items present the client situation followed by a table in which you will select one choice (Matrix Multiple Choice), or one or more choices (Matrix Multiple Response). Box 1.10 shows an example of a Matrix Multiple Choice test item and its answers.

The Matrix Multiple Choice test item example in Box 1.10 measures the ability to *Generate Solutions*. The nurse reviews the assessment findings in the Nurses Notes and identifies possible actions that may be needed to help meet the client's needs.

BOX 1.10 **Example of Matrix Multiple Response Test Item**

The nurse is caring for a 45-year-old client in the ED.

History and Physical	**Nurses Notes**	**Orders**	**Laboratory Results**

1420: Client admitted to ED with report of burns to both hands and left side of face. Was burning leaves when a gust of wind blew sparks onto the nearby grass. Client used blankets and water from hose to control fire but sustained burns. Second-degree burns on both palms of hands; first- and second-degree burns to left cheek and chin for total of 4% burn to body. Hair near cheek slightly singed. States facial burns much more painful than hand burns; reports pain level is 9/10 on a 0–10 pain scale. Alert and oriented ×4. Lung sounds clear throughout all fields; no adventitious breath sounds. S_1 and S_2 present. Bowel sounds present ×4. Moves all extremities freely. VS: T 98.8°F (37.1°C); HR 86 BPM; RR 22 bpm; B/P 114/70 mmHg; SpO_2 98% on RA.

1510: Partner present with client. Client alert and oriented ×4. Has nonproductive cough and states feeling "a little short of breath." VS: T 98.6°F (37°C); HR 90 BPM; RR 26 bpm; B/P 126/78 mmHg; SpO_2 94% on RA.

Determine whether the following potential nursing actions are indicated or not indicated for the client at this time.

Potential Nursing Actions	**Indicated**	**Not Indicated**
Maintain client in flat side-lying position		
Monitor respiratory rate and SpO_2 every 15–30 min		
Administer supplemental oxygen therapy		
Consult with respiratory therapy for treatment plan		

Answers:

Potential Nursing Actions	**Indicated**	**Not Indicated**
Maintain client in flat side-lying position		X
Monitor respiratory rate and SpO_2 every 15–30 min	X	
Administer supplemental oxygen therapy	X	
Consult with respiratory therapy for treatment plan	X	

Standalone Test Items

In addition to new item types used as part of unfolding cases, the NGN includes two types of Standalone test items—the Bowtie and Trend items. For both types of items, the client information is presented in one or more medical record tabs and does not unfold or evolve over time. An example of a Bowtie item with answers is presented in Box 1.11.

As you probably realized, the Bowtie test item typically measures more than one of the six clinical judgment thinking skills. To correctly answer the Bowtie item in Box 1.11, you need to

BOX 1.11   Example of an NGN Bowtie Test Item

The nurse is caring for a 75-year-client admitted this morning with an exacerbation of chronic heart failure.

| Health History | Nurses Notes | Orders | Laboratory Results |

1310: Client alert and oriented ×1 (person only). Visiting family members state that client has become very confused since being admitted to the hospital. Restless, anxious, and picking at bedcovers. Course crackles in both lung bases; dyspnea at rest; moist, productive cough when getting out of bed with assistance to the BR. S_3 present. Bowel sounds present ×4. Moves all extremities freely. Bilateral ankle and foot 3+ pitting edema. VS: T 98.8°F (37.1°C); HR 104 BPM; RR 26 bpm; B/P 164/90 mmHg; SpO_2 90% on O_2 3 L/min.

Complete the diagram by identifying from the choices below to specify what potential condition the client is likely experiencing, **two** nursing actions that are appropriate to take, and **two** parameters the nurse should monitor to assess the client's progress.

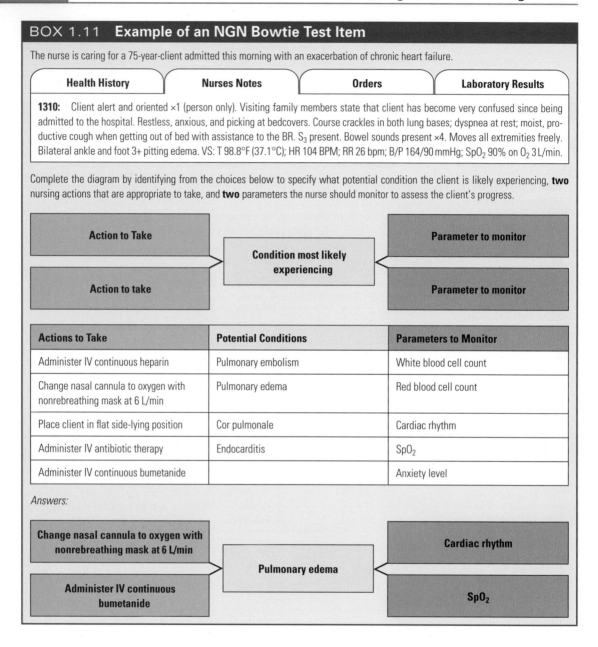

Actions to Take	Potential Conditions	Parameters to Monitor
Administer IV continuous heparin	Pulmonary embolism	White blood cell count
Change nasal cannula to oxygen with nonrebreathing mask at 6 L/min	Pulmonary edema	Red blood cell count
Place client in flat side-lying position	Cor pulmonale	Cardiac rhythm
Administer IV antibiotic therapy	Endocarditis	SpO_2
Administer IV continuous bumetanide		Anxiety level

Answers:

first determine what condition the client is likely experiencing by recognizing relevant cues and analyzing those findings (middle column). Then decide what possible actions would be needed to care for the client and meet expected outcomes (left column). Finally, select the findings you would want to monitor to determine whether the planned actions were effective (right column).

The Trend item is the second type of NGN Standalone format. This item type presents the client's findings over time in one or more medical record tabs such as the Laboratory Results shown in Box 1.6. The test item that accompanies the presented client findings may be any of the types listed in Box 1.7. Therefore, unlike the Bowtie item, the Trend item most often measures only one of the six clinical judgment thinking skills.

Chapters 2 through 7 discuss each of the six clinical judgment thinking skills in detail and include multiple Thinking Exercises to help you develop each skill. Chapter 8 provides you the opportunity to put all of the clinical judgment skills together by answering items as part of unfolding cases and Standalone test items. The answers and rationales for all Thinking Exercises are located in Appendix A of this book.

REFERENCES

AlMekkawi, M., & El Khalil, R. (2021). New graduate nurses' readiness to practice: A narrative literature review. *Health Professions Education, 3*(1), 304–316.

American Association of Colleges of Nursing (AACN). (2023). *Clinical judgment concept.* Retrieved from https://www.aacnnursing.org/Essentials/Concepts/Clinical-Judgment.

American Nurses Association (ANA). (2021). *Nursing scope and standards of practice* (4th ed.). Silver Spring, MD: ANA.

*Benner, P. (2001). *From novice to expert.* Upper Saddle River, NJ: Prentice Hall.

*Benner, P., Sutphen, M., Leonard, V., & Day, L. (2010). *Educating nurses: A call for radical transformation.* San Francisco, CA: Jossey-Bass.

Cheraghi, M. A., Pashaeypoor, S., Mardanian Dehkordi, L., & Khoshkesht, S. (2021). Creativity in nursing care: A concept analysis. *Florence Nightingale Journal of Nursing, 29*(3), 389–396.

Clemett, V. J., & Raleigh, M. (2021). The validity and reliability of clinical judgement and decision-making skills assessment in nursing: A systematic literature review. *Nurse Education Today, 102*: Article 104885.

Connor, J., Phil, M., Flenady, T., Massey, D., & Dwyer, T. (2022). Clinical judgement in nursing—An evolutionary concept analysis. *Journal of Clinical Nursing, 32*(13–14), 3328–3340.

Doane, G. H., & Varcoe, C. (2021). *How to nurse: Relational inquiry with individuals and families in changing health and health care contexts* (2nd ed.). Philadelphia, PA: Wolters Kluwer.

Ignatavicius, D. D. (2024). *Developing clinical judgment for professional nursing practice and the Next-Generation NCLEX-RN® Examination* (2nd ed.). St. Louis, MO: Elsevier.

Jacobs, S., Taylor, C., Dixon, K., & Wilkes, L. (2018). Consensus of the characteristics of clinical judgement utilised by nurses in their practice: Results of a survey. *Open Journal of Nursing, 8*(10), 746–757.

Joplin-Gonzales, P., & Rounds, L. (2022). The essential elements of clinical reasoning. *Nurse Educator, 47*(5), E145–E149.

*Kalisch, B. J., Landstrom, G. L., & Hinshaw, A. S. (2009). Missed nursing care: A concept analysis. *Advances in Nursing Science, 265*(7), 1509–1517.

Kavanagh, J. M., & Szweda, C. (2017). A crisis in competency: The strategic and ethical imperative to assessing new graduate nurses' clinical reasoning. *Nursing Education Perspectives, 38*(2), 57–62.

*Levett-Jones, T., Hoffman, K., Dempsey, J., Yeun-Sim Jeong, S., Noble, C. A. N., et al. (2010). The 'five rights' of clinical reasoning: An educational model to enhance nursing students' ability to identify and manage clinically 'at risk' patients. *Nurse Education Today, 30*(6), 515–520.

*Lunney, M. (2010). Use of critical thinking in the diagnostic process. *International Journal of Nursing Terminologies and Classifications, 21*(2), 82–88.

Manetti, W. (2019). Sound clinical judgment in nursing: A concept analysis. *Nursing Forum, 54*(1), 102–110.

Mirza, N., Manankil-Rankin, L., Prentice, D., Hagerman, L.-A., & Draenos, C. (2019). Practice readiness of new nursing graduates: A concept analysis. *Nurse Education in Practice, 37*(5), 68–74.

National Council of State Boards of Nursing (NCSBN). (2018). NCLEX-RN® examination analysis and research. *NGN News* Winter.

National Council of State Boards of Nursing (NCSBN). (2023). *Next-Generation NCLEX®: NCLEX-RN® Test Plan.* Chicago, IL: NCSBN.

*National League for Nursing (NLN). (2012). *Outcomes and competencies for graduates of practical/vocational, diploma, baccalaureate, master's practice doctorate, and research doctorate program in nursing.* Washington, DC: NLN.

*Saintsing, D., Gibson, L. M., & Pennington, A. W. (2011). The novice nurse and clinical decision-making: How to avoid errors. *Journal of Nursing Management, 19*(3), 354–359.

*Tanner, C. A. (2006). Thinking like a nurse. A research-based model of clinical judgment in nursing. *Journal of Nursing Education, 45*(6), 204–211.

*Denotes classic reference.

2

How to Recognize Cues

LEARNING OUTCOMES

1. Distinguish objective and subjective clinical cues.
2. Describe the variables that affect how nurses determine normal versus abnormal cues.
3. Explain the need for nurses to identify relevant cues to help prevent failure to rescue.
4. Outline how to perform a situational assessment to ensure timely and accurate cue recognition.
5. Identify the most common clinical cues used by nurses to detect changes in the client's condition.
6. Discuss strategies for cue recognition as the initial skill needed to make safe, appropriate clinical judgments.

KEY TERMS

Clinical cues: Objective findings (signs) and subjective findings (symptoms) that indicate client deterioration and improvement.

Clinical deterioration: A dynamic state in which the client progresses to a worsened clinical condition of increasing morbidity, body organ dysfunction, prolonged hospital or agency length of stay, and/or death.

Cognitive biases: Flaws or distortions in judgment and clinical decision-making, often contributing to sentinel events.

Cognitive load: The amount of information within one's working (short-term) memory.

Comprehensive health assessment: A client assessment that provides information about each of the client's body systems; also called a head-to-toe assessment.

Cue recognition: The mental process involved in extracting and identifying *relevant* and important information from the presenting client's situation.

Delegated responsibility: A nursing task or skill that is transferred from a licensed nurse to a delegate in a selected client care situation.

Early warning scoring system (EWSS): A client monitoring system that tracks multiple parameters at the same time and triggers more frequent assessments based on early changes in vital signs; it is a guide for the health care team to quickly determine a client's condition on the basis of a physiologic scoring matrix.

Failure to rescue (FTR): The inability of nurses or other interprofessional health team members to save a client's life in a timely manner when a health care issue or medical complication occurs.

Focused health assessment: A client assessment that provides information related to a client's change in clinical state or specific client symptom(s).

Intuition: The ability to predict client situations facilitated by a strong knowledge base; also called intuitive thinking.

Logic: Rational thinking based on evidence.

Objective findings: Client observations made by the nurse or other member of the interprofessional health care team; also called signs.

Observation: The purposeful gathering of information from clients and/or significant others/family members to inform clinical judgments.

Rapid response team: A group of health care professionals within a hospital, who save lives and decrease the risk for harm by providing care *before* a medical emergency occurs by rapidly intervening when needed for clients who are *beginning* to clinically decline.

Sentinel event: A *severe* variation in the standard of care is caused by human or system error that results in avoidable patient death or major harm.

Signs: Objective clinical cues that are usually measurable.

Situational awareness (SA): An essential client safety skill consisting of a nurse's ability to perceive the clinical situation accurately and completely, understand the meaning of the clinical situation, and rapidly predict the outcome of the clinical situation.

Subjective findings: Self-reports of the client's condition or significant others'/family's reports of client changes; also called symptoms.

Symptoms: Subjective clinical cues that may or may not be measurable.

IDENTIFYING CLINICAL CUES

As described in Chapter 1, identifying or recognizing relevant clinical cues is an essential cognitive or clinical reasoning skill. This chapter explores how to recognize cues as a basis for making safe, appropriate clinical judgments and the elements that can affect the ability to effectively use this skill.

Definitions

The clinical status or state of a client requiring health care typically fluctuates between improvement and deterioration during a hospital or other health care agency stay. Clinical deterioration is a dynamic state that occurs when the client progresses to a worsened clinical condition of increasing morbidity, body organ dysfunction caused by decompensation, prolonged hospital or agency length of stay, and/or death (Al-Moteri et al., 2020; Burdeu et al., 2021; Padilla & Mayo, 2018). Indicators of clinical deterioration are called clinical cues.

Clinical cues include both objective findings and subjective client findings and can indicate both deterioration and improvement in clients. These findings provide information for the nurse as the basis for making clinical judgments. Objective findings, also called signs, are client observations made by the nurse or another member of the interprofessional health care team. In addition to physical assessment data, these findings include diagnostic test results. Subjective findings are self-reports of the client's condition or significant others'/family's reports of client changes. These reported findings are also called symptoms. One way to remember the difference between objective and subjective findings is that objective data are *observable*, and subjective data are *stated* by the client, a significant other, or the family.

CLINICAL JUDGMENT TIP

Remember: **O**bjective client findings = **O**bservable data from the nurse or other interprofessional health care team member.

Subjective client findings = **S**tated data communicated by the client, a significant other, or a family member.

Some client findings, such as pain, can be both subjective and objective. If able to communicate effectively, the client can self-report pain and rate its intensity, quality, onset, and location using a pain assessment tool. If the client is *not* able to communicate these data, the nurse should observe for client behaviors such as gritting teeth, wincing, and yelling. Be sure to notice these nonverbal indicators of pain and intervene appropriately to manage pain.

Acute pain can also result in changes in vital signs, especially an elevated heart rate and blood pressure resulting from the stress response. By contrast, the body adapts to persistent (chronic) pain, so persistent pain may not affect vital sign values. The heart rate and blood pressure of some clients may be lower than normal when they experience persistent pain (Ignatavicius et al., 2024).

Distinguishing Objective and Subjective Clinical Cues

Client **signs** are measurable objective findings assessed through a variety of tools. For example, body temperature is a commonly measured vital sign that is assessed using various types of thermometers. The normal range for body temperature has been established such that a temperature higher than "normal" is assessed as hyperthermia or fever, and a temperature lower than "normal" is assessed as hypothermia. However, determining whether a temperature is within normal limits depends on the *context* of the client's situation. When identifying cues in a client situation, be sure to consider the context of the client or situation. Contextual considerations for identifying cues are discussed later in this chapter.

Some client **symptoms** are also measurable. For example, a client's self-report of pain is a subjective finding but can be quantified by the client using a variety of pain intensity scales, such as the 0–10 scale used for alert and oriented adults. The most intense pain is rated as a 10 using this scale. A client's self-report of anxiety, however, is more difficult to measure, although it may be described by the client as mild, moderate, or severe.

Some client signs indicate or support client symptoms. For example, an irregular heart rate (sign) may support a client's report of chest pain (symptom). If a client has an irregular heart rate, ask the client about any pain or discomfort being experienced. In other situations, client symptoms indicate or support client signs. For instance, a client's report of feeling warm or hot (symptom) may indicate or support the client's elevated body temperature (sign). Therefore, if the client reports feeling warm or hot, obtain the client's temperature to determine if a fever is present.

CLINICAL JUDGMENT TIP

Remember: If you notice the client presents with a new or changed sign (objective finding), assess for associated symptoms to support the measurable sign. If the client reports a new or changed symptom (subjective finding), assess for associated signs to support the stated symptom.

Client Changes Indicating Clinical Deterioration

Health care situations involving an emergency or acute change in the client's condition or clinical state require the nurse to think critically and use clinical reasoning (cognitive) skills to make safe clinical judgments. An acute change in a client's condition occurs when signs or symptoms differ from those of the last assessment of the client's objective and subjective findings. These changes often occur 24 hours or more *before* a client presents with an emergency or a medical complication. Therefore, your early recognition of relevant cues is essential to prevent clinical deterioration and possible death. The clients most at risk for clinical deterioration include the following (Padilla & Mayo, 2018):

- Emergency client admissions
- Clients with acute or preexisting health conditions
- Clients who have had recent surgeries
- Clients recovering from critical illnesses

Anticipate that any of these clients are at *high risk* for deterioration; report and document any subtle or beginning changes in their clinical state. Plan to assess these clients more frequently if clinical changes begin.

Client Changes Indicating Clinical Improvement

After the nurse and interprofessional health care team respond to the client's needs, emergency, or clinical deterioration, the client is carefully monitored and assessed. Continuing to recognize objective and subjective clinical cues helps determine whether the client is improving as an expected result of safe, evidence-based nursing actions. For example, a client who receives supplemental oxygen while in a semi-Fowler's position to help relieve dyspnea would be expected to report decreasing dyspnea as a result of these actions. If the client's dyspnea did not decrease, the nurse would take additional actions to achieve the expected outcome. Chapter 7 discusses, in detail, using the *evaluate outcomes* cognitive skill.

CLINICAL JUDGMENT TIP

Remember: Identify relevant cues when a client's condition changes to indicate clinical deterioration or clinical improvement.

Cues for Recognizing Changes in Client Condition

Recognizing changes in the client's condition or clinical state depends on your ability to identify relevant objective and subjective clinical cues. Box 2.1 briefly summarizes the findings of a systematic review to determine which cues are used by acute care nurses to assess changes in clients' clinical states.

BOX 2.1   Evidence-Based Practice

Which Clinical Cues Are Used by Nurses to Recognize Changes in Clients' Clinical States?

Based on Burdeu, G., Lowe, G., Rasmussen, B., & Consedine, J. (2021). Clinical cues used by nurses to recognize changes in patients' clinical states: A systematic review. *Nursing and Health* Science, *23*(1), 9–28.

The authors conducted a systematic review of nursing research literature to identify specific objective and subjective clinical cues acute care nurses use to detect acute client changes—either client deterioration or improvement. The 38 included studies reported 173 total clinical cues grouped into nine distinct objective clinical categories and four categories of subjective clinical cues. Examples of the nine objective clinical categories are physiological, function/activity, respiratory, and urinary/elimination.

The four categories of subjective clinical cues are the following:

1. Self-report of the presence or absence of pain
2. Clinical tools to describe the quantity and quality of pain
3. Self-report of changes, such as dyspnea, heartburn, anxiety, dizziness
4. Significant others' report of client changes, such as decreasing level of function, cognition, and/or activity

The authors also reported that nurses most often used objective clinical cues such as vital signs to assess acute client changes rather than subjective cues.

A variety of objective clinical cues may be identified and interpreted to determine a client's condition. Table 2.1 lists examples of clinical cues organized by objective categories that could indicate client deterioration.

TABLE 2.1   Examples of Clinical Cues Indicating Possible Client Deterioration

Objective Categories	Examples of Clinical Cues
Physiologic	• Tachypnea • Hypotension • Fever
Neurologic	• Weakness • Decreased level of consciousness • Numbness
Respiratory	• Adventitious breath sounds • Decreased peripheral oxygen saturation (SpO_2) • Increased respiratory secretions
Gastrointestinal	• Vomiting • Hypoglycemia • Absent bowel sounds
Urinary/Elimination	• Oliguria • Diuresis • Diarrhea
Skin	• Clammy and cool • Pale • Cyanotic or darker
Function/Activity	• Decreased ADL ability • Decreased energy • Decreased strength
Observed pain	• Gritting teeth • Screaming or yelling • Restlessness
Cognition	• Agitation • Hallucinations • Incomprehensible speech

Adapted from Burdeu, G., Lowe, G., Rasmussen, B., & Consedine, J. (2021). Clinical cues used by nurses to recognize changes in patients' clinical states: A systematic review. *Nursing and Health Science, 23*(1), 9–28.

Nurses and other members of the interprofessional health care team have multiple clinical encounters with clients in a variety of health care settings. The first few minutes of each encounter are particularly important because many clients share crucial information that could be missed. To ensure that you notice and recognize relevant subjective cues, follow these simple but essential guidelines:

1. Take time to actively listen, carefully and in a caring manner, to what the client, significant other, or family member is communicating to you.
2. Listen for the feelings and needs of the client by recognizing both verbal and nonverbal cues.
3. Remain present and attentive rather than performing tasks that could be distracting and cause you to miss an important subjective cue.
4. Ask questions to clarify or provide additional information about the client's subjective clinical cue(s) or symptom(s).

Thinking Exercise 2.1 will help you practice what you've learned in this chapter. The answer and rationale for the exercise are located at the end of the book.

THINKING EXERCISE 2.1

The nurse is caring for an 81-year-old client in the emergency department (ED).
Highlight the client findings below that require **immediate** follow-up.

History and Physical	Nurses Notes	Orders	Laboratory Results

1930: Brought to ED after slipping on wet floor. Family reports client fell on left side and avoided hitting head. Alert but unable to answer questions; holding left outer leg and yelling. Experiencing shortness of breath at times. No adventitious breath sounds; S_1 and S_2 present. Bowel sounds present ×4. Left leg externally rotated and shorter than right leg. Capillary refill <3 seconds bilaterally. Pedal pulses 1+ and equal; feet equally cool without swelling. Able to move all other extremities. H/O diabetes mellitus and hyper-cholesteremia controlled by drug therapy and diet. VS: T 98.4°F (36.9°C); HR 108 beats per minute; RR 26 breaths per minute; B/P 164/98 mmHg; SpO_2 90% on RA.

DIFFERENTIATING CLINICAL CUES

Client findings may be recognized in the form of cues that are normal or abnormal, relevant or not relevant, and expected or not expected. Be aware that many factors can influence how cues are recognized and interpreted. One of the most important factors influencing cue recognition and communication is the impact of cultural values, beliefs, and preferences.

Identifying relevant cues during client assessment requires effective and respectful communication with clients, their significant others, and/or family members. The American Nurses Association's (ANA) most recent standards of practice include competencies related to communication as part of client assessment. One assessment competency states the nurse "identifies enhancements and barriers to effective communication based on personal, cognitive, physiological, psychological, literacy, financial, and cultural considerations" (ANA, 2021, p. 76).

Cultural factors are further addressed as part of a separate ANA standard on respectful and equitable practice. Box 2.2 lists examples of competencies you need to utilize when communicating to identify cues in a culturally sensitive manner.

BOX 2.2 Examples of Competencies for ANA Standard 9: Respectful and Equitable Practice

- Uses appropriate skills and tools for the culture, literacy, and language of the individuals and population served.
- Communicates with appropriate language and behaviors, including the use of qualified health care interpreters and translators in accordance with [client] needs and preferences.
- Identifies the cultural-specific meaning of interactions, terms, and content.
- Applies knowledge of differences in health beliefs, practices, and communication patterns without assigning value to the differences.
- Reflects upon personal and cultural values, beliefs, biases, and heritage.

From the American Nurses Association (ANA). (2021). *Nursing: Scope and standards of practice* (4th ed.). ANA.

Distinguishing Normal Versus Abnormal Clinical Cues

Detecting relevant signs and symptoms requires you to use knowledge of what are considered normal findings. If your client's findings are outside the normal range, then you have identified abnormal clinical cues. Use all of your senses (sight, hearing, touch, and smell) to collect all of the relevant client information.

The ability to recognize cues requires knowing (1) how to perform accurate health assessments and (2) how to distinguish normal from abnormal clinical cues (signs and symptoms). Some textbooks use the term "usual" rather than "normal" for these client findings.

Nursing competence in performing health assessments is essential for making safe, appropriate clinical judgments for clients in any health care setting (Liyew et al., 2021). Generalist nurses most often perform two types of health assessments as required by the clinical situation. A comprehensive health assessment, often called a head-to-toe assessment, provides information about each of the client's body systems. This assessment is commonly performed by a nurse on admission to a health care setting and at the beginning of a work shift to serve as a baseline and provide an overall picture of the client. Fig. 2.1 highlights the key components of a body systems assessment.

BODY SYSTEMS ASSESSMENT

QUICK PRIORITY ASSESSMENT
General appearance • Vital signs • Communication • Allergies • Medical Problems • Medications • Drug/Alcohol Use • Skin/Circulation • Pain • Infection/Safety Risks • Age • Height • Weight

Musculoskeletal
- Range of motion
- Body alignment
- Bone alignment
- Pain

Genitourinary/reproductive
- Breasts, vulva, vagina, uterus
- Penis, prostate gland
- Urinary meatus
- Urine (color, odor, amount)
- Itching, burning

Gastrointestinal
- Mouth, teeth, gums, tongue, gag reflex, stomach, abdomen, bowel sounds, liver, spleen
- Pain

Integumentary
- Skin color, condition, and temperature
- Itching
- Pain

Neurological
- Level of consciousness
- Cognitive status
- Pupil, ocular movement
- Motor and sensory coordination
- Gag and other reflexes
- Pain

EE (vision, hearing)
- Eyes, ears, nose
- Pain

Respiratory
- Airway (mouth, throat, nose)
- Respiratory rate, rhythm, breath sounds
- Cough
- Pain

Cardiovascular
- Apical, radial, popliteal, and pedal pulses
- B/P, PMI
- Heart sounds
- Peripheral pulses
- Pain

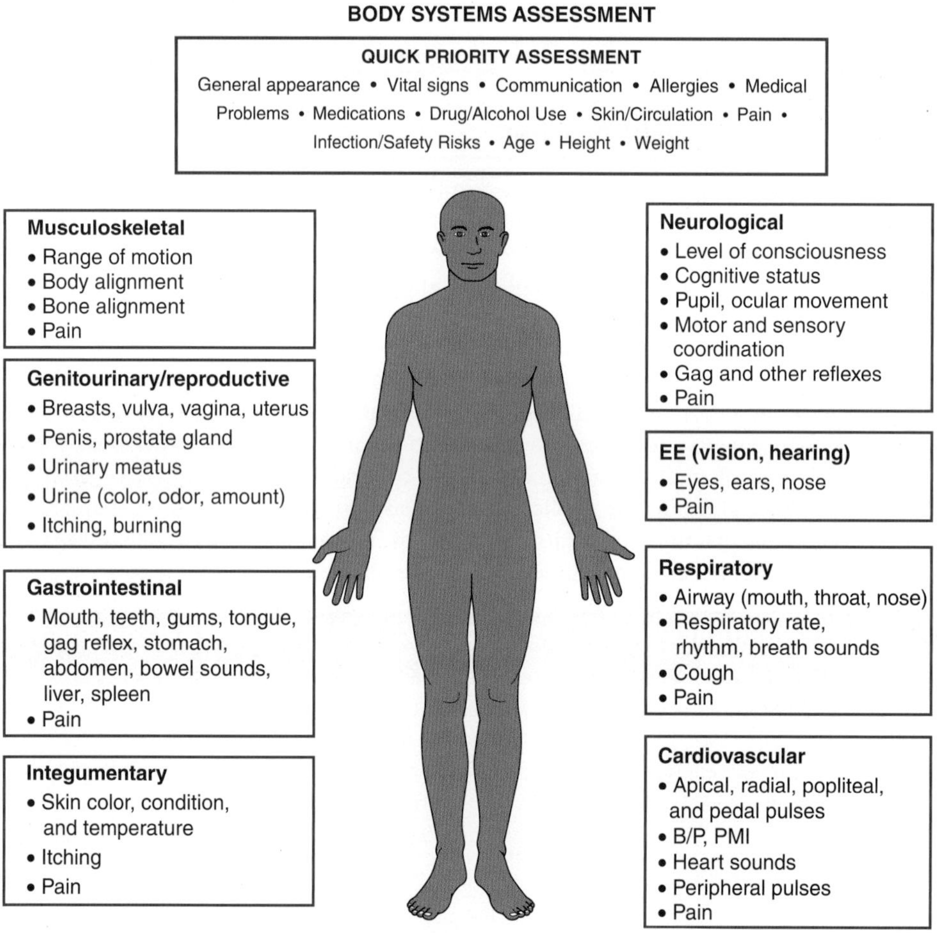

FIG. 2.1 Body systems assessment. To prioritize client assessment, go clockwise starting with the Quick Priority Assessment.

When a client's condition or clinical state changes, you must be able to perform relevant focused health assessments. A focused health assessment provides information related to a client's change in clinical state or specific client symptom(s). For example, if a client reports new-onset abdominal pain, you will want to perform an abdominal assessment. If the client has a new productive cough, you will want to perform a respiratory and possibly a cardiovascular assessment. When performing any type of health assessment, be aware that several variables, including age, sex, and race/ethnicity, affect cue recognition and analysis. These contextual considerations can affect your ability to effectively and safely make clinical judgments.

> ## CLINICAL JUDGMENT TIP
> *Remember:* Perform a focused health assessment when you notice a client's change in clinical state or specific client symptom(s). Be sure to use all of your senses (sight, hearing, touch, and smell) to collect all of the relevant client information.

Age Considerations

Nurses care for individuals across the life span in a variety of health care settings and, therefore, need knowledge of normal findings for each developmental age to identify urgent or emergent changes in client conditions. For example, the usual heart rate of a newborn is 120–140 beats per minute; the usual resting heart rate for an adult is 60–100 beats per minute (Hockenberry et al., 2024; Ignatavicius et al., 2024). A heart rate of 96 beats per minute for a newborn is an emergent clinical change (bradycardia) but would be within the normal range for an adult. Considering the age of the client you are caring for allows you to better determine what is normal and what is not.

As adults become older, they experience many normal physiologic changes associated with the aging process. These changes can make older adults more susceptible to rapid clinical deterioration and emergent medical complications. For example, the amount of water in the adult body typically decreases after age 65 as a normal physiologic change. This change places older adults at a higher risk for dehydration and hypovolemic shock than younger adults (Touhy & Jett, 2022).

Older adults may also present with signs and symptoms that differ from those of their younger counterparts. For example, the clinical presentation of infections in older clients may be different from that in younger clients. Older adults with severe infections tend to have fewer symptoms but are more susceptible to developing sepsis and septic shock. Fever is absent or low-grade in 20%–30% of older adults experiencing infection. Signs of infection in older adults can be nonspecific and include falls, delirium, anorexia, or generalized weakness (Touhy & Jett, 2022).

In some cases, usual physiologic changes of aging affect the normal ranges of laboratory tests. For instance, the normal blood glucose level for adults over 60 years of age is higher (82–115 mg/dL [4.6–6.4 mmol/L]) than the level for adults under 60 years of age (74–106 mg/dL [4.1–5.9 mmol/L]) (Pagana et al., 2022). The major reason for this increase in older adults is that the pancreas produces less insulin as individuals age. This change makes older adults more susceptible than young or middle-aged adults to developing type 2 diabetes mellitus (Touhy & Jett, 2022).

Sex Considerations

The normal ranges for selected laboratory tests may also vary because of the client's sex. For example, the normal findings for hemoglobin differ based on the sex the client was assigned at birth (natal sex) as specified below:
Male: 14–18 g/dL (8.7–11.2 mmol/L)
Female: 12–16 g/dL (7.4–9.9 mmol/L)

Older adult normal values are slightly less than those stated above. Clients who are pregnant are expected to have a hemoglobin value of less than 11 g/dL (6.8 mmol/L) because of hemodilution as blood volume increases (Pagana et al., 2022).

When reviewing laboratory test data, be sure to note the client's sex to distinguish what is normal from what is not. More research is needed to identify whether natal sex affects other objective client findings.

Race and Ethnicity Considerations

Clients present with varying skin tones and consequently have variable clinical findings that may require specific assessment techniques. For example, jaundice (icterus) is best assessed in the corner sclera of the eyes of clients who have light skin. Jaundice is best detected in the sclera of the eyes closest to the iris of clients who have dark skin (brown or black) (Jarvis & Eckhardt, 2024). Decreased blood flow to the skin causes brown skin to appear yellow-brown, and very dark brown or black skin to appear ash gray. Decreased blood flow in clients who have light skin manifests as pallor (Jarvis & Eckhardt, 2024).

Other objective client findings can also be influenced by race or ethnicity. For example, the normal laboratory reference ranges for prostate-specific antigen (PSA) are affected by age and can vary with the client's race or ethnicity. Table 2.2 lists the normal range of PSA for White and Black individuals assigned male at birth.

TABLE 2.2 Differences in Normal Reference Ranges for Serum PSA		
Age Range (Years)	**Blacks**	**Whites**
40–49	0.0–2.0	0.0–2.5
50–59	0.0–4.0	0.0–3.5
60–69	0.0–4.5	0.0–4.5
70–79	0.0–5.5	0.0–6.5

Adapted from Pagana, K.D., Pagana, T.J., & Pagana, T.N. (2022). *Mosby's manual of diagnostic and laboratory tests* (7th ed.). Elsevier.

In addition to laboratory test results, other objective clinical cues are influenced by race and ethnicity. Most recently, the COVID-19 pandemic revealed disparities between White individuals and people of color. A large study by Fawzy et al. (2022) showed that pulse oximetry readings are affected by skin pigmentation (see Box 2.3).

BOX 2.3   Evidence-Based Practice

Are Pulse Oximetry Readings Affected by Skin Pigmentation?
Based on Fawzy, A., Wu, T. D., Wang, K., Robinson, M. L., Farha, J., et al. (2022). Racial and ethnic discrepancy in pulse oximetry and delayed identification of treatment eligibility among patients with COVID-19. *JAMA Internal Medicine, 182*(7), 730–738.

The researchers conducted a large retrospective cohort study of 7126 clients who were diagnosed with COVID-19 during the pandemic. An analysis of 1216 clients whose arterial oxygen saturation was measured by pulse oximetry and arterial blood gas demonstrated that pulse oximetry overestimated oxygen saturation among Asian, Black, and Hispanic clients compared with White clients. The inaccurate data caused a delay or failure in initiating COVID-19 therapy protocols for people of color which could help explain why they had worse clinical outcomes compared with White clients.

More research is needed to identify if race and ethnicity affect other measurements of objective client findings.

> **CLINICAL JUDGMENT TIP**
>
> *Remember:* When performing any type of health assessment, be aware that several variables, including age, sex, and culture, affect how normal versus abnormal client findings are determined.

Distinguishing Relevant Versus Not-Relevant Clinical Cues

Cue recognition has been defined as "the mental process involved in extracting and identifying *relevant* and important information from the presenting [client] situation" (Betts et al., 2019). This information includes both objective and subjective clinical cues.

Relevant information matters because it has a bearing on what is going on with your client by adding or providing support for the clinical situation. Distinguishing relevant from irrelevant (not relevant) cues can be described as deciding what client information is important to understanding specific health concerns and what information is not important.

Distinguishing relevant from not relevant is especially difficult for novice nurses because this task is influenced by knowledge and experience. A few strategies that can help you determine what's relevant even though you have limited knowledge and experience at this point include:

1. List the clinical cues you collected about a presenting client situation. Then compare these cues with your knowledge of the normal or usual ranges for cues. Which cues are unexpected or not within the normal or usual ranges?
2. Then ask yourself "What is the connection between these abnormal cues and other client findings?" For example, what is the connection (if any) between a client's dyspnea and increased heart rate?
3. Ask the client, significant other, or family member to help identify relationships among signs (objective findings) and symptoms (subjective findings). For example, can you think of any relationship between your (the client's) decreased activity and fatigue levels?
4. When recognizing cues in a presenting client situation, ask yourself, "*What matters most* for the client at this time?" Which cues are outside normal limits and potentially life-threatening? To illustrate how to answer this question, let's review Thinking Exercise 2.1 below:

The nurse is caring for an 81-year-old client in the Emergency Department (ED).

History and Physical	Nurses Notes	Orders	Laboratory Results

1930:   Brought to ED after slipping on wet floor. Family reports client fell on left side and avoided hitting head. Alert but unable to answer questions; holding left outer leg and yelling. Experiencing shortness of breath at times. No adventitious breath sounds; S_1 and S_2 present. Bowel sounds present ×4. Left leg externally rotated and shorter than right leg. Capillary refill <3 seconds bilaterally. Pedal pulses 1+ and equal; feet equally cool without swelling. Able to move all other extremities. H/O diabetes mellitus and hypercholesteremia controlled by drug therapy and diet. VS: T 98.4°F (36.9°C); HR 108 beats per minute; RR 26 breaths per minute; B/P 164/98 mmHg; SpO_2 90% on RA.

In this situation, the client presents to the ED following a fall with an injury. Although the client has a history of diabetes mellitus and hypercholesteremia controlled by drug therapy and diet, these data do not provide information that is helpful about the current injury. Therefore, the information is *not* relevant and would not require immediate follow-up. However, the client's left leg is externally rotated and shorter than the right leg which is apparently causing the client extreme pain as evidenced by yelling. The nurse would want to follow up and manage the client's pain during the evaluation of the left leg deformity. These findings are relevant and require follow-up. The client's heart rate, respiratory rate, and blood pressure are elevated, which further supports the client's acute pain and matter in this situation. The client's vital sign abnormalities and shortness of breath may be caused by anxiety related to the situation and admission to an unfamiliar environment, but they are relevant findings for this client requiring immediate follow-up.

Some of the findings in the client situation are within the normal range, such as a capillary refill of less than 3 seconds and a temperature of 98.4°F (36.9°C), and are therefore irrelevant in the presenting client situation. The client's pedal pulses are equal at 1+ which is diminished in strength compared with a normal expected value of 2+. However, the client is an older adult. The process of aging causes arteries to become stiff and harden. These normal physiologic changes typically cause vasoconstriction and decreased distal perfusion. If the right pedal pulse was 1+ or 2+ and the affected left leg was absent, this finding would be relevant indicating that the leg injury may be affecting perfusion to the left foot. However, the client's pedal pulses are equal in both feet.

Another typical finding for clients of advanced age is acute confusion that can occur when they are injured, experience an illness, or are physically relocated. The client in this clinical scenario is alert (awake) but not able to respond to questions. This finding is *not* relevant because it does not support or add any information to help identify cues related to the injured leg.

CLINICAL JUDGMENT TIP

Remember. Relevant information *matters* because it has a bearing on what is going on with your client by adding or providing support for the clinical situation. When recognizing cues in a presenting client situation, ask yourself, *"What matters most* for this client at this time?"

Distinguishing Expected Versus Not-Expected Clinical Cues

Some client findings are expected in clinical situations, such as the effect of aging on older adults as previously discussed. In other situations, the client may have a chronic illness or disease that explains the assessment findings. For example, a client's shakiness may be caused by Parkinson disease. A client's inability to communicate coherently may be the result of advanced Alzheimer disease. An A_1C of 7.0 may be the normal or usual level for a client with long-term diabetes mellitus, especially if the client's levels have been much higher in the past. Be sure to obtain a reliable medical history from the client, significant other, or family member to help you distinguish expected from unexpected cues.

As part of the client's history, determine what medications the client has been taking. Clients may have therapeutic or side/adverse effects from drug therapy that could be misinterpreted as relevant clinical cues in a presenting clinical situation. Examples include:

1. Unequal pupil size caused by mydriatic (dilating) drops to treat cataract in one eye
2. Decreased level of consciousness (drowsiness) caused by analgesic or psychoactive drugs
3. Increased urinary output (diuresis or incontinence) caused by diuretic drug therapy
4. Bradycardia or low pulse rate caused by beta-adrenergic blocking agents used for hypertension or cardiac dysrhythmias

Thinking Exercise 2.2 will help you practice what you've learned in this chapter. The answer and rationale for the exercise are located at the end of this book.

⚡ THINKING EXERCISE 2.2

The nurse is caring for a 48-year-old client following surgery this morning.

History and Physical	Nurses Notes	Orders	Laboratory Results

1245: Returned from PACU at 1215 after an anterior cervical discectomy and fusion (ACDF). Client alert and oriented; able to speak but barely audible. Can move all extremities but left arm remains slightly weaker than right arm. No numbness in either arm or fingers. Hand strength equal; capillary refill <3 seconds bilaterally. Pulses present and bilaterally equal. Breath sounds clear throughout lung fields. S_1 and S_2 present. Bowel sounds diminished ×4. Left anterior neck surgical dressing dry and intact. No swelling noted around surgical area. VS: T 98.6°F (37°C); HR 86 beats per minute; RR 20 breaths per minute; B/P 120/78 mmHg; SpO_2 99% on O_2 at 3 L/min via NC. Pain reported at 3/10 on a 0–10 pain scale.

1410: O_2 discontinued. SpO_2 95% on RA. No dyspnea reported at this time. Voided ×1; no nausea or vomiting. IV infusing until tolerating fluids. Clear liquids offered.

1520: Reports having difficulty swallowing apple juice even though sitting upright in bed. Small amount of new swelling noted in left neck area. States feeling "a little short of breath."

Select **3** client findings that require **immediate** follow-up by the nurse:
- Speech quality
- Heart rate
- Shortness of breath
- Peripheral oxygen saturation
- Neck swelling
- Respiratory rate
- Pain level
- Left arm weakness
- Difficulty swallowing fluids

PREVENTING FAILURE TO RESCUE

As discussed in Chapter 1, inappropriate, inadequate, or "poor" clinical judgment skills result in negative outcomes that can pose a risk to client safety. The worst outcome of poor clinical judgment is client death.

Definition

Failure to rescue (FTR) is a term adopted by the Joint Commission which accredits acute care hospitals and other types of health care agencies. While there are several definitions in the literature, most of them center on the inability to prevent client death. For this book, failure to rescue is the inability of nurses or other interprofessional health team members to save a client's life in a timely manner when a health care issue or medical complication occurs (Ignatavicius et al., 2024). FTR occurs when early or subtle signs and symptoms are not noticed (*failure to recognize cues*) or accurately interpreted and therefore action to improve the client's condition is not implemented (*failure to escalate*).

While individual factors contribute to these events, organizational or health system factors can influence the incidence of FTR. For example, inadequate nursing staffing levels and a lack of a reliable patient monitoring system can increase the risk of client death.

A classic concept analysis by Mushta et al. (2018) found that FTR as a nurse-sensitive indicator has four key attributes or causes:
1. Failure to recognize changes in the client's condition (cues)
2. Failure to communicate changes in the client's condition
3. Errors of omission in nursing care (sometimes referred to as "missed" nursing care)
4. Failure to make safe, appropriate clinical decisions (clinical judgments)

A systematic review conducted by Burke et al. (2020) validated the concept analysis and found that the most common cause of FTR is the failure to recognize cues (see Box 2.4).

What are the Causes of Failure to Rescue for Clients Experiencing Clinical Deterioration?
Based on Burke, J. R., Downey, C., & Almoudaris, A. M. (2020). Failure to rescue deteriorating patients: A systematic review of root causes and improvement strategies. *Journal of Patient Safety, 18*(1), 140–155.
 The researchers conducted a systematic review of 1486 articles to determine the root causes for and ways to improve the incidence of failure-to-rescue (FTR) events when clients experience clinical deterioration. Fifty-two research studies were fully assessed as part of the review. As a result of data analysis, the authors proposed the 3Rs of FTR: recognize, relay, and react. Nurses and other health care professionals need to be vigilant when caring for clients in acute care settings to ensure early recognition of subtle signs and symptoms (cues), communication of relevant cues to the health care provider, and prompt and appropriate response to the presenting cues in a clinical deterioration situation.

How to Prevent Failure to Rescue

The first approach to preventing FTR events is to anticipate which clients are most likely to experience clinical deterioration as described earlier in this chapter. In addition to these factors, older adults are more likely than younger or middle-aged clients to clinically deteriorate.

 For the past 15–20 years, two new systems have been developed to help reduce the incidence of FTR for clients experiencing clinical deterioration: Rapid Response Teams (RRT) and Client Monitoring Systems. Rapid Response Teams began as part of the Institute for Healthcare Improvement's (IHI's) 100,000 Lives Campaign in 2005.

Rapid Response Teams and Client Monitoring Systems

Today most hospitals have an RRT, also called the Medical Emergency Team (MET). **Rapid Response Teams** save lives and decrease the risk of harm by providing care *before* a medical emergency occurs by intervening rapidly when needed for clients who are *beginning* to clinically decline. Members of the RRT are critical care experts who are on-site and available at any time. Although membership varies among agencies, the team may consist of an intensive care unit (ICU) nurse, respiratory therapist, intensivist (a physician who specializes in critical care), and/or hospitalist (physician, physician assistant, or nurse practitioner employed by the hospital) (Fig. 2.2).

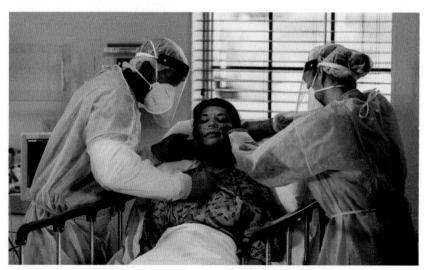

FIG. 2.2 Rapid Response Team members assessing a clinically deteriorating client. (From iStock.com/kali9)

The team responds to emergency calls, usually from clinical staff nurses, according to established agency protocols and policies. One abnormal parameter or a feeling that "something is just not right" can trigger a response from the RRT. Clients' families or significant others may also activate the RRT. A systematic review by Hall et al. (2020) showed that the use of RRTs has reduced client mortality, unplanned intensive care transfers, and unexplained cardiac arrests.

Although RRTs have helped to improve clinical outcomes, they usually respond when there is a report of a significant client change, such as low blood pressure or respiratory rate. Client monitoring systems like **Early Warning Scoring Systems (EWSS)** track multiple parameters at the same time and trigger more frequent assessments based on early changes in vital signs. An EWSS is a guide for the health care team to quickly determine a client's condition based on a physiologic scoring matrix. Keep in mind that this guide is meant to guide clinical judgment and not replace it. Although used for more than 20 years for adult clients admitted to general acute care units, tailored EWSS to include specific triggers associated with laboring clients is now used extensively on obstetric units.

The most commonly used matrix is the Modified Early Warning System (MEWS), which was developed in the United States, and the National Early Warning System, which was developed in the United Kingdom. Each of these systems monitors vital signs, level of consciousness, and urinary output by assigning a score for each parameter. A total score of 4 or more requires observation of the client every 30 minutes and triggers assessment by the RRT (see https://www.ihi.org/resources/Pages/ImprovementStories/EarlyWarningSystemsScorecardsThatSaveLives.aspx).

CLINICAL JUDGMENT TIP

Remember: An early warning scoring system is a guide for the health care team to quickly determine a client's condition based on a physiologic scoring matrix. Keep in mind that this tool is meant to guide or assist you in making clinical decisions and not replace them!

Although the MEWS and other early warning scoring systems encompass multiple clinical cues, several limitations have been documented. These limitations include:
1. The data are collected at intervals, often every 2–4 hours. Urine output must be documented every hour.
2. Mathematical calculations can be inaccurate.
3. Nurses often experience "alarm fatigue" which decreases sensitivity to critical triggers.

The most common clinical deterioration situations in general medical-surgical nursing units are sepsis and acute hypoxic respiratory failure. Stellpflug et al. (2021) conducted a quality improvement project to prevent negative outcomes from these medical complications. Staff nurses working on a 27-bed acute care medical unit were already using an evidence-based protocol for early identification of changes indicating clinical deterioration of clients. This protocol included:
1. MEWS monitoring
2. Use of the RRT
3. Structured evening rounds by the charge nurse with the on-call provider
4. Standardized subjective terminology to describe a client's condition
5. Criteria to determine the need to obtain a serum lactate level to detect sepsis

While there was clinical improvement as a result of this protocol, some clients experienced clinical deterioration in the hours between vital sign (VS) measurements.

As a result, a QI project was developed and implemented to improve client surveillance by adding a digital device for *continuous* VS monitoring. All clients on the unit wore this device on their wrist; alarms were set for VS parameters and the process for communicating VS data to the provider was established. The three primary results of these newly implemented interventions included:

1. Earlier identification of client deterioration
2. High nurse satisfaction
3. High client satisfaction

Although acute care hospital administration may be concerned about the costs of continuous monitoring, this project demonstrated the achievement of improved clinical outcomes for all clients.

While early warning systems can help nurses quickly identify clients who are clinically deteriorating, nurses in all health care settings are accountable for monitoring clients. Be sure to carefully and frequently observe clients and collect objective and subjective cues that are relevant to any clinical situation.

Role of Delegation in Failure to Rescue

As a nurse, you will delegate selected nursing tasks to assistive personnel (AP) such as certified nursing assistants (CNAs). In some countries, these staff members are referred to as unregulated health care workers (UHCW). A delegated responsibility is a nursing activity, skill, or procedure that is transferred from a licensed nurse to a delegate in a selected client care situation (NCSBN-ANA, 2019). Delegation is a skill that is developed over time with experience. This process requires precise and accurate *two-way* communication to prevent clinical errors, including FTR.

For instance, consider this clinical situation: *An acute care nurse working as the shift charge nurse on a general surgical unit started an infusion of packed red blood cells for an 89-year-old client at 0200. The nurse took and recorded the first several sets of vital signs after the infusion began and then delegated the remaining vital sign assessments to an experienced CNA. Approximately 30 minutes later, the nurse asked the CNA what the client's most recent vital sign findings were. The CNA responded that the blood pressure was unobtainable the last time it was taken. The nurse then found the client unresponsive and pulseless. The client died despite medical intervention.*

The decision of whether or not to delegate is based upon the nurse's judgment concerning the medical condition of the client, the competence of all members of the nursing team, and the degree of supervision that is required by the nurse if a task is delegated (NCSBN-ANA, 2019). In this situation, the nurse mistakenly delegated a nursing activity to the CNA for a client who was not medically stable. This client required the assessment skills of a professional nurse and not an unlicensed nursing staff member. Although the nurse is always *accountable* for delegated tasks and skills, the CNA has a responsibility to promptly report the inability to obtain blood pressure.

CLINICAL JUDGMENT TIP

Remember: You are always responsible and accountable for delegated tasks and skills; the delegatee is always responsible for performing the task or skill as needed or expected.

In the example clinical situation, the nurse failed to prevent an FTR event related to inadequate cue recognition. When delegating any nursing task, activity, or skill, follow these guidelines to ensure the ability to recognize cues in any clinical situation:

1. Do not delegate vital signs for a medically unstable client; the professional nurse should take vital signs to determine if they are abnormal and relevant.
2. Communicate clear expectations regarding the task and supervise the AP as needed to validate that the task is completed as expected.
3. Teach AP to report selected signs and symptoms based on the clinical situation to the nurse. For instance, a client who has total hip or knee arthroplasty is at risk for venous thromboembolism

despite preventive interventions. Ask the AP to immediately report any chest discomfort, difficulty breathing, or redness and swelling in either lower leg.

Box 2.5 summarizes safe practices for delegating nursing skills to help recognize cues and prevent FTR events.

BOX 2.5 Practices for Delegating Safely and Effectively

Delegate When
- the client is medically stable
- the task or skill is within the staff member's (delegatee's) capabilities
- you are able and have the time to do the teaching and supervision the delegate needs
- you have planned how and when to monitor client results yourself.

Do not Delegate When
- complex client assessment, thinking, and judgments are required
- the outcome of the task or skill is unpredictable
- there is an increased risk for harm.

Thinking Exercise 2.3 will help you practice what you've learned in this chapter. The answer and rationale for the exercise are located at the end of this book.

⚡ THINKING EXERCISE 2.3

The nurse is caring for a 9-year-old client in the Urgent Care Center.
Highlight the findings below that require follow-up during this visit.

History and Physical	Nurses Notes	Orders	Laboratory Results

1615: Parent visited center for child's nasal congestion, coughing, and low-grade fever for the past 2 days. Today the child seems much more tired, has a sore throat, and is beginning to feel achy. VS taken by certified medical assistant (CMA): T 101°F (38.3°C); HR 92 beats per minute; RR 20 breaths per minute; B/P 114/58 mmHg; SpO$_2$ 98% on RA. CMA reports observing various stages of old bruising on chest and back. Child states bruises resulted from playing sports, but would not make eye contact when answering. Throat slightly reddened. No adventitious breath sounds. Plan to test for strep, flu, and COVID-19.

ENSURING SITUATIONAL AWARENESS

The ability to notice changes in a client's condition and intervene appropriately is a sign of strong clinical reasoning to make safe clinical judgments. Failure to recognize these cues in a timely manner is often the result of inadequate situational awareness.

Definition

The most commonly cited definition of situational awareness in nursing is the result of the classic concept analysis conducted by Fore and Sculli (2013). These authors defined situational awareness (SA) as an essential client safety skill that consists of the nurse's ability to do the following:
- Perceive a clinical situation accurately and completely
- Understand the meaning of the clinical situation
- Rapidly predict the outcome of the clinical situation

This skill requires you to demonstrate the art of keen observation. Observation is the purposeful gathering of information from clients and/or significant others/family members to inform clinical judgments. It includes using all of your senses to collect subjective and objective data to determine the client's immediate and long-term needs. Depending on the severity or complexity of those needs, the client may require either intermittent or continuous observation or monitoring. Table 2.3 lists core principles of client observation with nursing practice examples.

TABLE 2.3   Core Principles of Client Observation With Examples

Core Principles	Examples
Observation is comprehensive.	Use your senses to collect information about the client, including sight, hearing, and smell (such as the smell of foul wound drainage to indicate infection); be aware and report any "gut feeling" about a client.
Observation is a critical part of client assessment.	Recall that observation is the initial activity during assessment and often the most important in providing assessment data; quickly develop trust in clients who are clinically deteriorating.
Observation requires interactive communication with the client.	Develop excellent communication skills to accurately and thoroughly collect both subjective and objective data, e.g., pain assessment.
Observation is affected by the health care environment.	Use quick and deliberate observation in emergent/urgent settings like the emergency department or other urgent care settings; remember that you may have only one opportunity for observation in these settings compared with hospitalized clients.
Observation needs to be communicated and documented.	Communicate client information from observation with health care team members; document findings promptly, accurately, and completely.

Being able to perceive a clinical situation in which the client experiences changes in condition or deterioration is the most important aspect of SA. This information is essential to identify client needs and prevent missed nursing care. It is equally important in assisting the health care provider in making an accurate diagnosis and initiating treatment. Therefore, SA is a critical component in reducing medical errors. Research has shown that nurses have inadequate knowledge to make prompt and accurate client observations when clinical deterioration occurs (Alastalo et al., 2022).

In addition to ensuring accuracy when recognizing cues, adequate SA enables nurses to perceive the situation completely or from a wholistic view. Nurses and other health care professionals may have "tunnel vision" when assessing a client's condition which could lead to negative clinical outcomes.

For instance, consider this clinical situation: *A 68-year-old client admitted to a neuroscience unit from the critical care unit had a surgical evacuation of a subdural hematoma following a fall almost 2 weeks ago. The client was treated with IV antibiotics for aspiration pneumonia but became increasingly lethargic, anorexic, and febrile 4 days ago. The client then developed diarrhea and severe abdominal distention. The neurosurgeon suspected meningitis or encephalitis which was ruled out by multiple diagnostic tests. The client's daughter-in-law visited the client for the first time in a week and noted the client's rapid, shallow respirations of over 50 breaths per minute. Additionally, the client could only be aroused by using painful stimuli. After the charge nurse reported these findings to the neurosurgical senior resident, the client was reexamined by the resident and transferred to the critical care unit where a central line was placed for IV fluids to treat severe dehydration. An emergency exploratory laparotomy that evening revealed a completely gangrenous colon. The client died from sepsis 2 days later.*

In this clinical situation, significant changes in the client's condition were assumed to be the result of a neurological health problem. Both the neuroscience staff nurses and the neurosurgical provider's team had "tunnel vision" and missed the obvious clinical cues indicating a nonneurological cause for the client's clinical deterioration. In other words, they had inadequate SA. For some older adults, antibiotic therapy can cause pseudomembranous colitis leading to toxic megacolon and subsequently gangrene and sepsis. Diarrhea combined with a lack of fluid intake further complicated this client's condition, causing severe dehydration. The client's decreasing level of consciousness, fever, tachypnea, abdominal distention, and diarrhea should have alerted the nurses on the unit that the client's basic needs were not being met. The result of inadequate SA in this clinical situation was the loss of a client's life.

CLINICAL JUDGMENT TIP

Remember. SA is an essential client safety skill that enhances your ability to recognize cues and prevent missed nursing care when making clinical decisions.

How to Perform a Situational Awareness Assessment

Follow these ABCs for performing an SA assessment:
1. **A**wareness of the environment
2. **B**elief in your gut feelings
3. **C**hanging what is wrong (follow-up)

Completing an SA assessment during your first client encounter or at the beginning of an inpatient shift allows you to establish a baseline and anticipate any potential medical complications. Once you practice this assessment and gain experience with multiple clients, you should be able to complete it in about 60 seconds.

Begin *awareness of the environment* by assessing the client's ABCs without touching the client. Observe the client's breathing and general behavior first. What is the client's color and respiratory rate? If you have cared for the client earlier, are the color and respiratory rate the same or different?

Then, check all tubes, lines, and respiratory equipment and support. Is the client's nasal cannula or mask correctly positioned? Is the oxygen flowmeter set for the appropriate rate? Are the IV solutions ready to be replaced because their levels are low? If the client has a urinary catheter, is the drainage bag off the floor and the tubing correctly positioned to promote gravity flow?

Assess the client's surroundings. For example, is the call light within reach? Are there any barriers or problems in the environment that can cause harm to the client, such as a wet floor? If the client uses an ambulatory aid, is the cane, walker, or crutches placed where the client can reach them?

Next, determine whether the client's situation seems "right." Do you have a *gut feeling* that the client's condition is deteriorating or that the client is developing a medical complication? This intuitive feeling is often the trigger for calling the RRT or health care provider and develops with increased experience and confidence.

If you note a problem or change in the client's condition, be prepared to *follow up*. For example, if the client is having difficulty breathing, be sure the client is in an upright sitting position, initiate supplemental oxygen, and/or increase the existing oxygen flow rate unless contraindicated.

Implementing SA helps prevent errors, missed nursing care, and potential FTR. Box 2.6 provides examples of common questions to use when performing an SA assessment.

BOX 2.6   Examples of Questions When Performing a Situational Awareness Assessment

ABC (Without Touching the Client)
- What information, if any, leads you to suspect any problem with airway, breathing, or circulation?
- If there is a suspected problem or need, is the problem or need urgent or not urgent?
- What clinical data would indicate the situation needs immediate action and why?
- Does anyone need to be contacted to assist with any client problem or need?
- If the client is receiving supplemental oxygen, what would you need to continue to monitor the client?
- Do you have any recommendations or suggestions regarding any client problem or need to be noted?

Tubes and Lines
- Does the client have any tubes or IV access?
- Is the IV infusion solution the correct one per orders?
- Does the client need the current tubes? If so, why?
- Do you notice any complications related to tubes and lines?
- What additional assessment is needed?

Client Safety Survey
- What are your safety concerns with this client, if any?
- Do you need to report this problem and, if so, to whom?

Environmental Survey
- Is there anything about the environment that could cause a client problem?
- If there is an actual or potential problem, how will you plan to manage the problem?

Sensory Assessment
- What are your senses telling you?
- Do you hear, smell, see, or feel something that needs to be explored?
- Does the client's situation seem or feel "right?"

Adapted from Struth, D. (2009). TCAB in the curriculum: Creating a safer environment through nursing education. *American Journal of Nursing, 109*(Suppl. 11), 55–58.

CLINICAL JUDGMENT TIP

Follow these ABCs for performing an SA assessment:
1. **A**wareness of the environment
2. **B**elief in your gut feelings
3. **C**hanging what is wrong (follow-up)

Thinking Exercise 2.4 will help you practice what you've learned in this chapter. The answer and rationale for the exercise are located at the end of this book.

RECOGNIZING CHANGES IN CLIENTS' CLINICAL CONDITIONS

Making timely appropriate clinical judgments is a priority skill that you will need to ensure client safety in any health care setting. Early recognition of changes in clients' clinical conditions is essential to make timely and safe decisions.

Factors That Influence the Ability of Nurses to Recognize Changes

Several factors influence the ability of nurses to recognize cues, the first step in making safe clinical judgments. Being aware of these factors can help you understand their impact on how you

---

⚡ THINKING EXERCISE 2.4

The nurse is caring for an 88-year-old client in a skilled nursing facility.

History and Physical	Nurses Notes	Orders	Laboratory Results

0900: Client remains in bed and not eating breakfast as usual in the recliner every morning. States having severe pain in right leg which worsened during the night. Reports pain at 10 on a 0–10 pain intensity scale. Describes pain as diffuse involving the entire leg. Right leg cooler than left; mottled appearance with pallor. Right pedal and popliteal pulses not palpable; left pedal pulse 1+; left popliteal pulse 2+. VS: T 98.6°F (37°C); HR 90 beats per minute; RR 18 breaths per minute; B/P 110/64 mmHg; SpO$_2$ 93% on RA.

0815: Charge nurse notified about client condition.

Select **4** findings below that require **immediate** follow-up:
- ○ Anorexia
- ○ Pain level and location in the right leg
- ○ Color of right leg
- ○ Temperature of right leg
- ○ Heart rate
- ○ Blood pressure
- ○ Distal pulses
- ○ SpO$_2$

recognize clinical cues and make decisions. These factors can be categorized into nurse factors, client factors, and system factors (Fig. 2.3).

Nurse Factors

The *work experience* of nurses and how it influences decision-making has been one of the most explored factors. Orique et al. (2019) found that new nursing graduates were technically competent but missed clinical cues that could have prevented client harm due to lack of work experience. The authors concluded that nursing experience matters because expert nurses have a higher

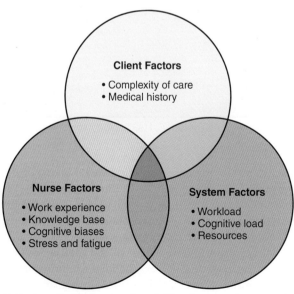

FIG. 2.3 Factors that influence the ability of nurses to recognize cues.

capacity for cue recognition and processing. Experienced nurses learn from each client interaction and can transfer that learning from one clinical situation to another.

A classic integrative literature review showed that experienced acute care nurses have the following characteristics that enhance their ability to recognize cues and make safe appropriate clinical judgments (Nibbelink & Brewer, 2018):

- Understanding of client status
- Intuitive thinking
- Protocol application
- Collaboration with colleagues

Experienced nurses understand their clients' clinical states by developing relationships with clients and spending time with them. Knowing clients helps nurses develop a gut feeling or "sixth sense" when changes in client conditions occur (Massey et al., 2017). A physical nurse presence is vital to noticing client changes and recognizing clinical cues as part of SA. Knowing the client includes (1) performing and documenting frequent assessments, especially client observations and vital signs (Nibbelink & Brewer, 2018), and (2) recognizing the client's pattern of responses.

Experienced expert nurses also use intuition to help recognize cues to make appropriate clinical judgments. Intuition, also called intuitive thinking, is the ability to predict client situations facilitated by a strong knowledge base. Sometimes referred to as "knowing without evidence," intuitive thinking includes the ability to recognize similarities between previous and current clinical situations, which is important for cue recognition (Table 2.4).

TABLE 2.4 Elements of Intuition With Descriptions

Element	Description
Pattern recognition	The ability to recognize patterns of responses and changes of behavior, e.g., nausea and vomiting after every meal
Similarity recognition	Recognizing client characteristics seen previously and using them as part of interpreting the current client situation
Common sense understanding	Recognizing and using commonly accepted practice
Skilled know-how	Making judgments about what seems to be the appropriate care for a client
Sense of salience	Recognizing the importance of a particular information source, even though it may be contradicted by another source
Deliberating rationality	Maintaining a broad view of the situation

Adapted from Benner, P., & Tanner, C. (1987). How expert nurses use intuition. *American Journal of Nursing, 87*(1), 23–24.

By contrast, novice nurses rely on rule-based thinking or step-by-step logic, which is defined as rational thinking based on evidence (Orique et al., 2019). With work experience and ongoing development of nursing expertise, you will be able to use intuitive thinking when needed.

Intuitive thinking is also called fast thinking which is predisposed to errors in clinical judgment. Nurses often make false assumptions about clients and develop *cognitive biases*. Cognitive biases are flaws or distortions in judgment and clinical decision-making; these biases often contribute to adverse or sentinel events (The Joint Commission, 2023). A sentinel event is a *severe* variation in the standard of care that is caused by human or system error and results in an avoidable patient death or major harm.

Cognitive biases may be influenced by the nurse's feelings and values. Consider this example: *A young adult with a history of substance abuse is admitted to the Emergency Department with a report of severe abdominal pain. The triage nurse assumes that the client is drug-seeking rather than focusing on relevant subjective and objective cues that help determine the client's actual needs.* In this example, the nurse assumed the young client was drug-seeking because of the client's substance abuse history. Be sure not to make assumptions without adequate clinical evidence to support cue recognition and processing.

CLINICAL JUDGMENT TIP

Nurses often make false assumptions about clients when recognizing cues and develop *cognitive biases*. Be sure not to make assumptions without adequate clinical evidence to support cue recognition and processing!

Client safety may be jeopardized when nurses have symptoms of burnout due to the high demand and complexity of care. This problem worsened during the pandemic when nurses cared for large volumes of critically ill patients, watched countless patients die without the presence of their loved ones, and often managed complex care without adequate supplies and equipment. The result was a decline in the well-being of many nurses and extreme fatigue and stress (Munn et al., 2021; Trinkoff et al., 2021). Extreme *fatigue and stress* can negatively affect the ability to perform cue recognition and processing. Fatigue and stress can also promote the development of cognitive biases. Be sure to take care of yourself at work and at home to help prevent burnout and poor well-being to ensure client safety.

Client Factors

In addition to nurse factors, several client factors can affect your ability to make appropriate clinical judgments, including the *complexity of client care* and *client history*. Hospitalized and older clients typically have numerous comorbidities that complicate care and impact decision-making when changes in condition occur. For example, a client who becomes dehydrated due to hypovolemia from bleeding needs fluid replacement as soon as possible. However, the client may have diabetes mellitus, heart disease, and chronic kidney disease which could influence the client's presenting cues. The nurse may identify peripheral edema as a relevant clinical cue and suspect hypervolemia or fluid overload rather than hypovolemia.

In some cases, the nurse may not have access to a complete client history. This lack of cues may result in a clinical judgment that is poor or inadequate, possibly causing client harm.

System Factors

Client harm can also occur as a result of system factors. Decision-making in acute care, for instance, is highly demanding because staff nurses are usually assigned to five or more clients each shift. As a result of this heavy *workload*, nurses are often overworked, have insufficient time to recognize early or subtle changes in client conditions, experience *cognitive overload*, and have minimal opportunity for self-care.

Cognitive load is the amount of information within one's working (short-term) memory while performing a variety of activities. Three types of cognitive load have been identified (Collins, 2020):

1. Intrinsic cognitive load: The level of cognitive effort needed for a nurse to complete a task or resolve a problem
2. Extrinsic cognitive load: The level of cognitive effort required of nurses by the work setting

3. Germane (relevant and appropriate) cognitive load: The level of cognitive effort needed for a nurse to make sense of new information

Nurses can become overwhelmed by the large amount of complex information received from multiple individuals, technological devices, and clinical systems causing cognitive overload (Collins, 2020). Cognitive overload can impact the nurse's mental, emotional, and physical well-being, which leads to errors in cue recognition and processing.

To ensure nurses' well-being, collaborate with leaders in your health care organization to help reduce stress and fatigue from cognitive overload. For example, during the COVID-19 pandemic, nurses formed support groups to share their feelings and brainstorm strategies to help each other. Some hospitals allow nurses to take turns resting or napping to help restore their energy and reduce complications from cognitive overload (Munn et al., 2021).

Technological and human *resources* can also impact the ability to recognize relevant clinical cues. For instance, the lack of available pulse oximeters in settings such as assisted living and long-term care facilities prevents assessment of a client's oxygenation status. The lack of adequate nursing staff in any health care setting prevents nurses from having the time to carefully observe clients to identify relevant or beginning changes in their condition.

Common Clinical Cues Used by Nurses

A large systematic study by Burdeu et al. (2021) found that nurses use body temperature, heart rate, and blood pressure as the most common clinical cues to determine changes in client conditions. However, changes in other vital signs are the most accurate signs of critical health problems. For example, tachypnea, hypoxemia, and decreased Glasgow Coma Scale scores are the most sensitive indicators of impending clinical deterioration. For many clients, these changes begin to occur 24–48 hours *before* a significant decline in client condition.

Some studies indicate that nurses do not always take and record a *complete* set of vital signs. Descriptions of what vital signs include differ among agencies in the same country or across countries. For example, in the United States, most health care agencies define vital signs as assessments of body temperature, heart rate, respiratory rate, and blood pressure. Some agencies also include peripheral oxygenation saturation rate (SpO_2). In other countries like Australia, the level of consciousness is added to this definition. Omitting some of the vital sign parameters suggests nurses may be tailoring their assessments to client needs or clinical conditions (Burdeu et al., 2021).

A study by Elliott and Endacott (2022) concluded that vital signs are simple to assess, take about 5 minutes to collect, and are the most important clinical cues to determine a client's condition. However, nurses often do not take a complete set of vital signs as part of their assessments, especially respiratory rate and level of consciousness. Additionally, the researchers found that abnormal vital signs are not always interpreted or responded to in a timely manner. This lack of essential data can result in client harm and missed nursing care.

Several factors may explain the actions of nurses in failing to collect and record complete vital sign data, including the following (Elliott & Endacott, 2022):

- Lack of knowledge about the importance of taking vital signs
- Inadequate staff and lack of time to take complete vital signs
- Absence of formal guidelines on taking vital signs, including definition
- Assuming that vital signs are not needed for low-risk clients

Another factor is the use of AP (or UHCWs) to take vital signs. Overworked nurses may feel they do not have time to supervise these health care staff. In some cases, nurses fail to follow up if vital signs are abnormal or unexpected. In other cases, the nurses note abnormal vital signs but may fail to interpret them as key clinical cues indicating an urgent or emergent change in the client's condition.

CLINICAL JUDGMENT TIP

Remember: Be sure you know the definition of vital signs in your health care setting. Take and record a *complete* set of vital signs or delegate this activity with follow-up supervision. Review vital sign findings and identify relevant clinical cues.

In addition to recognizing cues, especially vital signs, to detect clinical deterioration or other changes in client conditions, use these data to determine when the client improves. Cues to indicate improved clinical condition have been underreported in the literature. Decreasing pain is the most common cue used to identify client improvement, but other data such as improving vital signs, are more useful in determining whether a client's condition has improved or worsened (Burdeu et al., 2021). Chapter 7 discusses cues for evaluating outcomes in more detail.

Thinking Exercise 2.5 will help you practice what you've learned in this chapter. The answer and rationale for the exercise are located at the end of this book.

⚡ THINKING EXERCISE 2.5

The nurse is caring for a 30-year-old client who had an emergency Caesarean section 2 hours ago.

History and Physical	Nurses Notes	Orders	Laboratory Results

0245: Alert and oriented ×4. Abdominal pain 5/10; uterus massaged. Minimal vaginal bleeding on peri-pad. Abdominal dressing dry and intact. VS: T 98°F (36.7°C); HR 92 beats per minute; RR 18 breaths per minute; B/P 106/64 mmHg; SpO$_2$ 97% on RA.

0415: Abdominal pain increased to 8/10 although given analgesic an hour ago. Slight abdominal distention. Minimal vaginal bleeding on peri-pad. Abdominal dressing dry and intact. VS: T 98.6°F (37°C); HR 110 beats per minute; RR 20 breaths per minute; B/P 92/50 mmHg; SpO$_2$ 96% on RA.

Which of the following client findings require **immediate** follow-up? **Select all that apply:**
- Body temperature
- Heart rate
- Respiratory rate
- Blood pressure
- SpO$_2$
- Abdominal pain
- Vaginal bleeding

RECOGNIZING CUES TO MAKE SAFE CLINICAL JUDGMENTS

As discussed in this chapter, being able to recognize cues is the most important cognitive skill needed to make safe and appropriate clinical judgments as a nurse. Having a strong *knowledge base* is essential when making clinical judgments, especially when recognizing cues.

Role of Knowledge

Nursing knowledge is drawn from a multifaceted, complex base, and can be categorized into four major sources as described in Table 2.5 (Smith et al., 2021).

TABLE 2.5 **Sources of Knowledge Used by Practicing Nurses**	
Knowledge Source	**Knowledge Source Description**
Scientific knowledge	Knowledge generated through research to inform nursing practice
Aesthetic knowledge	Knowledge about the art of nursing to provide empathic care
Ethics knowledge	Knowledge about the moral principles of nursing practice
Personal knowledge	Knowledge gained through experiences in clinical situations

Nurses have been encouraged to abandon traditional ways of practice and adopt *scientific knowledge*, or current empirical evidence, to guide practice. For example, to be able to accurately recognize cues in a clinical situation, you must have a thorough understanding of pathophysiology. Knowledge of pathophysiology is particularly important to distinguish normal versus abnormal client findings and relevant versus irrelevant findings.

However, many nursing experts have questioned relying *solely* on empirical evidence as the guide for the complexity and wholistic nature of professional practice. Smith et al. (2021) state that "the purpose of evidence-based practice and clinical guidelines is to promote standardization of approaches to care, rather than individualization. For this reason, applying general evidence to a particular situation may be inappropriate, and at times might even be harmful" (p. 13). The knowledge that guides nurses to be physically present for clients and understand what matters to them comes from the philosophies, values, and theories of the nursing profession, not from research (Smith et al., 2021). For that reason, nurses use other sources of knowledge, sometimes referred to as patterns of knowing.

CLINICAL JUDGMENT TIP

Remember. Recall your knowledge of pathophysiology to help you recognize relevant clinical cues by differentiating normal/usual versus abnormal/unusual client findings.

Aesthetic knowledge guides nurses to provide compassionate, empathic, and individualized care. Caring nurses strive to identify the most relevant clinical cues to determine a client's condition while providing emotional support and establishing trust. Nurses also use *ethics as moral knowledge* by embracing key ethical principles when caring for clients (Table 2.6).

TABLE 2.6 **Key Ethical Principles Used in Practicing Nurses**	
Ethical Principle	**Description of Ethical Principle**
Autonomy	Advocating for clients who cannot self-manage or make their own decisions
Beneficence	Doing good for and helping clients
Nonmaleficence	Preventing harm and ensuring the client's well-being
Fidelity	Keeping obligations and promises to clients
Veracity	Telling the truth (which helps build trust) and avoiding providing incorrect information
Social justice	Treating all clients equally and fairly

Strategies for Recognizing Cues

This chapter has explored factors that affect your ability as a nurse to recognize cues. This discussion summarizes the strategies you will need to correctly identify relevant cues as a client's condition changes or deteriorates (Box 2.7).

BOX 2.7   **Strategies for Recognizing Cues**

- Carefully review all client findings (both objective and subjective data) in the clinical situation while ensuring SA.
- Identify the clients most at risk for clinical deterioration or medical complications.
- Anticipate common medical complications that are associated with or could occur as a result of the client's current condition.
- Determine which client findings are normal/usual or abnormal/unusual in the clinical situation.
- Consider contextual factors that influence if client findings in the clinical situation are expected or unexpected.
- Determine which assessment findings in the clinical situation are relevant or not relevant.
- Determine which relevant findings require **immediate** follow-up.

Carefully Review All Client Findings

Whether you are caring for a client in clinical practice or reading a clinical situation in a Thinking Exercise or NCLEX® test item, be sure to review all client assessment findings carefully and thoroughly. That means that you need to review various parts of the client's medical record and assess the client directly if you are practicing in an actual clinical setting or at home. Recall that clinical cues include both objective findings (signs) and subjective findings (symptoms) indicating client deterioration and improvement. During initial encounters with health care professionals, clients often share a significant amount of information that can provide meaningful insight into their condition. Be sure to engage in active listening and follow up with questions to elicit additional information as needed. Be aware of all aspects of the client's situation, including environmental factors such as the health care setting and available health care technologies.

Identify Clients Most at Risk for Clinical Deterioration

To effectively recognize cues, anticipate which clients are most at risk for clinical deterioration or medical complications. As identified earlier in this chapter, clients most at risk for clinical deterioration include those with the following characteristics (Padilla & Mayo, 2018):
- Are admitted to the Emergency Department
- Present with acute or preexisting health conditions
- Had recent surgeries
- Are recovering from critical illnesses

Anticipate that any of these clients are at *high risk* for deterioration or medical complications; report and document any subtle or beginning changes in their clinical state.

Anticipate Common Medical Complications

Consider the client's current condition and past medical history, if available, to help anticipate for which complications the client may be at risk. For example, clients who have had recent surgeries are often at risk for multiple postoperative complications, including wound infection which could progress to sepsis. Some surgeries are associated with specific complications for which the nurse would anticipate, such as venous thromboembolism (deep vein thrombosis or pulmonary embolism) in clients who have total hip or knee arthroplasty. Clients who have open abdominal surgery are at risk for different complications, including evisceration, peritonitis, and paralytic ileus.

Complications or client conditions are not always biologic or physical. For instance, clients who have a history of severe depression may be at risk for or attempt suicide. Children or older adults may be at risk for physical or emotional abuse or neglect. Identify clients at risk and assess for verbal and/or nonverbal cues that confirm these conditions.

Sometimes a client can experience a normal life event like birthing a baby but complications can occur. For example, postpartum hemorrhage can occur in clients who have normal spontaneous vaginal deliveries. Postpartum depression or posttraumatic stress disorder can also develop as a result of newborn delivery.

Recall your knowledge of pathophysiology to help anticipate these possible complications. Then ask yourself: For what complications or conditions might this client be at risk? What clinical cues could indicate the client is experiencing one or more of these complications or conditions?

Determine Which Client Findings Are Normal/Usual or Abnormal/Unusual

Client findings within the usual expectations or range are "normal." As discussed earlier in this chapter, if you determine the client's findings are outside the normal or usual range, then you have identified abnormal or unusual clinical cues. However, not all abnormal findings are significant in a presenting client situation. In some client scenarios, abnormal findings are expected due to the nature of the clinical situation. For instance, a client experiencing acute pain typically has an elevated heart rate and blood pressure due to the stress response. Remember, if you notice the client presents with a new or changed sign (objective finding), assess for associated symptoms to support the measurable sign. If the client reports a new or changed symptom (subjective finding), assess for associated signs to support the stated symptom.

Consider Client Contextual Factors

As discussed earlier in this chapter, demographic factors such as age can affect which cues are perceived as normal versus abnormal. Be sure to notice the client's age which can assist you in determining developmental stage. Knowledge of a client's developmental stage helps to identify clinical cues that may be abnormal or unusual. For example, a school-age child who is reluctant to answer questions and avoids eye contact may be developmentally delayed, afraid of health care professionals, or the victim of abuse and/or neglect.

Knowledge of normal physiologic and psychological changes associated with aging is also essential. Many nurses make incorrect assumptions about older adults, expecting confusion, ADL dependence, and incontinence to be normal findings for this age group. These changes are *not* normal or usual as people age and often indicate underlying health conditions that are frequently treatable.

Determine Which Client Findings Are Relevant

As introduced earlier in this chapter, relevant information matters because it has a bearing on what is going on with your client by adding or providing support for the clinical situation. Distinguishing relevant from irrelevant (not relevant) cues can be described as deciding what client information is pertinent to understanding specific health needs and what information is not pertinent. For example, a client who is admitted to the Emergency Department with stab wounds in both arms may also have slightly elevated serum glucose. This laboratory result is abnormal but is not important or pertinent at this time. The client may be experiencing glucose elevation because of increased production of epinephrine from the adrenal glands as part of the "flight or fight response." Or the client may have undiagnosed diabetes mellitus or some other endocrine condition. Whatever the cause of hyperglycemia, this client finding is not relevant when managing the client's injuries.

Determine Which Relevant Findings Require Immediate Follow-Up

In some clinical situations, client findings are relevant but do not need immediate follow-up. When recognizing cues, you need to determine which abnormal, unexpected, and/or relevant client findings need to be followed up immediately. These findings are often life-threatening or potentially life-threatening, and therefore, are the priority for client care. Given that nurses often do not take a complete set of vital signs and that vital sign changes, including level of consciousness (LOC), typically occur hours or days before clinical deterioration, be sure to pay particular attention to these findings.

Thinking Exercise 2.6 will help you practice what you've learned in this chapter. The answer and rationale for the exercise are located at the end of this book.

THINKING EXERCISE 2.6

The nurse is caring for a 17-year-old client in the Emergency Department (ED).
Highlight the findings below that require **immediate** follow-up.

History and Physical	Nurses Notes	Orders	Laboratory Results

1048:   Brought to ED by family for severe abdominal pain, fever, and vomiting which started last night. Has not eaten for almost 24 hours due to anorexia. History of fractured humerus and severely sprained ankle from participating in multiple high school sports. Alert and oriented ×4; reports pain at 10/10 especially in right lower quadrant radiating to mid-abdomen. Hypoactive bowel sounds ×4 with abdominal distention. VS: T 100.8°F (38.2°C); HR 94 beats per minute; RR 22 breaths per minute; B/P 124/86 mmHg; SpO$_2$ 96% on RA. Prepared for abdominal ultrasound.

END-OF-CHAPTER EXERCISES

Additional End-of-Chapter Exercises will help you apply what you've learned in this chapter. The answers and rationales for these exercises are located at the end of this book.

END-OF-CHAPTER EXERCISE 2.1

The nurse reviews recent laboratory results for a 39-year-old client who is 31 weeks pregnant and has gestational diabetes mellitus.

History and Physical	Laboratory Results	Orders	Nurses Notes
Serum Laboratory Test/ Reference Range	Yesterday	2 Weeks Ago	4 Weeks Ago
Uric acid (<6 mg/dL [<0.36 mmol/L])	7.8 mg/dL (0.46 mmol/L)	6.4 mg/dL (0.38 mmol/L)	5.7 mg/dL (0.34 mmol/L)
Creatinine (0.5–1.1 mg/dL [44.2–97.3 µmol/L])	2.3 mg/dL (203.4 µmol/L)	2.1 mg/dL (185.7 µmol/L)	1.3 mg/dL (115 µmol/L)
Hematocrit (>33%)	34%	35%	35%
Platelets (150,000–400,000/ mm^3 [150–400 × 10^9/L])	100,000/mm^3 (100 × 10^9/L)	145,000/mm^3 (145 × 10^9/L)	158,000/mm^3 (158 × 10^9/L)
Fasting blood glucose (74–106 mg/dL [4.1– 5.9 mmol/L])	110 mg/dL (6.1 mmol/L)	104 mg/dL (5.8 mmol/L)	100 mg/dL (5.6 mmol/L)

Which of the following client findings require **immediate** follow-up? **Select all that apply.**
- Uric acid
- Creatinine
- Hematocrit
- Platelets
- Fasting blood glucose

END-OF-CHAPTER EXERCISE 2.2

The nurse is caring for a 59-year-old client following an open exploratory laparotomy late yesterday afternoon.

History and Physical	Nurses Notes	Orders	Laboratory Results

0750:   Alert and oriented ×4; reports abdominal pain worsening for the past few hours even though using patient-controlled analgesia as instructed. States feeling nauseated and unable to try clear liquids. Does not feel like getting out of bed this morning. Using incentive spirometer 1–2 hours; compression stockings in place. Able to move all extremities. Cap refill <3 seconds. No abnormal or adventitious breath sounds. S_1 and S_2 present. Abdominal dressing dry and intact with small amount of dried blood. Bowel sounds absent ×4; abdomen moderately distended. VS: VS: 99.4°F (37.4°C); HR 98 beats per minute; RR 20 breaths per minute; B/P 116/72 mmHg; SpO_2 95% on RA.

Complete the following sentence by selecting from the lists of options below.
The nurse recognizes that the client's _____**1 [Select]**_____, _____**2 [Select]**_____, and ____**3 [Select]**____ require **immediate** follow-up.

Options for 1	Options for 2	Options for 3
Elevated temperature	Tachycardia	Nausea
Worsening abdominal pain	Tachypnea	Presence of S_1 and S_2
Absent bowel sounds	Abdominal distension	Blood on abdominal dressing

END-OF-CHAPTER EXERCISE 2.3

The nurse is screening a 16-year-old client visiting the primary health care provider office prior to the client's annual physical examination.

Nurses Notes	History and Physical	Orders	Laboratory Results

1015:   Client states the past year has been very difficult because of mandatory remote learning instead of in-person education during the COVID-19 pandemic. Has missed friends and social events; has no interest in participating in virtual activities. Client appears very thin and tired; reports insomnia, very dry skin, and hair loss that have worsened over the past few months. Height 68 in (172.7 cm); weight 98 lb (44.5 kg); BMI 14.9. BMI a year ago 18.7. VS: 97.6°F (36.4°C); HR 100 beats per minute and irregular; RR 20 breaths per minute; B/P 88/48 mmHg; SpO_2 95% on RA.

Select **4** of the following findings that require **immediate** follow-up:
○ Lack of interest in activities
○ Hair loss
○ Insomnia
○ BMI
○ Body temperature
○ Heart rate
○ Blood pressure
○ SpO_2

END-OF-CHAPTER EXERCISE 2.4

The nurse is caring for a 40-year-old client in the Urgent Care Center.

History and Physical	Nurses Notes	Orders	Laboratory Results

1955: Client states coming to center due to heart palpitations that have lasted for over an hour. History of two similar episodes in the past 3 years. Has had diabetes mellitus for almost 20 years. Alert and oriented ×4. No abnormal or adventitious breath sounds; skin cool and clammy. No report of chest pain or discomfort. FSBG 76 mg/dL (4.21 mmol/L). VS: 98.6°F (37°C); HR 188 beats per minute and irregular; RR 22 breaths per minute; B/P 144/92 mmHg; SpO$_2$ 97% on RA.

Complete the following sentence by selecting from the list of Word Choices below.
The nurse identifies that the client's **[Word Choice]** and **[Word Choice]** require *immediate* follow-up.

Word Choices	
Heart rate	Palpitations
Blood glucose	Blood pressure
Respiratory rate	

Answers and Rationales for Thinking Exercises

CHAPTER THINKING EXERCISES

THINKING EXERCISE 2.1

Answer:

History and Physical	Nurses Notes	Orders	Laboratory Results

1930: Brought to ED after slipping on wet floor. Family reports client fell on left side and avoided hitting head. Alert but unable to answer questions; holding left outer leg and yelling. Experiencing shortness of breath at times. No adventitious breath sounds; S$_1$ and S$_2$ present. Bowel sounds present ×4. Left leg externally rotated and shorter than right leg. Capillary refill <3 seconds bilaterally. Pedal pulses 1+ and equal; feet equally cool without swelling. Able to move all other extremities. H/O diabetes mellitus and hypercholesteremia controlled by drug therapy and diet. VS: T 98.4°F (36.9°C); HR 108 beats per minute; RR 26 breaths per minute; B/P 164/98 mmHg; SpO$_2$ via pulse ox 90% on RA.

Rationale: In this situation, the client presents to the ED following a fall with an injury. Although the client has a history of diabetes mellitus and hypercholesteremia controlled by drug therapy and diet, these data do not provide information that is helpful about the current injury. Therefore, these findings would not require immediate follow-up. However, the client's left leg is externally rotated and shorter than the right leg which is apparently causing the client extreme pain as evidenced by yelling. The nurse would want to follow up and manage the client's pain during the evaluation of the left leg deformity. These findings are relevant and require follow-up. The client's heart rate, respiratory rate, and blood pressure are elevated which further supports the client's acute pain. The client's vital sign abnormalities and shortness of breath may be caused by anxiety related to the situation and admission to an unfamiliar environment, but they are relevant findings for this client requiring immediate follow-up. Some of the findings in the client situation are within normal range, such as the capillary refill of less than 3 seconds and a temperature of 98.4°F (36.9°C), and are therefore irrelevant in the presenting client situation. The client's pedal pulses are equal at 1+, which is diminished in strength compared with a normal expected value of 2+. However, the client is an older adult. The process of aging causes arteries to become stiff and harden. These normal physiologic changes typically cause vasoconstriction and decreased distal perfusion. If the right pedal pulse was 1+ or 2+ and the affected left leg was absent, this finding would be relevant indicating that the leg injury may be affecting perfusion to the left foot. However, the client's pedal pulses are equal in both feet.

THINKING EXERCISE 2.2

Answer:
Select **3** client findings that require **immediate** follow-up by the nurse:
- ○ Speech quality
- ○ Heart rate
- **X** Shortness of breath
- ○ SpO$_2$
- **X** Neck swelling
- ○ Respiratory rate
- ○ Pain level
- ○ Left arm weakness
- **X** Difficulty swallowing fluids

Rationale: The client had an anterior neck surgical approach to fuse the cervical spine. The normal expected physiologic response to tissue injury is inflammation, including swelling and pain. Swelling of the neck can cause difficulty breathing (shortness of breath) or swallowing and needs to be followed up immediately. A hoarse or quieter speech is expected immediately after this type of surgery due to the proximity of the larynx to the surgical area. The client's arm weakness was likely present before surgery due to spinal nerve compression and will improve during the surgical recovery. The client's pain level is appropriate because the client is receiving postoperative analgesia. The client's respiratory rate, heart rate, and SpO$_2$ are within normal or usual ranges for an adult.

THINKING EXERCISE 2.3

Answer:

History and Physical	Nurses Notes	Orders	Laboratory Results

1615:   Parent visited center for child's nasal congestion, coughing, and low-grade fever for the past 2 days. Today the child seems much more tired, has a sore throat, and is beginning to feel achy. VS taken by certified medical assistant (CMA): T 101°F (38.3°C); HR 92 beats per minute; RR 20 breaths per minute; B/P 114/58 mmHg; SpO$_2$ 98% on RA. CMA reports observing various stages of old bruising on chest and back. Child states bruises resulted from playing sports, but would not make eye contact when answering. Throat slightly reddened. No adventitious breath sounds. Plan to test for strep, flu, and COVID-19.

Rationale: The child has respiratory signs and symptoms including nasal congestion, coughing, sore throat, achiness, fatigue, and an elevated temperature. These findings need to be addressed because respiratory infections are common in children and can lead to pneumonia or other complications. In addition, the client has various stages of old bruising on the trunk which could indicate physical abuse. The child would not make eye contact which could indicate fear or anxiety. Vital signs, except for temperature, are within normal or usual limits.

THINKING EXERCISE 2.4

Answer:
Select **4** findings below that require **immediate** follow-up:
- ○ Anorexia
- **X** Pain level and location in the right leg
- **X** Color of the right leg
- **X** Temperature of the right leg
- ○ Heart rate
- ○ Blood pressure
- **X** Distal pulses
- ○ SpO$_2$

THINKING EXERCISE 2.4—cont'd

Rationale: The client's report of severe pain diffuse pain in combination with mottling, coolness, and absent palpable distal pulses indicates an acute impairment of arterial blood flow (perfusion) in the right leg. These findings need immediate follow-up to prevent tissue necrosis and possible loss of the affected leg. Vital signs are normal or usual for a client who is 88 years old. Although the SpO_2 is below 95% which is considered the lower range of the "normal" peripheral oxygen saturation level, older clients often have values between 90%–94%. This client is not experiencing respiratory distress or tachypnea and, therefore, there is no need for immediate follow-up. The client's heart rate and blood pressure are within normal limits. The client's anorexia and desire to stay in bed are likely the result of being in severe pain and would not require follow-up. Once the pain is managed, the client's appetite and mobility will likely improve.

THINKING EXERCISE 2.5

Answer:

Which of the following client findings require **immediate** follow-up? **Select all that apply.**

- ○ Body temperature
- X Heart rate
- ○ Respiratory rate
- X Blood pressure
- ○ SpO_2
- X Abdominal pain
- ○ Vaginal bleeding

Rationale: The client's blood pressure decreased significantly (hypotension) while the heart rate increased (tachycardia) following childbirth via a C-section. These acute changes suggest a decrease in blood volume, and along with increased abdominal pain and distention indicate possible retroperitoneal bleeding. Therefore, these findings require immediate follow-up. The amount of vaginal bleeding is expected; the client's other vital signs, including SpO_2, are within the normal or usual range.

THINKING EXERCISE 2.6

Answer:

History and Physical	Nurses Notes	Orders	Laboratory Results

1048: Brought to ED by family for severe abdominal pain, fever, and vomiting which started last night. Has not eaten for almost 24 hours due to anorexia. History of fractured humerus and severely sprained ankle from participating in multiple high school sports. Alert and oriented ×4; reports pain at 10/10 especially in right lower quadrant radiating to midabdomen. Hypoactive bowel sounds ×4 with abdominal distention. VS: T 100.8°F (38.2°C); HR 94 beats per minute; RR 22 breaths per minute; B/P 124/86 mmHg; SpO_2 96% on RA. Prepared for abdominal ultrasound.

Rationale: The client has acute severe abdominal pain, nausea, vomiting, anorexia, fever, and diminished bowel sounds. These changes are abnormal and need immediate follow-up to prevent fluid and electrolyte imbalances or other complications. The other vital signs are normal; the client's history is not relevant to the current situation.

END-OF-CHAPTER THINKING EXERCISES

END-OF-CHAPTER THINKING EXERCISE 2.1

Answer:
Which of the following client findings require **immediate** follow-up? **Select all that apply:**

X Uric acid
X Creatinine
○ Hematocrit
X Platelets
○ Fasting blood glucose

Rationale: Serum uric acid levels usually decrease in early pregnancy and increase to about 4–5 mg/dL (237.9 mmol/L) by the third trimester. This client's uric acid level is much higher than expected and could indicate preeclampsia, low birth weight, and other complications. Therefore, this lab finding is of requires immediate follow-up. The platelet count in pregnancy typically decreases due to hemodilution. However, a count of less than 100,000/mm³ (100×10⁹/L) could indicate preeclampsia, a dangerous pregnancy complication. The client's current platelet count has decreased and could be significant requiring immediate follow-up. The client's serum creatinine also requires follow-up at this time because it suggests kidney impairment. The client's hematocrit is within the normal reference range and the glucose level is only slightly elevated, which does not require follow-up at this time.

END-OF-CHAPTER THINKING EXERCISE 2.2

Answer:
The nurse recognizes that the client's **worsening abdominal pain**, **abdominal distention**, and **nausea** require ***immediate*** follow-up.

Rationale: The client had surgery yesterday and should be taking liquids today if possible. However, the client's abdominal pain has intensified despite analgesia and the abdomen is moderately distended. These findings are not expected or usual for clients having an exploratory laparotomy. Nausea and refusal to try fluid intake are also not typical postoperatively and would require immediate follow-up, especially given increased abdominal pain and distention.

END-OF-CHAPTER THINKING EXERCISE 2.3

Answer:
Select **4** of the following findings that require **immediate** follow-up.

○ Lack of interest in activities
○ Hair loss
X Insomnia
X BMI
○ Body temperature
X Heart rate
X Blood pressure
○ SpO$_2$

Rationale: This client has lost significant weight over the past year and is now considered severely underweight. The client is also likely to experience a decreased blood volume as evidenced by tachycardia and hypotension. These vital sign changes are significant and require immediate follow-up. The client's mood has been affected by a lack of socialization as a result of remote learning. Hair loss, dry skin, and insomnia are not expected findings but indicate inadequate nutrition. Lack of sleep is the most serious of these findings because it can cause multiple physical or mental health conditions. Therefore, insomnia is a finding that requires immediate follow-up.

↯ **END-OF-CHAPTER THINKING EXERCISE 2.4**

Answer:
The nurse identifies that the client's **heart rate** and **blood pressure** require ***immediate*** follow-up.

Rationale: The assessment findings that require immediate follow-up are the client's tachycardia (causing palpitations) and hypertension. The client is at risk for complications like stroke or myocardial infarction if these findings are not followed up immediately. Although the client's respiratory rate is slightly elevated, the client is not in respiratory distress. This increase could be caused by anxiety about the situation or compensation for tachycardia. The other vital signs are within normal limits.

REFERENCES

Alastalo, M., Salminen, L., Vahlberg, T., & Leino-Kilpi. (2022). Subjective and objective assessment in skills evaluation: A cross-sectional study among critical care nurses. *Nordic Journal of Nursing Research.* https://doi.org/10.1177/20571585221089145.

Al-Moteri, M., Cooper, S., Symmons, M., & Plummer, V. (2020). Nurses' cognitive and perceptual bias in the identification of clinical deterioration cues. *Australian Critical Care, 33*(4), 333–342.

American Nurses Association (ANA). (2021). *Nursing: Scope and standards of practice* (4th ed.). Silver Spring, MD: ANA.

Betts, J., Muntean, W., Kim, D., Jorion, N., & Dickison, P. (2019). Building a method for writing clinical judgment items for entry-level nursing exams. *Journal of Applied Technology, 20*(S2), 21–36.

Burdeu, G., Lowe, G., Rasmussen, B., & Consedine, J. (2021). Clinical cues used by nurses to recognize changes in patients' clinical states: A systematic review. *Nursing and Health Science, 23*(1), 9–28.

Burke, J. R., Downey, C., & Almoudaris, A. M. (2020). Failure to rescue deteriorating patients: A systematic review of root causes and improvement strategies. *Journal of Patient Safety, 18*(1), 140–155.

Collins, R. (2020). Clinician cognitive overload and its implications for nurse leaders. *Nurse Leader, 18*(1), 44–47.

Elliott, M., & Endacott, R. (2022). The clinical neglect of vital signs' assessment: An emerging patient safety issue? *Contemporary Nurse, 58,* 249–252.

Fawzy, A., Wu, T. D., Wang, K., Robinson, M. L., Farha, J., et al. (2022). Racial and ethnic discrepancy in pulse oximetry and delayed identification of treatment eligibility among patients with COVID-19. *JAMA Internal Medicine, 182*(7), 730–738.

Fore, A. M., & Sculli, G. L. (2013). A concept analysis of situational awareness in nursing. *Journal of Advanced Nursing, 69*(12), 2613–2621.

Hall, K., Lim, A., & Gale, B. (2020). The use of rapid response teams to reduce failure to rescue events: A systematic review. *Journal of Patient Safety, 16*(3), S3–S7.

Hockenberry, M. J., Duffy, E. A., & Gibbs, K. (2024). *Wong's nursing care of infants and children* (12th ed.). St. Louis, MO: Elsevier.

Ignatavicius, D. D., Rebar, C. R., & Heimgartner, N. M. (2024). *Medical-surgical nursing: Concepts for interprofessional collaborative care* (11th ed.). St. Louis, MO: Elsevier.

Institute for Healthcare Improvement. (2019). *Early warning systems: Scorecards that save lives.* Retrieved from https://www.ihi.org/resources/Pages/ImprovementStories/EarlyWarningSystemsScorecardsThatSaveLives.aspx.

Jarvis, C., & Eckhardt, A. (2024). *Physical examination and health assessment* (9th ed.). St. Louis, MO: Elsevier.

Liyew, B., Tilahun, A., & Kassew, T. (2021). Practices and barriers towards physical assessment among nurses working in intensive care units. *BioMed Research International, 2021,* 5524676. https://doi.org/10.1155/2021/5524676.

*Massey, D., Chaboyer, W., & Anderson, V. (2017). What factors influence ward nurses' recognition of and response to patient deterioration? An integrative review of the literature. *Nursing Open, 4*(1), 6–23.

Munn, L. T., Liu, T. L., Swick, M., Rose, R., Broyhill, B., New, L., et al. (2021). Well-being and resilience among health care workers during the COVID-19 pandemic: A cross-sectional study. *AJN, 121*(8), 24–34.

*Mushta, J., Rush, K., & Andersen, E. (2018). Failure to rescue as a nurse-sensitive indicator. *Nursing Forum, 53*(1), 84–92.

NCSBN-ANA. (2019). *National guidelines for nursing delegation.* Retrieved from https://www.nursingworld.org/~4962ca/globalassets/practiceandpolicy/nursing-excellence/ana-position-statements/nursing-practice/ana-ncsbn-joint-statement-on-delegation.pdf.

*Nibbelink, C. W., & Brewer, B. B. (2018). Decision-making in nursing practice: An integrative literature review. *Journal of Clinical Nursing, 27*(5–6), 917–928.

Orique, S. B., Despins, L., Wakefield, B. J., Erdelez, S., & Vogelsmeier, A. (2019). Perception of clinical deterioration cues among medical-surgical nurses. *Journal of Advanced Nursing, 75*(11), 2627–2637.

*Padilla, R. M., & Mayo, A. M. (2018). Clinical deterioration: A concept analysis. *Journal of Clinical Nursing, 27*, 1360–1368.

Pagana, K. D., Pagana, T. J., & Pagana, T. N. (2022). *Mosby's manual of diagnostic and laboratory tests* (7th ed.). St. Louis, MO: Elsevier.

Smith, M. C., Chinn, P. L., & Nicoll, L. H. (2021). Knowledge for nursing practice: Beyond evidence alone. *Research and Theory for Nursing Practice, 35*(1), 7–23. https://doi.org/10.1891/RTNP-D-20-00095.

Stellpflug, C., Pierson, L., Roloff, D., Mosman, E., Gross, T., Marsh, S., et al. (2021). Continuous physiological monitoring improves patient outcomes. *AJN, 121*(4), 40–46.

*Struth, D. (2009). TCAB in the curriculum: Creating a safer environment through nursing education. *AJN, 109*(Suppl. 11), 55–58.

The Joint Commission. (2023). *Quick safety 28: Cognitive biases in health care.* Retrieved from https://www.jointcommission.org/resources/news-and-multimedia/newsletters/newsletters/quick-safety/quick-safety--28/cog.

Touhy, T. A., & Jett, K. (2022). *Ebersole and Hess' gerontological nursing & healthy aging* (6th ed.). St. Louis, MO: Elsevier.

Trinkoff, A. M., Baldwin, C. M., Chasens, E. R., Dunbar-Jacob, J., Geiger-Brown, J., Imes, C. C., et al. (2021). Nurses are more exhausted than ever: What should we do about it? *AJN, 121*(12), 18–29.

*Denotes classic reference

How to Analyze Cues

THIS CHAPTER AT A GLANCE...

Organizing and Linking Identified Clinical Cues
- Using Higher Order Thinking
- Organizing Cues to Identify Patterns
- Making Inferences

Interpreting Clinical Cues
- Identifying Assumptions
- Recognizing Implicit Biases

Anticipating Common Medical Conditions
- Role of Predictive Models
- Common Medical Conditions

Determining Client Conditions
- Actual Client Conditions
- Potential Client Conditions

Analyzing Cues to Make Safe Clinical Judgments

- Factors that Influence the Ability of Nurses to Analyze Cues
- Role of Nursing Knowledge

Strategies for How to Analyze Cues
- Organize Identified Relevant Clinical Cues
- Compare the Relevant Clinical Cues with Nursing Knowledge
- Determine whether Inconsistencies or Gaps Exist
- Make an Inference Based on Cue Interpretation
- Identify Potential Client Conditions

End-of-Chapter Exercises

LEARNING OUTCOMES

1. Identify the role of higher order thinking in the clinical judgment skill of analyzing cues.
2. Describe how to identify patterns from clinical cues and make inferences about a client's condition.
3. Discuss the need to recognize assumptions and be aware of implicit bias that can affect the ability to analyze clinical cues.
4. Explain how predictive models can inform clinical decision-making.
5. Identify examples of potential client conditions that nurses need to anticipate as part of care.
6. Describe nurse and system factors that can affect the ability to analyze cues.
7. Discuss strategies for analyzing cues to make safe, appropriate clinical judgments.

KEY TERMS

Assumptions: Preconceived beliefs, biases, and suppositions without supporting clinical cues.

Client condition: Medical disorder or complication that may place the client at risk for clinical deterioration.

Clustering cues: Scientific principle of classifying data to enhance the ability to determine relationships between and among those data.

Differential diagnosis: Creating a list of possible client conditions, and weighing the probability of one condition against others that are closely related.

Higher order thinking: Complex level of thinking that entails analyzing and classifying or organizing perceived qualities and relationships, meaningfully combining concepts and principles, and then synthesizing ideas into supportable thoughts or generalizations that hold true for many situations.

Implicit bias: Associated with attitudes (either positive or negative) and involves unintentional assumptions about individuals or groups that occur involuntarily without a person's awareness; also called unconscious or hidden bias.

Inference: Conclusion or interpretation based on analysis of client cues.

Pattern recognition: Ability to compare a client's clinical cues with information retrieved from the nurse's knowledge.

Predictive analysis: Computer data interpretation to extract valuable client patterns to inform clinical decision-making.

Predictive model: A proactive approach that aims to predict and manage risk factors *before* problems arise, and is based on current research and best practices.

Recognizing clinical cues involves much more than collecting and documenting client findings. Unfortunately, nurses are often busy and may not take the time to adequately interpret or analyze relevant clinical cues, which can lead to errors or missed nursing care (see Chapter 1).

Sound clinical judgment requires nurses to be competent in recognizing and analyzing clinical cues. As defined in Chapter 2, clinical cues are objective findings (signs) and subjective findings (symptoms) that can indicate both client deterioration and improvement. Although recognizing changes in a client's clinical state depends on your ability to identify relevant cues, making decisions about what actions are needed depends on your ability to determine what those cues mean.

This chapter focuses on how to analyze the clinical cues that nurses identify when clients experience changes in their clinical situation. Analyzing cues involves three major components (Fig. 3.1):

- Clustering or organizing relevant clinical cues
- Identifying actual and/or potential client conditions based on relevant clinical cues
- Determining if inconsistencies or gaps exists related to the relevant clinical cues

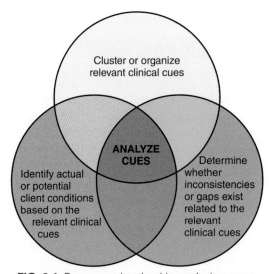

FIG. 3.1 Processes involved in analyzing cues.

ORGANIZING AND LINKING IDENTIFIED CLINICAL CUES

Analyzing cues is the ability to organize and link recognized cues to the client's presenting clinical situation to determine probable client conditions. This clinical skill requires higher order thinking to interpret or make sense of relevant clinical cues and what they mean.

Using Higher Order Thinking

Higher order thinking is needed when encountering problems, questions, or dilemmas; it requires many types of thinking, including critical, logical, reflective, and creative thinking (see Chapter 1). Although higher order thinking is beyond basic facts and memorization, it is based on lower order skills linked to prior knowledge. Therefore, nurses need a strong knowledge base to effectively use higher order thinking when analyzing cues.

Higher order thinking generally can be defined as "a complex level of thinking that entails analyzing and classifying or organizing perceived qualities and relationships, meaningfully combining concepts and principles …, and then synthesizing ideas into supportable … thoughts or generalizations that hold true for many situations" (IGI Global, 2023). Consider the following key points in this definition and how higher order thinking is used by nurses:

- Higher order thinking is complex thinking which suggests a large amount of interrelated client information is involved.
- Higher order thinking requires analyzing, classifying, and/or organizing the interrelated client information.
- Higher order thinking results in synthesizing (creating) ideas or inferences supported by sound generalizations about the client's condition.

Therefore, when analyzing cues, nurses use higher order thinking to organize and link a large amount of client information or clinical cues to make inferences about what the cues mean within the context of a client situation.

Organizing Cues to Identify Patterns

Organizing cues begins by clustering or grouping similar clinical cues together to identify patterns. Clustering cues is the scientific principle of classifying data to enhance the ability of determining relationships between and among those data. This process helps you get a picture of patterns of health or illness. A good way to remember the importance of clustering related data is to think about how to put together a picture puzzle: you probably put all the edges of the picture in one pile, all the pieces of a certain color in another pile, and so on. Putting the pieces in piles helps you begin to recognize patterns. The same principle applies to client findings, but in health care you need to recognize relationships based on your knowledge and put together (cluster) signs and symptoms (cues) by body system or client condition.

CLINICAL JUDGMENT TIP

Remember: To accurately analyze cues, you need to recognize relationships based on your knowledge and put together (cluster) signs and symptoms (cues) by body system or client condition.

At times some clinical cues may contradict each other. For example, imagine you are caring for a client after chest surgery who reports having no pain. However, the client moves very little and barely breathes when you ask the client to take a deep breath. The way the client is moving is inconsistent with statements about being pain free.

Recognizing inconsistencies indicates a need to probe more deeply to validate client findings. It also helps focus your assessment to clarify the client's condition. Compare what the client states (subjective data) with what you observe (objective data). If what the client states is not supported by what you observe, this inconsistency needs to be investigated further by collecting additional assessment data.

Once all the data you need are collected, cluster the relevant clinical cues to identify a pattern. A pattern expresses a relationship among three components—context (circumstance), problem, and conclusion. Be sure to keep contextual factors in mind when identifying the pattern as discussed in Chapter 2.

To identify a pattern, first analyze the cues you put together and decide which of the following patterns they represent:

- Normal pattern (*clinical cues* consistent with a normal pattern are present)
- Risk for abnormal pattern (*risk factors* consistent with a potential client problem are present)
- Abnormal pattern (*clinical cues* consistent with an actual client problem are present)

After you get a beginning idea of the pattern, look for gaps in data collection by asking, "What other information might clarify my understanding of this pattern?"

Pattern recognition, then, is the ability to compare a client's clinical cues with information retrieved from the nurse's knowledge. The differences among nurses in their ability to recognize patterns largely depends on nursing knowledge. When compared to novice or beginning nurses, expert nurses are better at recognizing patterns because they are similar to those encountered during years of practice; previous experiences help increase nursing knowledge (Al-Moteri et al., 2020).

Making Inferences

Inferences are based on evidence and reasoning. Analyzing cues requires you to make inferences about the client's condition that follow logically based on organizing those cues. In nursing practice, an **inference** is your conclusion or interpretation based on client cues. Making inferences is sometimes referred to as *generating hypotheses* or drawing valid conclusions. The ability to interpret data and draw valid conclusions is key to making sound clinical judgments. If you draw incorrect conclusions, your clinical judgments will be flawed, which may cause the plan of care to be flawed. Therefore, it is important to identify and analyze all relevant cues to make a valid conclusion.

Think about alternative conclusions (hypotheses). What other issues could the clinical cues suggest? Consider worst-case scenarios, such as "Could a client's headache be related to impending stroke rather than tension?" Anticipating what could happen in a clinical situation within a given context is important in your ability to interpret clinical cues.

Table 3.1 lists examples of common clinical cues with potential inferences. Each of these cues is consistent with more than one condition, requiring additional client assessment to narrow the conclusion about what the cue means.

TABLE 3.1   Examples of Common Clinical Cues and Potential Inferences

Common Clinical Cues	Potential Inference	Alternative Inference
Elevated white blood cell count	Infection	Severe inflammation from systemic disorder
Yelling out and combative	Delirium	Acute pain
Chest pain	Angina or myocardial infarction	Gastroesophageal reflux disorder
Oliguria	Acute kidney injury or chronic kidney disease	Urinary retention caused by obstruction
Acute confusion	Delirium	Hypoxia

Making correct inferences requires knowledge of:

- Signs and symptoms of common complications and health problems
- The common needs of certain age groups (e.g., young vs. older adults)
- Cultural and spiritual influences
- Knowledge of the client as a person

- Anatomy, pathophysiology, pharmacology, medical-surgical nursing, and specialty nursing practice (e.g., pediatrics)

Inferences are sometimes made based on analysis of diagnostic results such as laboratory tests and imaging studies. Sometimes these objective data can help support your inference. When reviewing laboratory or other diagnostic test results, ask yourself:

- Which test results indicate the presence of a client problem (such as a medical complication) or clinical deterioration?
- Are any test results consistent with or do they support a medical complication or clinical deterioration?

The most difficult inferences to make may be those related to changes in a client's mental condition. Observe nonverbal cues such as client facial expression, emotional demeanor, and behavior. Listen carefully to what the client says and note changes in the client's voice. For example, clients who sustain a severe traumatic brain injury often become aggressive and potentially violent. By interpreting changes in a client's voice and facial expression, you may be able to detect impending aggressive behaviors and prepare to manage them.

CLINICAL JUDGMENT TIP

Remember: Making inferences is sometimes referred to as *generating hypotheses* or drawing valid conclusions. The ability to interpret data and draw valid conclusions is key to making sound clinical judgments.

Once you have enough evidence to support your inference, you can feel confident that you are probably correct. Avoid making inferences based on only one cue or only one source. The more facts and sources you have to support your inference, the more likely it is that your inference is correct.

Thinking Exercise 3.1 will help you practice what you've learned in this chapter about analyzing cues. The answer and rationale for the exercise are located at the end of this book.

THINKING EXERCISE 3.1

The nurse is caring for a 39-year-old client in the prenatal clinic.

History and Physical	Nurses Notes	Orders	Laboratory Results

1620: Being seen today for routine 32-week prenatal visit. Labs within normal limits except for elevated WBCs of 20,300/mm³ (20.3×10^9/L). (Normal reference range 5000–10,500/mm³ [$5.0–10.5 \times 10^9$/L].) Denies urinary frequency or burning, but sometimes feels pressure over bladder. Reports increased fatigue since last visit 4 weeks ago due to difficulty sleeping and "can't get comfortable in bed." Stops drinking fluids about 2 hours prior to bedtime to reduce number of times needed for bathroom at night. Lung sounds clear with no adventitious breath sounds; S_1 and S_2 present. Bowel sounds present ×4. Capillary refill <3 seconds bilaterally. VS: T 99.6°F (37.6°C); HR 88 beats per minute; RR 20 breaths per minute; B/P 140/92 mmHg; SpO₂ 97% on RA.

Complete the following sentence by selecting from the lists of options below.
The client likely has ___1 [Select]___ as evidenced by ___2 [Select]___ and ___3 [Select]___.

Options for 1	Options for 2	Options for 3
Preeclampsia	Elevated blood pressure	Bladder pressure
Urinary tract infection	Low-grade fever	Increased fatigue
Anemia	Insomnia	Elevated WBC count

INTERPRETING CLINICAL CUES

Cue perception and processing involve detecting, selecting, organizing, and interpreting relevant cues to understand a clinical situation. Verifying that the identified relevant clinical cues are accurate and complete helps you avoid making inferences or judgments based on incorrect or incomplete data. Misinterpreting clinical cues can also lead to poor judgment (Al-Moteri et al., 2020).

> ### CLINICAL JUDGMENT TIP
> *Remember:* Verify that relevant clinical cues are accurate and complete to help avoid making judgments based on incorrect or misinterpreted data.

Identifying Assumptions

Assumptions are preconceived beliefs, biases, and suppositions without supporting evidence. As humans, we all have preconceived notions and tend to make assumptions, especially in unfamiliar circumstances. Sound clinical reasoning requires that you make judgments based on the best available evidence. This means double-checking your thinking to overcome your brain's natural tendency to grasp things at an intuitive ("gut") level. By identifying assumptions, you apply logic and avoid jumping to incorrect conclusions and making judgment errors.

The best way to identify assumptions is to answer questions like, "What is being taken for granted here?" and "How do I know that I have recognized the most relevant clinical cues?" Make sure you have a complete picture of what is going on with the client. Be aware of any bias or belief *you* may have that could positively or negatively affect how you process the meaning of clinical cues. For example, do not assume that an older adult's acute confusion or urinary incontinence represents normal patterns for the client's age.

Recognizing Implicit Biases

Everyone has various biases, beliefs, and assumptions shaped by their life experiences from childhood through adulthood. Biases in health care often occur in predictive patterns, especially when nurses use intuitive ("fast") thinking (see Chapter 2 for discussion of intuition) (Thirsk et al., 2022).

As defined in Chapter 2, cognitive bias is a flaw or distortion in judgment and clinical decision-making (thinking). By contrast, implicit bias, also called unconscious or hidden bias, is associated with *attitudes* (either positive or negative) and involves unintentional assumptions about individuals or groups that occur involuntarily without a person's awareness (Narayan, 2019; Sabin, 2022; Thirsk et al., 2022). Research indicates that health care professionals exhibit the same levels of implicit bias as the general population (FitzGerald & Hurst, 2017). Unconscious biases by nurses and other members of the health care team can contribute to adverse clinical outcomes and health care disparities for members of groups that face discrimination. As a result, members of these groups often lack trust in the health care system.

To manage implicit bias, nurses and other health care professionals need to recognize that they have implicit bias. Increased knowledge about vulnerable populations and empathy for all individuals promotes client-centered care. Treating each client as an individual rather than making broad generalizations or assumptions is especially important when analyzing clinical cues to determine the client's needs, concerns, and conditions. Thirsk et al. (2022) conducted an important study on the effect of cognitive and implicit bias on clinical judgment (Box 3.1).

BOX 3.1   Evidence-Based Practice

What is the Effect of Implicit Bias on Nurses' Clinical Judgment?

Based on Thirsk, L. M., Panchuk, J. T., Stahlke, S., & Hagtvedt, R. (2022). Cognitive and implicit bias in nurses' judgment and decision-making: A scoping review. *International Journal of International Studies, 133.* https://www.doi.org/10.1016/j.ijnurstu.2022.104284.

Few studies have been conducted on the effect of cognitive and implicit bias on the ability of nurses to make safe, appropriate clinical judgments. The researchers performed a thorough literature search and selected 77 studies for review to answer the research questions. A number of studies (16) found that nurses were not consistent in how they managed pain; i.e., pain management varied based on the age or gender of their clients. For example, the pain experienced by older adults and women often was not managed as aggressively or perceived to be as severe as that in younger adults or men. Six studies found that ED triage scoring varied based on race/ethnicity. For example, Black children presenting with a fever were given a lower priority score when compared to White children.

When analyzing cues, be sure to be nonjudgmental about the client's health care behaviors and what they mean. For example, a client may have waited to seek medical attention for weeks or months after relevant clinical cues began. This delay may have been the result of lack of access to health care, lack of health insurance, lack of knowledge, or cultural belief or practice. Additional information about these social determinants of health is provided in Chapter 5 of this book.

CLINICAL JUDGMENT TIP

Remember. When analyzing cues, be sure to be nonjudgmental about the client's health care behaviors and what they mean.

Thinking Exercise 3.2 will help you practice what you've learned in this chapter about analyzing cues. The answer and rationale for the exercise are located at the end of this book.

⚡ THINKING EXERCISE 3.2

The nurse is caring for a 45-year-old veteran in the Emergency Department (ED).

History and Physical	Nurses Notes	Orders	Laboratory Results

0355: Brought to ED by EMS after found shivering in ditch in crouched position with old bloody bandages on both wrists. Yelling at cars going by to "get out of the IED field." Alert and oriented ×1 to person only. Emergency family contact information located in client's pocket; notified them client admitted to ED. Has healed left above-the-knee amputation with prothesis. Dressed in torn clothes inappropriate for weather. VS: T 97.6°F (37.6°C); HR 90 beats per minute; RR 20 breaths per minute; B/P 130/86 mmHg; SpO$_2$ 95% on RA.

0440: Family states client has been homeless for about 3 months after being unable to pay for rent. Has a history of severe insomnia and nightmares about IED explosion causing leg amputation during Afghanistan war. Client usually visits family about once a week for hot meal and sometimes stays at local shelter.

Complete the following sentence by selecting from the list of word choices below.
Based on the history and current findings, the client is at ***high*** risk for **[Word Choice]**.

Word Choices	
Schizophrenia	Depression
Suicide	Frostbite

ANTICIPATING COMMON MEDICAL CONDITIONS

Nurses are most effective in providing safe client care when they are proactive and thinking ahead to expect problems that could occur in any clinical situation. This type of thinking is sometimes referred to as *anticipatory thinking* and helps nurses be better prepared for potential complications or changes in a client's condition. Unfortunately, nurses are often so busy or short-staffed that they are unable to find the time to put clinical cues together to determine what they mean. To help predict changes in a client's condition or a medical complication, electronic predictive models are used in many hospitals.

Role of Predictive Models

A predictive care model requires moving from a diagnose and treat (DT) approach—which implies waiting for problems to occur to generate solutions and take actions—to a predictive model: predict, prevent, manage, and promote (PPMP). Generally speaking, a predictive model is a proactive approach that aims to predict and manage risk factors *before* problems arise, and is based on current research and best practices.

Most hospitals use one or more predictive models in which data from the electronic health record are analyzed to identify clients at risk for a selected condition or death. Predictive analysis is defined as computer data interpretation to extract valuable client patterns to inform clinical decision-making. This application of artificial intelligence (AI) to improve health care does not replace clinical judgment but rather uses the nurses' documented assessment findings to alert nurses and other health care professionals about the risk for potential client problems.

Most predictive models are designed to identify specific client conditions and are customized based on the health care setting, such as:

- Pressure injuries
- Heart failure
- Postoperative complications
- Sepsis
- Fall risk
- Hospital readmissions

A systematic review found that about 50% of reviewed studies demonstrated that predictive models improved clinical outcomes (Box 3.2).

BOX 3.2   Evidence-Based Practice

What is the Effectiveness of Predictive Models?

Lee, T. C., Shah, N. U., Haack, A., & Baxter, S. L. (2020). Clinical implementation of predictive models embedded within electronic health record systems: A systematic review. *Informatics, 7*(3), 25. https://www.doi.org/10.3390/informatics7030025.

The researchers selected 44 studies for data extraction and analysis to answer the research question of whether predictive models in hospitals are effective. About 50% of the analyzed studies showed improvement in clinical outcomes. However, client condition-specific predictive models that were customized based on health care setting had better outcomes than those not customized and used across settings. The researchers found several problems with predictive models regardless of customization, including:

- Alert fatigue (frequent alerts become ignored)
- Inadequate responses to alerts
- Increased work and burden for nurses and other health care professionals
- Lack of staff training

The study concluded that best practices for implementing predictive models are still evolving.

Common Medical Conditions

A client condition is a medical disorder or complication that may place the client at risk for clinical deterioration. Nurses need a strong knowledge of common medical conditions and associated signs and symptoms to accurately analyze cues. Being able to cluster relevant clinical cues, recognize a pattern, and compare the pattern to a pathophysiologic condition enables you to identify *actual* client conditions. Being able to assess for subtle changes in a clinical situation and predict possible medical complications or clinical deterioration enables you to identify *potential* client conditions. When caring for your clients, ask yourself, "What could go wrong with this client today?" "What could place your client at risk for adverse outcomes or even death?" Being able to anticipate medical complications or clinical deterioration can help you be better prepared to analyze cues and respond appropriately. Box 3.3 lists some of the most common conditions your clients may experience.

BOX 3.3   Examples of Common Potential Client Conditions

Cardiovascular Conditions
Dysrhythmias
Heart failure/pulmonary edema
Severe fluid imbalances
Cardiogenic shock
Cardiac tamponade
Hypertensive crisis
Cardiac arrest
Venous thromboembolism
Sickle cell crisis

Respiratory Conditions
Acid–base and electrolyte imbalances
Respiratory failure
Pneumonia
Sepsis/septic shock
Pulmonary hypertension
Pneumothorax/hemothorax
Atelectasis
Status asthmaticus

Neurologic Conditions
Traumatic brain injury
Increased intracranial pressure
Spinal cord injury
Spinal shock
Neurogenic shock
Autonomic dysreflexia
Status epilepticus
Stroke

Endocrine Conditions
Hypoglycemia
Hyperglycemia (diabetic ketoacidosis or hyperglycemic hyperosmolar syndrome)

Elimination Conditions
Acute kidney injury
Electrolyte/acid–base imbalances

Anemia
Pyelonephritis
Urinary tract obstruction
Urinary tract infection
Chronic kidney disease
Intestinal obstruction
Upper/lower gastrointestinal bleeding
Peritonitis

Immune Conditions
Allergic response/anaphylactic shock
Opportunistic infections
Oncologic emergencies

Fractures and Other Trauma
Compartment syndrome
Venous thromboembolism
Wound infection/osteomyelitis
Internal bleeding/hypovolemic shock
Sepsis/septic shock

Perioperative Complications
Internal bleeding/hypovolemic shock
Paralytic ileus
Venous thromboembolism
Wound infection
Wound evisceration/dehiscence

Mental Health/Behavioral Health Conditions
Psychoses
Dehydration
Malnutrition
Suicide
Violence (against self or others)
Self-mutilation
Substance use disorder/overdose

CLINICAL JUDGMENT TIP

Remember. Being able to cluster relevant clinical cues, recognize a pattern, and compare the pattern to a pathophysiologic condition enables you to identify *actual* client conditions.

For some clients, drug therapy or another treatment modality can cause adverse effects or complications for which you need to monitor carefully. For example, many cardiovascular drugs have potential adverse effects including bradycardia and severe hypotension. Diuretics can result in severe electrolyte imbalances, especially hypokalemia, which can cause life-threatening cardiac dysrhythmias.

Treatment modalities can cause a variety of medical complications. For example, clients who have hemodialysis can become severely hypotensive. Clients receiving intravenous therapy can experience fluid overload, air embolus, or phlebitis. Be sure to observe clients who are being treated with invasive modalities for complications, especially when they are used for the first time.

Thinking Exercise 3.3 will help you practice what you've learned in this chapter about analyzing cues. The answer and rationale for the exercise are located at the end of this book.

DETERMINING CLIENT CONDITIONS

Ensuring that your clients' actual and potential conditions are correctly identified based on clinical cues from the nursing assessment and other sources of data is essential to make safe, appropriate clinical judgments. Recall that a client condition is a medical disorder or complication that may place the client at risk for clinical deterioration. As described in Chapter 2, clinical deterioration is a dynamic state in which the client progresses to a worsened clinical condition increasing morbidity, body organ dysfunction, prolonged hospital or agency length of stay, and/or death.

Analyzing cues includes (1) ensuring that clinical cues beyond your scope of practice are referred to the appropriate health care professional; (2) choosing the client condition that is consistent with the relevant clinical cues; (3) determining the cause(s) and contributing factors to the client's condition; and (4) identifying the clinical cues that lead you to believe the condition is present. It also includes differential diagnosis: creating a list of possible client conditions, and weighing the probability of one condition against others that are closely related. This process is also referred to as *generating hypotheses*.

Actual Client Conditions

Making definitive conclusions about the client's current condition is key to being able to prioritize hypotheses, generate solutions, and take action designed to prevent, manage, or resolve it. If you miss determining an accurate client condition or are too vague about the condition, you have made a diagnostic error that may cause you to:

- Initiate actions that aggravate the problems or waste time
- Omit essential actions required to prevent and manage the condition
- Allow the condition to go untreated
- Influence others to make the same mistake you did

If your knowledge and expertise are limited, you are at risk for making any one of the following diagnostic errors:

- Identifying the condition without considering whether the data may represent a different condition altogether (e.g., assuming the client's report of indigestion signifies gastric reflux rather than possible myocardial infarction).

THINKING EXERCISE 3.3

The nurse is caring for a 58-year-old female client in acute care following an open traditional exploratory laparotomy and colon resection yesterday morning.

History and Physical	Nurses Notes	Orders	Laboratory Results

2340:   Client alert and oriented ×4. Reports abdominal pain increased this evening, especially when moving in bed or getting OOB. Abdomen continues to be slightly distended with diminished BS ×4. New-onset hyperpigmentation and warmth around abdominal incision but intact. Lungs clear without adventitious breath sounds. States using incentive spirometer every 4–6 hours while awake. S_1 and S_2 heart sounds present. Able to move all extremities. Refuses to wear sequential compression stockings because they are "too hot." Cap refill <3 seconds bilaterally. VS: T 100.8°F (38.2°C); HR 100 beats per minute; RR 20 breaths per minute; B/P 116/69 mmHg; SpO_2 95% on RA.

History and Physical	Laboratory Results	Orders	Nurses Notes

Serum Laboratory Test and Reference Range	1800 Today	Preoperative
Red blood cell (RBC) count (M: $4.7–6.1 \times 10^6$ μL [$4.7–6.1 \times 10^{12}$/L]; F: $4.2–5.4 \times 10^6$/μL [$4.2–5.4 \times 10^{12}$/L])	4.2×10^6/μL (4.2×10^{12}/L)	4.9×10^6/μL (4.9×10^{12}/L)
Hemoglobin (M: 14–18 g/dL [8.7–11.2 mmol/L]; F: 12–16 g/dL [7.4–9.9 mmol/L])	12.2 g/dL (7.57 mmol/L)	14.1 g/dL (8.75 mmol/L)
Hematocrit (M: 42%–52% [0.42–0.52 volume fraction]; F: 37%–47% [0.37–0.47 volume fraction])	38% (0.38 VF)	44% (0.44 VF)
White blood cell (WBC) count (5000–10,000/mm³ [$5–10 \times 10^9$/L])	10,500/mm³ (10.5×10^9/L)	7200/mm³ (7.2×10^9/L)

Select **4** potential postoperative complications for which this client is **most** at risk.
- Atelectasis
- Wound infection
- Peptic ulcer
- Compartment syndrome
- Hypovolemic shock
- Venous thromboembolism
- Contractures
- Anemia

- Not considering all the relevant data because of a narrow focus (e.g., not looking for other cardiovascular cues because you decide that the person has indigestion).
- Failing to recognize personal biases or assumptions. *Example*: Thinking that the client is not in pain because the client doesn't appear to be in pain. Knowledgeable nurses know that people handle pain differently and that often outward signs of pain are not present, even though the person is experiencing significant discomfort. This is especially true for clients who experience persistent (chronic) pain.
- Overanalyzing the client's situation and delaying taking action which could result in a life-threatening clinical situation. For example, White et al. (2021) demonstrated newly licensed nurses had the knowledge needed to analyze clinical cues consistent with sepsis (recognize patterns) but were unable to prevent clients' progression to septic shock in a timely manner.

Potential Client Conditions

Predicting potential conditions helps you identify what signs and symptoms to look for when monitoring a client, anticipate what could happen if the client's condition worsens, and be prepared to manage the condition if it occurs. Some clients are more at risk for potential complications or clinical deterioration than others. For example, when caring for adult clients, older adults are often more at risk for complications than younger or middle-aged adults as a result of typical physiologic changes associated with aging (Table 3.2).

TABLE 3.2   Common Physiologic Changes of Aging which Increase Risk for Medical Complications

Body System	Physiologic Changes	Potential Complications
Integumentary	Increased healing time	Infection
	Thinning skin	Skin tears and other injury
Musculoskeletal	Decreased bone density	Fractures
	Decreased muscle strength and joint range-of-motion	Falls
Cardiovascular	Decreased body water	Dehydration
	Decreased arterial wall elasticity	Hypertension
	Stiffening and thickening of heart tissue	Heart failure
		Dysrhythmias
Respiratory	Decreased elasticity of chest wall and alveoli	COPD
		Pneumonia
Renal	Decreased glomerular filtration rate and nephrons	Fluid, electrolyte, and acid–base imbalances
Endocrine	Increased insulin resistance	Diabetes mellitus type II
Neurologic/sensory	Changes in brain causing decreased balance	Falls
	Increased farsightedness	
Gastrointestinal	Decreased esophageal motility	Gastroesophageal reflux disease
	Decreased stomach motility and bicarbonate	Peptic ulcer disease

From Touhy, T.A., & Jett, K. (2022). *Ebersole and Hess' gerontological nursing and healthy aging* (6th ed.). Elsevier.

Normal laboratory values are also affected by changes associated with aging. For example, as one ages, the high limits for normal serum glucose increase (Pagana et al., 2022):

- Adult through 59 years: 74–106 mg/dL (4.1–5.9 mmol/L)
- Adult 60–90 years: 82–115 mg/dL (4.6–6.4 mmol/L)
- Adult >90 years: 75–121 mg/dL (4.2–6.7 mmol/L)

In addition to age, some clients are more likely than others to develop medical complications or clinical deterioration as a result of one or more comorbid conditions. For example, the surgical client who has diabetes mellitus is at risk for slower healing and possible infection. The client who is obese is at risk for severe respiratory distress when developing respiratory infections, especially COVID-19. Be sure to become familiar with each client's coexisting health conditions and medications to better anticipate possible medical complications and clinical deterioration.

At times, clinical cues present differently in clients who are biologically female or male. For instance, normal reference ranges for some laboratory test results may differ based on natal sex. Examples are hemoglobin and hematocrit. Both of the normal ranges for these laboratory tests are higher in men than in women (Pagana et al., 2022). In other cases, certain client conditions present differently in women when compared to men. The signs and symptoms of myocardial infarction, for example, vary depending on natal sex. Therefore, the context of a situation, including demographic factors, often determines if clinical cues are relevant.

Regardless of age or other factors, some clients more readily develop medical complications or clinical deterioration as a result of one or more social determinants of health. According to Healthy People 2030, **social determinants of health (SDOH)** are the conditions in the environments where people are born, live, learn, work, play, worship, and age that affect a wide range of health, functioning, and quality-of-life outcomes and risks. These factors can cause health inequities that lead to negative clinical outcomes. Chapter 5 discusses the impact of SDOH on nursing care and clinical judgment.

CLINICAL JUDGMENT TIP

Remember. Anticipate potential medical complications or signs and symptoms of clinical deterioration based on your client's age, comorbidities, and social determinants of health.

Thinking Exercise 3.4 will help you practice what you've learned in this chapter about analyzing cues. The answer and rationale for the exercise are located at the end of this book.

⚡ THINKING EXERCISE 3.4

The nurse is caring for an 87-year-old client in the Urgent Care Center.

History and Physical	Nurses Notes	Orders	Laboratory Results

2010:   Brought to Urgent Care by family with report of extreme fatigue, shortness of breath, and worsening cough over the past 2 days. Client alert and oriented ×1 (person only). Family states client's mind is usually very sharp. Bilateral lower lobe crackles. Diffuse chest pain especially when moving. S_1 and S_2 heart sounds present; no murmurs or gallops. Able to move all extremities. Cap refill <3 seconds bilaterally. VS: T 100.2°F (37.9°C); HR 104 beats per minute and irregular; RR 24 breaths per minute; B/P 122/78 mmHg; SpO_2 89% on RA.

For each client finding listed below, determine if the finding is consistent with the health conditions of pneumonia, pulmonary embolism, or acute pulmonary edema. Each finding may support more than one condition.

Client Findings	Pneumonia	Pulmonary Embolism	Pulmonary Edema
Fever			
Crackles			
Mental status changes			
Cough			
Fatigue			
Chest pain			
Shortness of breath			
Irregular rapid heart rate			

ANALYZING CUES TO MAKE SAFE CLINICAL JUDGMENTS

Analyzing cues requires higher order thinking to cluster or organize relevant cues, identify actual or potential client conditions based on the cues, and determine if inconsistencies or gaps exist related to the cues. A number of factors can affect the ability of nurses to analyze cues when caring for clients who are experiencing medical complications or clinical deterioration.

Factors that Influence the Ability of Nurses to Analyze Cues

Nurses make clinical judgments that are affected by many factors in multilayered health care settings. Factors that influence your ability to analyze cues can be divided into nurse and system or organizational factors.

Nurse Factors

Personal nurse factors that can influence your ability to utilize higher order thinking when analyzing cues include:
- Work experience
- Education
- Communication ability
- Situational awareness
- Physical and mental health
- Knowledge

Nurses who have *work experience* typically have the cognitive skills needed to make safe, appropriate clinical judgments. As discussed in Chapter 2, nursing experience matters because expert nurses have a higher capacity for cue processing when compared to novice nurses. Experienced nurses learn from each client interaction and can transfer that learning from one clinical situation to another (Orique et al., 2019).

Education can affect the ability of nurses to utilize higher order thinking skills. For example, continuing education has been shown to improve the ability of nurses to analyze cues and deciding when to call the Rapid Response Team. Other studies have suggested that nurses with baccalaureate or higher degrees may have advanced clinical reasoning skills (Alaseeri et al., 2021).

Your ability to effectively *communicate* with clients and the interprofessional health care team can also influence your ability to accurately analyze cues and make safe clinical judgments (Afriyie, 2020). Establishing a trusting relationship with clients to enhance communication is essential when validating clinical cues or determining inconsistencies or gaps related to cues. When making inferences about the meaning of relevant clinical cues, you may need to communicate your conclusions to members of the health care team using SBAR or another reporting system. Communication with both clients and interprofessional health care team members can be positively or negatively affected by personal biases and beliefs as discussed earlier in this chapter.

Experienced nurses understand their clients' clinical status by developing relationships and spending time with them. These relationships are part of *situational awareness* in which nurses correctly perceive a client situation, accurately recognize patterns, and are able to predict the client outcome, sometimes in minutes. As described earlier in this chapter, when compared to novice or beginning nurses, expert nurses are better at recognizing patterns because they are similar to those encountered during years of practice (Al-Moteri et al., 2020).

The physical and mental health status of nurses can impact their ability to determine the meaning of relevant cues. As discussed in Chapter 2, extreme fatigue and stress can negatively affect the ability to perform cue recognition and processing (analyzing cues). Fatigue and stress can also promote the development of cognitive biases.

System Factors

System factors can also influence your ability to utilize higher order thinking when analyzing cues. Probably the most important factor is nurses' increasing workloads in most health care organizations. Several related factors to workload include (Alaseeri et al., 2021):

- Managing a high patient–nurse ratio
- Performing nonnursing jobs
- Handling multiple distractions and interruptions

These workload factors make it difficult to think due to time restrictions and cognitive overload. Additional system factors reported by nurses include lack of organizational support, lack of available technological resources, and inadequate policies and procedures (Alaseeri et al., 2021).

Role of Nursing Knowledge

Clinical reasoning requires that nurses integrate discipline-specific knowledge to make safe, appropriate clinical judgments. As you might recall from Chapter 1, the NCSBN defines clinical judgment as a process that *uses nursing knowledge* to observe and assess presenting situations. A strong knowledge base, then, helps you make (but does not guarantee) sound judgments in each client situation.

Classic work by Gillespie (2010) identified five components of the foundational knowledge nurses need to make appropriate situated clinical judgments (Table 3.3).

TABLE 3.3 Components of Foundational Nursing Knowledge Needed to Make Appropriate Situated Clinical Judgments

Nursing Knowledge Component	Nursing Knowledge Component Description
Knowing the profession	Knowledge of standards of practice, competencies, and skills of nurses
Knowing yourself	Knowledge of individual strengths, limitations, skills, experience, assumptions, and biases
Knowing the clinical situation	Knowledge of pathophysiology, patterns that exist in typical cases, predicted outcomes and client responses
Knowing the client	Knowledge of a client's baseline data, including laboratory results or other clinical findings
Knowing the person	Knowledge of a client's past experience related to health and illness, and patterns related to client's response to pathology and treatment, preferences, and resources

Data adapted from Gillespie, M., Paterson, B. (2009) Helping novice nurses make effective clinical decisions: the situated clinical decisionmaking framework. *Nursing Education Perspectives*, 30 (3), 164–170

STRATEGIES FOR HOW TO ANALYZE CUES

This chapter has explored the process for analyzing cues and the factors that affect your ability as a nurse to use this clinical judgment skill. This discussion summarizes the strategies you will need to accurately analyze relevant cues as a client's condition changes or deteriorates (Box 3.4).

BOX 3.4   Strategies for Analyzing Cues

- Organize identified relevant clinical cues to develop a pattern.
- Compare the relevant clinical cues with information retrieved from your knowledge.
- Determine if inconsistencies or gaps exist related to the relevant clinical cues.
- Make an inference (actual client condition) based on interpretation of relevant clinical cues.
- Identify potential client conditions based on the clinical situation.

Organize Identified Relevant Clinical Cues

Organizing or clustering relevant clinical cues is the first step in the process of analyzing cues. Determine which cues (signs and symptoms) could be linked together to form one or more patterns. For example, consider this list of clinical cues identified in a hypothetical adult client situation in the Emergency Department (nonsurgical client):

- Report of diffuse abdominal pain
- Abdominal distention
- Increased bowel sounds above umbilicus
- Diminished bowel sounds below umbilicus
- Hypotension
- Tachycardia
- Irregular heart rate
- Nausea and vomiting
- Muscle weakness
- Generalized fatigue

To accurately analyze cues, remember to recognize relationships based on your knowledge and put together (cluster) clinical cues (signs and symptoms) by body system or condition. Interpret the clinical cues to determine what they mean and decide which cues could be linked. For example, abdominal pain, distention, and bowel sound changes could be clustered to begin forming a pattern. Box 3.5 shows clusters of potentially related cues organized into two recognizable patterns for this client situation.

BOX 3.5   Clustering Clinical Cues

Possible Gastrointestinal Cues	Possible Fluid and Electrolyte Cues
• Report of diffuse abdominal pain	• Hypotension
• Abdominal distention	• Tachycardia
• Increased bowel sounds above umbilicus	• Irregular heart rate
• Diminished bowel sounds below umbilicus	• Muscle weakness
• Nausea and vomiting	• Generalized fatigue

Compare the Relevant Clinical Cues with Nursing Knowledge

Once the cues are clustered, compare the identified potential patterns with your own knowledge. The client likely has an actual gastrointestinal (GI) condition causing abdominal pain and distention. Many GI conditions cause these signs and symptoms. However, when interpreting bowel sound changes which vary by abdominal location, it is likely that the client has an intestinal obstruction. Bowel sounds above the obstruction increase in an attempt to get GI contents past the blockage; bowel sounds below the obstruction are absent or diminished because peristalsis decreases.

Nausea and vomiting occur because GI contents cannot flow forward as usual. The additional clinical cues are likely the result of fluid and electrolyte balances caused by losing GI contents and possible intestinal obstruction. Recall that:

- Vomiting causes loss of fluids and sodium, resulting in dehydration and hyponatremia.
- Hypotension and tachycardia are common clinical cues associated with dehydration.
- Muscle weakness and generalized fatigue are common clinical cues associated with hyponatremia.
- Muscle weakness and irregular heart rate are common clinical cues associated with potassium imbalance, especially hypokalemia.

Determine whether Inconsistencies or Gaps Exist

Additional assessments are needed to validate the patterns determined in this client situation. For example, laboratory testing would help validate fluid and electrolyte imbalances; an abdominal CT scan or ultrasound would help diagnose intestinal obstruction. Based on the list of clinical cues in the hypothetical client situation, there are no obvious inconsistencies in the assessment findings.

Make an Inference Based on Cue Interpretation

The ability to interpret data and draw valid conclusions is key to making sound clinical judgments. The clinical cues identified from the hypothetical situation can be concluded to be consistent with an intestinal obstruction with associated fluid and electrolyte imbalances. Cues were organized by body system to form patterns which were then compared to the nursing knowledge of pathophysiology. While laboratory and imaging tests would help validate this likely actual client condition, sufficient evidence exists to make this inference.

Identify Potential Client Conditions

In addition to determining one or more actual client conditions by interpreting relevant clinical cues, you want to anticipate potential client conditions to generate a complete list of hypotheses. As described earlier in this chapter, predicting potential conditions helps you identify what signs and symptoms to look for when monitoring a client, anticipate what could happen if the client's condition worsens, and be prepared to manage the condition if it occurs. Using your nursing knowledge to determine the potential conditions in the hypothetical clinical situation, think about what *could* happen to the client who has intestinal obstruction, dehydration, hyponatremia, and possibly hypokalemia. Box 3.6 lists common potential complications that could occur as a result of having these actual hypothetical conditions.

BOX 3.6 Potential Complications Associated with Actual Client Conditions

Intestinal Obstruction	Dehydration	Hyponatremia	Hypokalemia
Paralytic ileus	Hypovolemic shock	Seizures	Cardiac dysrhythmias
Perforation	Acute kidney injury	Decreased level of	Respiratory failure
Peritonitis	Cerebral edema	consciousness	Paresis/paralysis
Abdominal abscess		Respiratory failure	

Once you have analyzed the client's relevant clinical cues, the next challenge is to prioritize your hypotheses. The process for how to prioritize hypotheses is described in Chapter 4.

Thinking Exercise 3.5 will help you practice what you've learned in this chapter about analyzing cues. The answer and rationale for the exercise are located at the end of this book.

THINKING EXERCISE 3.5

The nurse is caring for a 20-month-old toddler in the Pediatric Urgent Care Center.

History and Physical	Nurses Notes	Orders	Laboratory Results

0835:   Family brought child to center with report of rhinorrhea, anorexia, coughing, and sneezing for the past 2 days. Started day care last week and is up to date with immunizations. Client crying softly and pulling on right ear. Mild wheezing auscultated throughout lung fields; coughing frequently. No pharyngeal redness or pustules. Cervical and periauricular lymph nodes enlarged. VS: T 103.6°F (39.8°C); HR 135 beats per minute; RR difficult to count while crying; B/P 92/50 mmHg; SpO$_2$ 95% on RA.

Which of the following client conditions are consistent with the client's current findings? **Select all that apply.**

- Otitis media
- Asthma
- RSV infection
- Streptococcal infection
- Kawasaki's disease
- Gastroenteritis

END-OF-CHAPTER EXERCISES

Additional end-of-chapter exercises will help you apply what you've learned in this chapter. The answers and rationales for these exercises are located at the end of this chapter.

END-OF-CHAPTER EXERCISE 3.1

The nurse is caring for a 61-year-old client with a history of cirrhosis admitted to the acute care medical unit.

History and Physical	Nurses Notes	Orders	Laboratory Results

1210:   Sitting upright in bed with O$_2$ at 3 L per minute via NC. Ate minimal food for lunch due to lack of appetite. Alert and oriented ×4. No adventitious breath sounds. Abdomen distended with ascites but breathing not labored. Reports having several diarrheal stools. Hyperactive bowel sounds in all quadrants. Moves all extremities freely; cap refill <3 seconds bilaterally. VS: T 98.6°F (37°C); HR 94 beats per minute; RR 22 breaths per minute; B/P 114/66 mmHg; SpO$_2$ 99% on supplemental O$_2$.

1555:   Family visiting and report client vomited red-tinged emesis ×2 since lunch. Client drowsy but easily awakened. Oriented ×4. Pale and clammy skin. VS: T 98.6°F (37°C); HR 106 beats per minute; RR 24 breaths per minute; B/P 96/58 mmHg; SpO$_2$ 95% on O$_2$ at 3 L per minute via NC.

Complete the following sentence by selecting from the lists of options below.
The client is likely experiencing ___1 [Select]___ as evidenced by ___2 [Select]___ and ___3 [Select]___ .

Options for 1	Options for 2	Options for 3
Respiratory failure	Anorexia	Tachycardia
Bleeding esophageal varices	Diarrhea	Hypoxemia
Encephalopathy	Hematemesis	Bradypnea

END-OF-CHAPTER EXERCISE 3.2

The nurse is caring for a 78-year-old client in the Emergency Department (ED).

History and Physical	Nurses Notes	Orders	Laboratory Results

1940: Brought to ED by family with report of acute confusion, extreme fatigue, and decreased voiding. H/O diabetes mellitus type II, hypertension, and osteoarthritis. Went to primary care provider last week with similar concerns which have worsened. Labs drawn and client sent home with instructions to drink more fluids. Usually cognitively intact and able to care for self independently at home. Currently alert and oriented ×2 (person and place). Breath sounds clear throughout lung fields. Abdomen slightly distended with diminished bowel sounds. Moves all extremities freely; cap refill 5 seconds bilaterally. 3+ nonpitting edema in both lower legs and feet. VS: T 100.6°F (37°C); HR 98 beats per minute; RR 20 breaths per minute; B/P 110/58 mmHg; SpO$_2$ 94% on RA. Stat labs drawn.

2125: Indwelling urinary catheter in place and draining scant amount of dark yellow urine. Lab results available.

History and Physical	Laboratory Results	Orders	Nurses Notes

Serum Laboratory Test and Reference Range	ED 1940 Today
Blood urea nitrogen (BUN) (10–20 mg/dL [3.6–7.1 mmol/L])	49 mg/dL (17.5 mmol/L)
Creatinine (M: 0.7–1.3 mg/dL [61.89–114. µmol/L]) (F: 0.5–1.2 mg/dL [44.21–106.1 µmol/L])	3.2 mg/dL (282.94 µmol/L)
Glucose (82–115 mg/dL [4.6–6.4 mmol/L])	276 mg/dL (15.32 mmol/L)
Sodium (136–145 mEq/L [136–146 mmol/L])	127 mEq/L (127 mmol/L)
Potassium (3.5–5 mEq/L [3.5–5 mmol/L])	5.6 mEq/L (5.6 mmol/L)

Complete the following sentence by selecting from the list of word choices below.
Due to the client's age and history of diabetes mellitus type II, the client is likely experiencing **[Word Choice]**.

Word Choices	
Hyperglycemia hyperosmolar syndrome	Acute kidney injury
Pyelonephritis	Diabetic ketoacidosis

END-OF-CHAPTER EXERCISE 3.3

The nurse is caring for a 21-year-old client in the Emergency Department (ED).

History and Physical	Nurses Notes	Orders	Laboratory Results

2250:   Brought to ED by ambulance after being found on sidewalk lying in vomitus. Stuporous when found by first responders but lethargic at present after IV fluid administration. Unable to answer questions or provide any information about what happened. Long-time friend accompanying client unaware of any significant medical history other than depression for which drug therapy has controlled for several years. Client doesn't usually drink but recently learned that the client's partner wanted to "break up." Client began drinking this morning and consumed several bottles of "hard liquor." Skin clammy with bluish-tinged fingers. Lung fields clear with no adventitious sounds. S_1 and S_2 present. Hypoactive bowel sounds in all quadrants. Cap refill <3 seconds bilaterally. VS: T 97.2°F (36.2°C); HR 58 beats per minute; RR 10 breaths per minute and shallow; B/P 96/54 mmHg; SpO_2 93% on RA.

Complete the following sentence by selecting from the lists of options below.
The client likely has ___**1 [Select]**___ as evidenced by the client's ___**2 [Select]**___ and ___**3 [Select]**___ .

Options for 1	Options for 2	Options for 3
Bipolar disorder	History of depression	Hypoxemia
Suicide ideation	Decreased level of consciousness	Hypothermia
Alcohol poisoning	Hypoactive bowel sounds	Antidepressant drug therapy

END-OF-CHAPTER EXERCISE 3.4

The nurse is caring for a 16-year-old client in the Emergency Room (ED).

History and Physical	Nurses Notes	Orders	Laboratory Results

1015:   Brought to ED by family with report of headache, nausea, trouble concentrating, and anxiety. Family states client was "sacked" several times during a high school football game 2 nights ago. Drowsy and oriented ×4. Frontal headache pain at 8/10. PERRLA; CNs intact. Can move all extremities freely. Lung fields clear with no adventitious sounds. S_1 and S_2 present. Bowel sounds present in all quadrants. Cap refill <3 seconds bilaterally. VS: T 98.6°F (37°C); HR 80 beats per minute; RR 18 breaths per minute; B/P 110/62 mmHg; SpO_2 98% on RA.

Select **1** client condition that the client is likely experiencing at this time.
- Migraine headache
- Malignant brain tumor
- Meningioma
- Traumatic brain injury
- Sinus infection

END-OF-CHAPTER EXERCISE 3.5

The nurse is caring for a 33-year-old client in the Urgent Care Center.

History and Physical	Nurses Notes	Orders	Laboratory Results

1755:   Client seen in center with report of headache, occasional nausea and vomiting, and muscle aches. Concerned that signs and symptoms are being caused by flu or COVID-19; did not have immunizations for these illnesses. History of diabetes mellitus type I and ADHD. Alert and oriented ×4. Lung fields clear with no adventitious sounds. S_1 and S_2 present. Bowel sounds present in all quadrants. Cap refill <3 seconds bilaterally. Skin dry and flushed. VS: T 98°F (36.7°C); HR 76 beats per minute; RR 16 breaths per minute; B/P 102/50 mmHg; SpO_2 98% on RA. FSBG 305 mg/dL (16.93 mmol/L). (Reference range 74–106 mg/dL [4.1–5.9 mmol/L].)

Complete the following sentence by selecting from the list of word choices below.
The client is most likely experiencing **[Word Choice]** based on the presenting client findings.

Word Choices	
Hyperglycemic hyperosmolar syndrome	Diabetic ketoacidosis
COVID-19 infection	Influenza

Answers and Rationales for Thinking Exercises

CHAPTER THINKING EXERCISES

THINKING EXERCISE 3.1

Answer:
The client likely has **urinary tract infection** as evidenced by **low-grade fever** and **elevated WBC count**.

Rationale: The client is in the third trimester of pregnancy and stops drinking fluids 2 hours before bedtime to prevent nocturia. Flushing of bacteria in the urinary tract is dependent on urinary flow. Therefore, fluid restriction can lead to concentrated urine that is prone to infection. Clients who are pregnant are at risk for silent UTIs in which the client has no obvious symptoms like urinary frequency and burning. However, the client's low-grade fever and elevated WBC count indicate a possible infection somewhere in the body. While it is normal for the WBC count to increase during pregnancy, this client's value is much higher than expected. There is no indication that the client has anemia. Increased fatigue is common in the third trimester. Other than an elevated blood pressure, the client has no other findings associated with preeclampsia. Insomnia and bladder pressure are common during the third trimester. The fetus moves frequently and can cause pelvic pressure and an inability to sleep well.

THINKING EXERCISE 3.2

Answer:
Based on the history and current findings, the client is at **_high_** risk for **suicide**.

Rationale: The client is a veteran who demonstrates disorientation, nightmares, and delusions because the client thinks there are IEDs outside, which can occur with posttraumatic stress disorder (PTSD). Given that the client may have PTSD and has old bandages on the wrists, the client is at high risk for suicide. Clients who are schizophrenic usually have hallucinations, delusions, and disorganized thinking. The client may be depressed but there are inadequate data to support that conclusion. Being unhoused at times can lead to frostbite during cold months, but the client has options such as family and local shelters to prevent this complication.

✸ THINKING EXERCISE 3.3

Answer:
Select **4** potential postoperative complications for which this client is **most** at risk.

X Atelectasis
X Wound infection
○ Peptic ulcer
○ Compartment syndrome
○ Hypovolemic shock
X Venous thromboembolism
○ Contractures
X Anemia

Rationale: The client has an abdominal incision that is warm and hyperpigmented (erythema in dark skin tone clients). In addition, the client has an elevated temperature and mild leukocytosis which could indicate the potential for or actual wound infection. The client is at risk for atelectasis because the client uses the incentive spirometer every 4–6 hours rather than every 1–2 hours as needed to expand the lungs. The client is also at high risk for venous thromboembolism because of refusing to wear SCDs while in bed. These devices improve venous flow which helps prevent deep vein thrombosis that could result in a pulmonary embolus, a life-threatening complication. The laboratory results show a decrease in RBC count, hemoglobin, and hematocrit, which indicates the client is at risk for anemia if these values continue to decline. There are no client findings that provide evidence for risks of peptic ulcer, compartment syndrome, or contractures.

✸ THINKING EXERCISE 3.4

Answer:

Client Findings	Pneumonia	Pulmonary Embolism	Acute Pulmonary Edema
Fever	X		
Crackles	X		X
Mental status changes	X	X	X
Cough	X	X	X
Fatigue	X		
Chest pain	X	X	
Shortness of breath	X	X	X
Irregular rapid heart rate	X	X	X

Rationale: The client findings are all consistent with pneumonia, which is a lung inflammation caused by a viral, bacterial, or fungal infection. The infection can be localized as a solid infiltrate or diffuse throughout both lungs. Having a fever and fatigue is common in the presence of any type of infection. In the presence of fever, the heart rate typically increases and can beat irregularly. Because the alveoli are usually filled with purulent material, oxygen diffusion is impaired causing mental status changes, shortness of breath, and chest pain in older adults. Crackles are common due to alveolar fluid. The body attempts to rid the lungs of the infected material by coughing. A pulmonary embolism (PE) occurs when a clot occludes a pulmonary artery decreasing lung perfusion. Classic signs and symptoms of PE are acute chest pain, shortness of breath, dysrhythmia (often atrial fibrillation), and cough, sometimes with blood. The client who has a PE typically does not have a fever, crackles, or fatigue. Acute pulmonary edema typically results from heart failure, but other causes are trauma and infection. In acute pulmonary edema, the client's alveoli fill with fluid and cause crackles, cough, shortness of breath, and irregular rapid heart rate. Chronic pulmonary edema can cause fatigue, but this finding is not common in clients with acute pulmonary edema.

THINKING EXERCISE 3.5

Answer:

Which of the following client conditions are consistent with the client's current findings? **Select all that apply.**

X Otitis media

○ Asthma

X RSV infection

○ Streptococcal infection

○ Kawasaki's disease

○ Gastroenteritis

Rationale: The toddler has a fever, mild wheezing, rhinorrhea, anorexia, coughing, and sneezing which are all consistent with a respiratory infection. Because the child does not have pharyngeal inflammation or pustules, the child likely has RSV infection rather than a streptococcal infection. The child is pulling on the right ear which is typical behavior for a toddler with an earache. Otitis media is common in this age group due to the short length of the eustachian tube connecting the middle ear with the pharynx. Asthma usually causes wheezing without fever. Gastroenteritis is a GI infection causing anorexia, nausea, vomiting, and diarrhea, which this client does not have. Kawasaki's disease is an autoimmune disorder that affects blood vessels primarily in children under 5 years of age. This disease causes fever, enlarged lymph nodes, swollen dry lips, and swollen reddened or hyperpigmented (in dark skin tones) hands. Joint and abdominal pain may also occur. This client does not have most of these assessment findings.

END-OF-CHAPTER THINKING EXERCISES

END-OF-CHAPTER THINKING EXERCISE 3.1

Answer:

The client is likely experiencing **bleeding esophageal varices** as evidenced by **hematemesis** and **tachycardia**.

Rationale: Clients who have cirrhosis are at risk for many complications as a result of portal hypertension and liver damage. The client experienced hematemesis, which is a common finding when varicosed esophageal blood vessels start to actively bleed. Because the client is losing fluid, the blood pressure decreases and the heart rate increases (tachycardia) to compensate for less blood volume. The client's peripheral oxygen saturation and respiratory rate do not support the client experiencing respiratory failure. Therefore, the client is likely not hypoxemic. The respiratory rate of 24 breaths per minute is tachypnea and not bradypnea. The client does not have signs and symptoms of encephalopathy as evidenced by being alert and oriented ×4. If this complication was occurring, the client would be disoriented and likely confused. Anorexia is common in clients who have chronic diseases. Diarrhea is not consistent with bleeding esophageal varices.

END-OF-CHAPTER THINKING EXERCISE 3.2

Answer:

Due to the client's age and history of diabetes mellitus type II, the client is likely experiencing **acute kidney injury**.

Rationale: The client has likely had dehydration for some time which resulted in decreased urinary output and increased BUN. Dehydration and a history of diabetes mellitus (DM) are risk factors for acute kidney injury (AKI). The client has dependent edema and acute confusion because the kidneys cannot excrete sufficient fluid and waste products that are toxic to the brain. In AKI, increased fluid retention dilutes serum sodium causing hyponatremia. However, potassium is retained when the kidneys' function decreases. The client's BUN and serum creatinine are markedly increased. While BUN can increase due to dehydration, kidney damage, and increased protein catabolism, creatinine is specific to kidney function. An increased creatinine level indicates kidney impairment. The client's low-grade fever is likely due to dehydration rather than pyelonephritis. Pyelonephritis causes flank pain, nausea and vomiting, frequent painful urination, high fever, and chills in most clients. This client does not have these findings. Although the serum glucose is elevated and the client is dehydrated, the client does not meet all the criteria for hyperglycemic, hyperosmolar syndrome, a complication of DM type II. Diabetic ketoacidosis is a complication of DM type I.

⚡ END-OF-CHAPTER THINKING EXERCISE 3.3

Answer:
The client likely has **alcohol poisoning** as evidenced by the client's **decreased level of consciousness** and **hypothermia**.

Rationale: There is no indication that the client has suicide ideation because the client has not verbalized the desire for suicide or a plan to commit suicide. The friend indicated a history of depression, which could be associated with bipolar disorder. However, the most likely condition that the client has is alcohol poisoning as supported by a decreased LOC, hypothermia, bradycardia, and slow shallow respirations. Hypoactive bowel sounds are not a common finding associated with alcohol poisoning. Although the client has an SpO_2 of 93% which is below the desired level of 95%, there is no other evidence of hypoxemia. Hypoxemia is usually accompanied by tachycardia rather than bradycardia.

⚡ END-OF-CHAPTER THINKING EXERCISE 3.4

Answer:
Select **1** client condition that the client is likely experiencing at this time.
- ○ Migraine headache
- ○ Malignant brain tumor
- ○ Meningioma
- **X** Traumatic brain injury
- ○ Sinus infection

Rationale: The client experienced a traumatic experience during a football game which can cause injuries, especially traumatic brain injury (TBI). Mild TBI or concussion is associated with headaches, nausea, anxiety, disorientation, trouble thinking, and feeling "foggy." There is no evidence that the client has an infection, including a sinus infection. Although the client could have a brain tumor, the client's history of being "sacked" at a football game as an acute event strongly supports TBI. Brain tumor signs and symptoms are usually more subtle or gradual in their presentation. The client has a severe headache but none of the other findings associated with migraine headache.

⚡ END-OF-CHAPTER THINKING EXERCISE 3.5

Answer:
The client is most likely experiencing **diabetic ketoacidosis** based on the presenting client findings.

Rationale: The client most likely has diabetic ketoacidosis (DKA) as evidenced by dry flushed skin, headache, nausea and vomiting, muscle aches, and a blood glucose (FSBG) of over 300 mg/dL (16.65 mmol/L). There is no evidence of infections such as COVID-19 or influenza because the client does not have the typical fever seen with these respiratory problems. Hyperglycemic, hyperosmolar syndrome is a complication of diabetes mellitus (DM) type II; this client has DM type I.

REFERENCES

Afriyie, D. (2020). Effective communication between nurses and patients: An evolutionary concept analysis. *British Journal of Community Nursing*, *25*(9), 438–445.

Al-Moteri, M., Cooper, S., Symmons, M., & Plummer, V. (2020). Nurses' cognitive and perceptual bias in the identification of clinical deterioration cues. *Australian Critical Care*, *33*(4), 333–342.

Alaseeri, R., Rajab, A., & Banakhar, M. (2021). Do personal differences and organizational factors influence nurses' decision making? A qualitative study. *Nursing Reports*, *11*(3), 714–727.

FitzGerald, C., & Hurst, S. (2017). Implicit bias in healthcare professionals: A systematic review. *BMC Medical Ethics*, *18*(1). https://www.doi:10.1186/s12910-017-0179-8.

*Gillespie, M. (2010). Using the situated clinical decision-making framework to guide analysis of nurses' clinical decision-making. *Nurse Education in Practice, 10*, 333–340.

Healthy People 2030. U.S. Department of Health and Human Services, Office of Disease Prevention and Health Promotion. *Social determinants of health.* Retrieved from https://health.gov/healthypeople/priority-areas/social-determinants-health.

IGI Global. (2023). *What is higher order thinking?*. Retrieved from https://www.igi-global.com/dictonionary/higher-order-thinking/13104.

Lee, T. C., Shah, N. U., Haack, A., & Baxter, S. L. (2020). Clinical implementation of predictive models embedded within electronic health record systems: A systematic review. *Informatics, 7*(3), 25. https://www.doi.org/10.3390/informatics7030025.

Narayan, M. C. (2019). Addressing implicit bias in nursing: A review. *AJN, 119*(7), 36–43.

Orique, S. B., Despins, L., Wakefield, B. J., Erdelez, S., & Vogelsmeier, A. (2019). Perception of clinical deterioration cues among medical-surgical nurses. *Journal of Advanced Nursing, 75*(11), 2627–2637.

Pagana, K. D., Pagana, T. J., & Pagana, T. N. (2022). *Mosby's Manual of diagnostic and laboratory tests* (*7th* ed.). Elsevier.

Sabin, J. A. (2022). Tackling implicit bias in health care. *New England Journal of Medicine, 387*, 105–107.

Thirsk, L. M., Panchuk, J. T., Stahlke, S., & Hagtvedt, R. (2022). Cognitive and implicit bias in nurses' judgment and decision-making: A scoping review. *International Journal of International Studies, 133.* https://www.doi.org/10.1016/j.ijnurstu.2022.104284.

Touhy, T. A., & Jett, K. (2022). *Ebersole and Hess' gerontological nursing and healthy aging* (6th ed.). Elsevier.

White, A., Maguire, M. B. R., Brannan, J., & Brown, A. (2021). Situational awareness in acute patient deterioration: Identifying student time to task. *Nurse Educator, 46*(2), 82–86.

*Denotes classic reference

4

How to Prioritize Hypotheses

LEARNING OUTCOMES

1. Briefly describe four common frameworks used for prioritizing hypotheses.
2. Identify key considerations and approaches for prioritizing hypotheses.
3. Explain the three levels of priority client conditions.
4. Differentiate two commonly used specialty triage systems.
5. Discuss the relationship of selected priority-setting models.
6. Describe nurse and system factors that can affect the ability to prioritize hypotheses.
7. Discuss strategies for prioritizing hypotheses to make safe, appropriate clinical judgments.

KEY TERMS

Disaster triage tag system: Mass casualty system that categorizes and ranks clients by their condition; priorities for client care are indicated by colored tags and numbers.

Emergency triage system: Ranking or classifying clients into priority levels depending on condition or condition severity, with the highest acuity conditions receiving the quickest evaluation and treatment.

Emergent condition: A *life-threatening situation* in which the client could suffer significant harm without rapid or immediate therapeutic and/or diagnostic action.

Ethnocentric: The application of one's own culture as the frame of reference to evaluate or judge the practices, beliefs, and culture of others.

Hypotheses: Suppositions, assumptions, or likely conclusions that are made based on client data (clinical cues).

Mental health crisis: Acute disruption of psychological homeostasis in which an individual's usual coping mechanisms fail, causing distress and functional impairment.

Missed nursing care: Nursing care left undone, rationed care, or unfinished care.

Nonurgent condition: Clinical situation that is not serious and does not require immediate medical care.

Prioritization: Process in which the nurse chooses to take a specific action instead of some other action based on the client's condition or primary need.

Priority setting: Process of deciding which client condition needs to be addressed first to then determine the preferred order for taking nursing actions.

Stable condition: State in which a client is not at high risk for or experiencing physiologic or psychologic cues that indicate clinical deterioration or medical complications.

Unstable condition: State in which a client is at high risk for or is experiencing physiologic or psychologic cues that indicate clinical deterioration or medical complications.

Urgent condition: A serious, *not* life-threatening situation requiring medical attention.

Chapter 3 described the process of analyzing relevant cues to generate hypotheses about a client's condition. This chapter discusses the process of prioritizing those hypotheses to help you determine which nursing actions may be needed in a clinical situation and in what sequential order.

PRIORITIZING HYPOTHESES

Prioritizing hypotheses is a clinical judgment cognitive skill that allows nurses to establish a preferred order for care. This skill is particularly important when a client has multiple physical and mental client conditions and needs. The new American Association of Colleges of Nursing (AACN) *Essentials* for nurse generalists include this competency as part of the Person-Centered Care Domain: "2.4. Prioritize [client] problems/health concerns" (AACN, 2021, p. 30).

Keep in mind that any client's priority for care can change in minutes or hours. The order of priorities often changes depending on the seriousness and relationship of the problems. For example, if abnormal lab values are at life-threatening levels, they could be the highest priority. If your client is having difficulty breathing because of acute rib pain, managing the pain may be a higher priority than dealing with a rapid pulse, because the pain is likely causing the rapid pulse.

Definitions

Hypotheses are suppositions, assumptions, or likely conclusions that are made based on presenting client data (clinical cues). In practice, the nurse recognizes relevant clinical cues in a client situation that need timely follow up, and interprets those assessment data to determine one or more hypotheses (actual or potential client conditions). These hypotheses are evaluated and ranked based on:

- Likelihood of occurrence
- Urgency
- Risk for complications

The nurse then decides which client condition needs to be addressed first to determine the preferred order for taking nursing actions (Potter et al., 2023). This process is known as priority setting.

Similar to other clinical judgment cognitive skills, prioritizing hypotheses is contextual and clinically situated. In other words, priorities for client care differ depending on where health care occurs and what type of care is needed. For example, priority setting for a client admitted to an acute care hospital unit would be different than that for a client at end-of-life in palliative/hospice care. The priority in acute care is managing a client's airway and breathing, but the priority for end-of-life care is promoting client comfort as part of ensuring a "good" death. Prioritizing hypotheses also depends on what the client expects or desires as a clinical outcome. Be sure to incorporate the client's or guardian's preferred priority to ensure person-centered care, also called client-centered care.

> **CLINICAL JUDGMENT TIP**
>
> *Remember:* Prioritizing hypotheses is contextual and clinically situated. In other words, priorities for client care differ depending on where health care occurs and what type of care is needed.

Prioritization of Client Conditions

Prioritization means that the nurse chooses to take a specific action instead of some other action based on the most important client condition or primary need (Suhonen et al., 2018). The overall purpose of prioritization is to maintain client safety and reduce risk to the client's well-being. Key components of prioritization include the importance, impact, and urgency of the client's conditions, and can be framed in several ways, including:

- Acute or chronic conditions
- Actual or potential conditions
- Stable or unstable conditions
- Urgent or nonurgent conditions

Acute Versus Chronic Client Conditions

Acute client conditions usually occur suddenly and can be very severe or possibly life-threatening. In most cases, they are treatable and can resolve quickly if they respond to treatment. Acute conditions may be unstable and emergent/urgent requiring immediate nursing and/or collaborative interventions. Examples of acute client conditions are myocardial infarction (MI), fracture, and respiratory syncytial virus (RSV) infection.

By contrast, *chronic* client conditions usually occur over a long period of time and are typically stable, nonurgent, and not life-threatening. While most chronic conditions can be managed, controlled, or possibly improve, they do not completely resolve. Examples of chronic client conditions are chronic obstructive pulmonary disease (COPD), osteoporosis, and diabetes mellitus.

Over time, chronic conditions can worsen and result in an urgent or emergent complication. For instance, clients who have COPD can develop acute respiratory failure and clients with diabetes mellitus can develop emergencies such as diabetic ketoacidosis (DKA).

Acuity and severity are foundational concepts for prioritization! Because these conditions can be severe and are usually treatable, acute conditions are usually considered a higher priority than chronic conditions. Clients who have acute exacerbations or complications of chronic conditions are also considered higher priority than those with more stable chronic conditions.

> **CLINICAL JUDGMENT TIP**
>
> *Remember:* Because acute client conditions can be severe and potentially life-threatening, prioritize these conditions higher than chronic stable conditions.

Actual Versus Potential Client Conditions

Nurses may assume that an actual client condition is a higher priority than a potential condition. In many client situations, this assumption is valid. However, in some instances, a potential condition is equally or more important and takes priority over an actual condition. For example, an older client who has COPD may be able to manage this actual condition at home independently. However, if that client also has severe osteoporosis, the client's priority potential condition is one or more fragility fractures, especially if the client is a high risk for falls. To help you decide whether an actual or potential client condition would be the priority for care, remember that the desired clinical outcome is to maintain safety and reduce risk to the client.

Another example of identifying a potential condition as a priority for care is the recognition of clients at risk for adverse outcomes like sepsis and surgical site infection. These conditions are complications that most often develop in clients admitted to acute care hospitals. Clients admitted to critical care units like an ICU are also at high risk for adverse outcomes *after* discharge, such as delirium and posttraumatic stress disorder. To improve client outcomes in these settings and after discharge, care bundles of evidence-based interventions have been developed and are discussed in detail in Chapter 6. As a nurse you are expected to follow these widely accepted standards of practice for selected potential client conditions as a priority for care.

Stable Versus Unstable Client Conditions

When communicating about the condition of clients, nurses frequently refer to clients as stable or unstable; however, there are no universally established definitions for these terms. Generally speaking, referring to a client as having a stable condition means that the client is *not* at high risk for or experiencing physiologic or psychologic cues that indicate clinical deterioration or medical complications. As defined in Chapter 2, clinical deterioration is a dynamic state in which the client progresses to a worsened clinical condition increasing morbidity, body organ dysfunction, prolonged hospital or agency length of stay, and/or death. A client in an unstable condition is at high risk for or is experiencing physiologic or psychologic cues that indicate clinical deterioration or medical complications. These cues are often potentially life-threatening and therefore become the priority for client care to ensure safety.

CLINICAL JUDGMENT TIP

Remember: When setting priorities, recall that the desired outcome is to maintain safety and reduce risk to the client.

Emergent, Urgent, and Nonurgent Client Conditions

Establishing priorities can also be based on the time and complexity of client conditions. An emergent condition is a *life-threatening situation* in which the client could suffer significant harm without rapid or immediate therapeutic and/or diagnostic action. Emergent conditions are most often managed in an Emergency Department of a tertiary health care system. Examples of emergent client conditions are status asthmaticus and severe traumatic brain injury (TBI).

By contrast, an urgent condition is a serious, but *not* life-threatening situation requiring medical care. Urgent conditions are usually managed in the Emergency Department, Urgent Care Center, or health care provider's practice office. Examples of urgent client conditions are serious respiratory infections like pneumonia and closed fractures. When prioritizing client conditions, emergent conditions are more important than urgent ones.

As the name implies, a nonurgent condition is not serious and does not require immediate medical care. These conditions are usually managed in a health care provider's office, other ambulatory care setting, or home setting. An example of a nonurgent client condition is eczema (atopic dermatitis). When prioritizing client conditions, remember that nonurgent conditions are the least important.

Thinking Exercise 4.1 will help you practice what you've learned in this chapter about prioritizing hypotheses. The answer and rationale for the exercise are located at the end of this book.

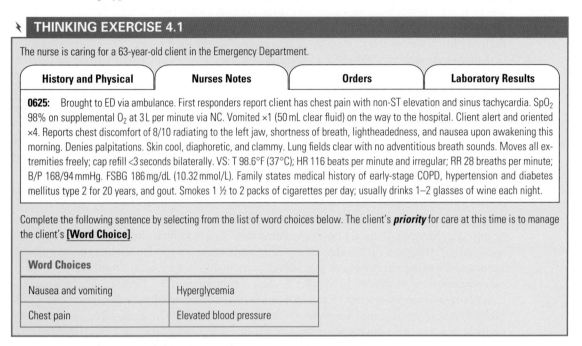

THINKING EXERCISE 4.1

The nurse is caring for a 63-year-old client in the Emergency Department.

History and Physical	Nurses Notes	Orders	Laboratory Results

0625: Brought to ED via ambulance. First responders report client has chest pain with non-ST elevation and sinus tachycardia. SpO$_2$ 98% on supplemental O$_2$ at 3 L per minute via NC. Vomited ×1 (50 mL clear fluid) on the way to the hospital. Client alert and oriented ×4. Reports chest discomfort of 8/10 radiating to the left jaw, shortness of breath, lightheadedness, and nausea upon awakening this morning. Denies palpitations. Skin cool, diaphoretic, and clammy. Lung fields clear with no adventitious breath sounds. Moves all extremities freely; cap refill <3 seconds bilaterally. VS: T 98.6°F (37°C); HR 116 beats per minute and irregular; RR 28 breaths per minute; B/P 168/94 mmHg. FSBG 186 mg/dL (10.32 mmol/L). Family states medical history of early-stage COPD, hypertension and diabetes mellitus type 2 for 20 years, and gout. Smokes 1 ½ to 2 packs of cigarettes per day; usually drinks 1–2 glasses of wine each night.

Complete the following sentence by selecting from the list of word choices below. The client's **_priority_** for care at this time is to manage the client's **[Word Choice]**.

Word Choices	
Nausea and vomiting	Hyperglycemia
Chest pain	Elevated blood pressure

APPROACHES TO PRIORITIZING CLIENT CONDITIONS

Prioritizing client conditions is a difficult skill for novice nurses to develop owing to their lack of clinical experience and the variety of approaches that could be used. Regardless of the approach or model used to establish priorities, incorporate these concepts to ensure person-centered care.

Key Considerations for Determining Priorities

Although the nurse considers multiple factors when prioritizing hypotheses, these two considerations are particularly important:
1. Priority setting should be guided by ethical principles of justice and equity.
2. Priority setting is most challenging for clients who require complex care and are at high risk for clinical deterioration.

Ethical Concepts for Priority Setting

Few studies examining how ethics affect priority settings have been published. Suhonen et al. (2018) conducted a scoping review to determine how ethical elements affect the priority-setting ability of practicing bedside nurses in acute care settings (Box 4.1). Although the study did not address how nurses prioritize among conditions for an individual client, it demonstrated trends that affect this level of priority setting.

BOX 4.1   Evidence-Based Practice

What Ethical Elements Impact the Priority Setting of Bedside Staff Nurses?
Suhonen, R., Stolt, M., Habermann, M., Hjaltadottir, I., Vryonides, S., et al. (2018). Ethical elements in priority setting in nursing care: A scoping review. *International Journal of Nursing Studies, 88,* 25–42.

The authors conducted a scoping review of current research articles to identify the ethical elements impacting the priority setting of nurses at the bedside in acute care settings. In general, the review of the selected 25 articles revealed that the values guiding priority setting by nurses are affected by organizational (system) policies, the client, and the nurse. More specific results of this study included that priorities in practice by nurses are made based on:
- Client group membership
- Client daily care needs
- Nurses' prioritization of their work by tasks
- Nurses' participation in priority setting

As nurses prioritize their tasks, caring interventions are often rationed or deprioritized. An inability to provide these interventions, including caring and empathy, often causes a feeling of inadequacy, powerlessness, guilt, dissatisfaction, and frustration by bedside nurses.

One of the major findings from the Suhonen et al. (2018) study was the inability of nurses to provide caring interventions at times. Caring interventions include listening to client concerns, providing emotional support and empathy, and promoting comfort.

More recently, during the height of the COVID-19 pandemic, nurses often did not have the time or resources to provide emotional support, empathy, or comfort. Specific ethical dilemmas related to priority setting during the pandemic included (Hossain & Clatty, 2021):
- *Justice and equity*: Nurses had to choose where and how to spend their time and energy given limited resources for multiple critically ill and often dying clients.
- *Duty to care*: Nurses had to sacrifice client-centered care ethics (greater good for clients) as they shifted to public health ethics (greater good for society).

Another finding of the Suhonen et al. (2018) study was that bedside nurses often make decisions about priorities based on client group membership. For example, postsurgical clients were prioritized over clients who had chronic conditions. The severity and acuity of conditions among postoperative clients were determined to be the highest priority. Older adults were given the lowest priority, demonstrating possible issues related to justice, fairness, and equity in client care related to priority setting.

Complex and High-Risk Clients

Clients who require complex care typically have two or more chronic conditions; each condition may affect or influence the care needed for another condition. These chronic conditions are usually a combination of physical, mental health, and social issues. Clients who are at an especially high risk for clinical deterioration or medical complications include newly admitted hospital clients, postoperative clients, older adults, and premature neonates. To prioritize hypotheses for clients in these high-risk categories, use an appropriate priority-setting model as discussed later in this chapter.

Keep in mind that acuity and severity are foundational concepts for prioritization. Box 4.2 lists examples of common clinical situations (conditions and treatments) that are high priority because they can place any client at high risk for complications or clinical deterioration. These situations are typically included as part of client acuity tools on medical-surgical nursing units (Ingram & Powell, 2018).

> **BOX 4.2   Examples of High-Priority Client Situations**
>
> - Unstable vital signs
> - New tracheostomy
> - Frequent bronchial suctioning
> - Chest tubes
> - CPAP/high-flow oxygen
> - Mechanical ventilation
> - Unstable dysrhythmias
> - Blood products or chemotherapy
> - Complicated IV medications (e.g., heparin, insulin)
> - Total parenteral nutrition
> - Frequently measured Jackson–Pratt or nephrostomy drainage
> - Uncontrolled pain

> **CLINICAL JUDGMENT TIP**
>
> *Remember:* Priority setting is most challenging for clients who require complex care and are at high risk for clinical deterioration. To prioritize hypotheses for these clients, use an appropriate priority-setting model (discussed later in this chapter).

Basic Hierarchy for Determining Priorities

In your nursing program, you probably learned how to prioritize client needs using the basic hierarchy developed by Abraham Maslow. In 1943, Maslow proposed that human beings are motivated by a five-step hierarchy of needs. Each step or level of the hierarchy has to be met or "satisfied" before an individual can progress to the next level. As shown in Fig. 4.1, the first and lowest level of the hierarchy is the survival level. Examples of *physiological needs* at this level include air (breathing), food, water, comfort, and sleep. The four highest levels with examples of needs are:

1. *Safety needs:* Personal security, health, employment, property
2. *Love and belonging needs:* Friendship, family, intimacy, sense of connection
3. *Esteem:* Self-esteem, respect, recognition, freedom, confidence
4. *Self-actualization:* Creativity, morality, meaning of life, quality of life

   In nursing, Maslow's basic hierarchy of needs can be applied to both nurses and their clients. For example, during the COVID-19 pandemic, sleep and food for nurses were needed to ensure safe practice. For clients who had severe COVID-19 infection, breathing was more important for life preservation than socializing with friends or being creative.

   Nurse educators often teach Maslow's hierarchy as the main method of priority setting to correctly answer NCLEX®-style test items. Relying on Maslow's needs as the main method of priority setting in nursing practice, however, presents several problems, including:

- The original hierarchy was published over 80 years ago and designed to explain how human beings are motivated; it was not designed to help prioritize the needs of a client requiring health care.
- The *physiological needs* within the lowest survival level are not prioritized. For example, if a client has difficulty eating, drinking, breathing, and sleeping, Maslow's hierarchy does not help you determine which of these needs are most important.

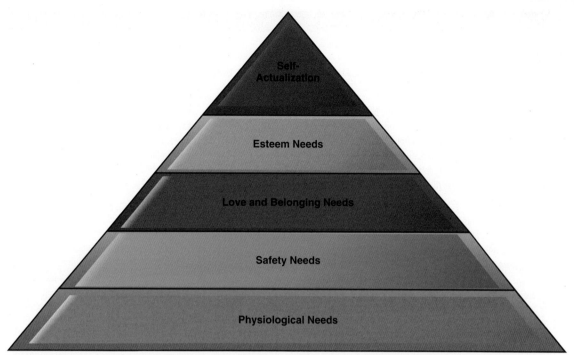

FIG. 4.1 Maslow's hierarchy of needs. (Modified from Maslow, A.H. (1943). A theory of human motivation. *Psychological Review, 50*, 370–396; Black, B. (2024). *Professional Nursing* (10th ed.). Elsevier.)

- The hierarchy is ethnocentric, which is defined as the application of one's own culture as the frame of reference to evaluate or judge the practices, beliefs, and culture of others. Maslow studied individuals in the United States and did not differentiate needs based on gender, age, or ethnicity. Therefore, individual diversity, culture, or equity are not considered when determining priorities using this model.
- Even though the use of Maslow's *revised* hierarchy was designed to be more flexible, an individual must meet most of the needs of any given level before progressing to a higher level. This guideline suggests that a person who has food insecurity would not be able to meet higher-level love and belonging needs. It also suggests that a person living in poverty could not be creative (self-actualization level). Both of these statements are false and, therefore, challenge the validity of Maslow's hierarchy for prioritizing hypotheses.

A number of alternative models are more appropriate to help you prioritize client conditions, and are described later in this chapter. Remember to consider the client's or guardian's priority to provide person-centered care.

Thinking Exercise 4.2 will help you practice what you've learned in this chapter about prioritizing hypotheses. The answer and rationale for the exercise are located at the end of this book.

⚡ THINKING EXERCISE 4.2

The nurse is caring for a 14-year-old client in the Emergency Department.

History and Physical	Nurses Notes	Orders	Laboratory Results

0240: Brought to ED via ambulance. First responders report client has two gunshot wounds (GSW) in abdomen and one in lower right leg. IV of NS infusing in left forearm. No other injuries, significant medical history, or known allergies. Client crying out in pain, but alert and oriented ×4. Very anxious and asking for family. Right upper quadrant abdominal GSW with right flank bullet exit wound; old blood on dressings. Mid-abdominal GSW without bullet exit wound. Abdominal pain reported at 10/10. Right lower leg compound fracture covered loosely with sterile dressing and inflatable splint. Skin cool, diaphoretic, and clammy. Right foot cooler than left foot; right LE distal pulses absent; left LE distal pulses 2+. Cap refill <3 seconds in left foot; cap refill >3 seconds in right foot. Reports pain in right lower leg as 7/10. VS: T 99.4°F (37.4°C); HR 112 beats per minute; RR 24 breaths per minute; B/P 92/48 mmHg; SpO$_2$ 98% on 4L O$_2$ via NC.

0255: POC abdominal US shows perforation in right ileum with probable active bleed. Stat blood work ordered.

Complete the following sentence by selecting from the lists of options below. The ***priority*** for nursing care is to manage the client's _____**1 [Select]**_____ as evidenced by _____**2 [Select]**_____ and _____**3 [Select]**_____ .

Options for 1	Options for 2	Options for 3
Anxiety	Hypoxia	Hypotension
Severe pain	Tachycardia	Tachypnea
Internal bleeding	Fever	Cool skin with diaphoresis
Leg fracture	Absent distal pulses	Decreased capillary refill

LEVELS OF PRIORITY FOR CLIENT CONDITIONS

Prioritizing hypotheses requires (1) differentiating between client conditions needing immediate attention and those requiring subsequent action, and (2) deciding what conditions must be addressed in the client health record. As a practicing nurse, you will need to quickly recognize when clients experience or are at risk of experiencing clinical deterioration, and determine which conditions require immediate action. If you do not know how to set priorities, you could cause life-threatening treatment delays. One commonly used method for priority-setting is to rank physiologic changes into three levels of importance. Table 4.1 lists examples of physiologic conditions for each of these levels.

First-Level Priorities

First-level priorities are client conditions that reflect clinical deterioration with critical findings and are life-threatening. These conditions require *emergent* action to prevent negative client outcomes, including possible death. Examples of first-level priority conditions include crushing chest pain and bradycardia (see Table 4.1). Although most changes in clinical findings are physiologic, planning suicide or verbalizing a desire to hurt others are mental health client conditions that are classified as first-level priorities because these behaviors are also life-threatening.

TABLE 4.1 **Levels of Priority and Examples of Physiologic Client Conditions**	
Levels of Priority	**Examples of Physiologic Client Conditions**

First-level priorities (emergent action)	➢ Cardiovascular compromise (hemodynamic instability):
	  - Crushing chest pain
	  - Bradycardia
	  - Pulselessness
	  - Severe hypotension
	  - Low peripheral oxygen saturation
	➢ Respiratory distress:
	  - Respiratory rate below 10 breaths per minute (adult); below 30 for neonate
	  - Tachypnea
	  - Labored breathing
	  - Nasal flaring
	  - Intercostal retractions

Second-level priorities (prompt action)	➢ Increasing pain level ➢ High fever ➢ Decreasing level of consciousness (LOC) ➢ Delirium ➢ Cold extremities ➢ Acute changes in lab values, such as hypo-/hyperkalemia, severe hyponatremia, and severe anemia ➢ New-onset infection
Third-level priorities (action can wait)	➢ Decreased functional ability ➢ Decreased mobility ➢ Lack of knowledge ➢ Insomnia

Second-Level Priorities

Second-level priorities are client conditions that *may lead* to clinical deterioration or become life-threatening without action. Therefore, these conditions require *prompt* action to prevent progression to clinical deterioration. Examples of second-level priority conditions include high fever and decreasing LOC (see Table 4.1).

CLINICAL JUDGMENT TIP

Remember: First-level priorities are client conditions that reflect clinical deterioration and are life-threatening; provide *emergent* action to prevent negative outcomes, including possible death. Second-level priorities are client conditions that may lead to clinical deterioration or become life-threatening without action. Therefore, provide *prompt* action to prevent progression to clinical deterioration.

Third-Level Priorities

Third-level priorities are nonurgent, not serious, and usually not acute. Having a nonurgent condition means that actions to meet the client's needs *can wait* without concern for negative outcomes. Examples of third-level priority conditions are decreased functional ability (such as inability to perform ADLs independently) and lack of knowledge about care after discharge from an inpatient unit (see Table 4.1).

Thinking Exercise 4.3 will help you practice what you've learned in this chapter about prioritizing hypotheses. The answer and rationale for the exercise are located at the end of this book.

THINKING EXERCISE 4.3

The nurse is caring for a 76-year-old client in a long-term care facility.

History and Physical	Nurses Notes	Orders	Laboratory Results

0700   FSBG 198 mg/dL (10.99 mmol/L). History of diabetes mellitus (DM) type 2, hypertension, osteoarthritis, incontinence, and peptic ulcer disease. Metformin dose increased 3 days ago.

0830 Drowsy but easily aroused this AM. Oriented to person only. Ate ¼ of breakfast and offered enteral supplement. Dry mucous membranes and skin. Reminded CNA to offer oral fluids frequently and apply skin lotion after shower. No adventitious breath sounds or respiratory distress. Hypoactive bowel sounds present ×4. Moves all extremities. Cap refill >3 seconds. Dependent 3+ edema in both feet and ankles. VS: T 100.2°F (37.4°C); HR 101 beats per minute; RR 20 breaths per minute; BP 98/54 mmHg. Waiting on lab results, including urine culture obtained 3 days ago.

1015 CNA reports client moaning and grimacing when preparing for and taking shower. Given acetaminophen for joint pain and general discomfort.

1200 FSBG 236 mg/dL (13.10 mmol/L) before lunch. Has not voided yet today. Refuses to drink water, but consumed ½ of enteral supplement. Not moaning or grimacing during care at this time. Registered dietitian nutritionist in for consult due to weight loss of 9 pounds (4.1 kg) in the last 3 days. Changed to daily weights with increased enteral supplements to 4 cans per day. VS: 100.8°F (38.2°C); HR 107 beats per minute; RR 18 breaths per minute; BP 95/50 mmHg.

History and Physical	Laboratory Results	Orders	Nurses Notes

Serum Laboratory Test and Reference Range	Today at 0600
Blood urea nitrogen (10–20 mg/dL [3.6–7.1 mmol/L])	67 mg/dL (23.93 mmol/L)
Creatinine (0.7–1.3 mg/dL [61.89–114.95 µmol/L])	1.5 mg/dL (132.63 µmol/L)
Fasting blood glucose (82–115 mg/dL [4.6–6.4 mmol/L])	195 mg/dL (10.82 mmol/L)
Prealbumin (15–36 mg/dL [150–360 mg/L])	13.8 mg/dL (138 mg/L)
Urine Laboratory Test and Reference Range Urine culture (negative: <10,000 bacteria/mL urine; positive: >100,000 bacteria/mL urine)	17,500 bacteria/mL urine

Select **2 *priority*** client conditions that require nursing action.
- Urinary tract infection
- Dehydration
- Malnutrition
- Hyperglycemia
- Osteoarthritis pain
- Fluid overload
- Decreased peristalsis

TRIAGE SYSTEMS

Triage is a sorting or ranking process to determine priorities. In health care, several triage systems are commonly used to determine priorities for client care. Two types of systems are briefly described in this section.

Emergency Triage Systems

Various triage systems are used by hospital emergency departments to rank clients by condition. Based on the severity of the client's condition, a well-known emergency triage system is the three-tiered model of "emergent, urgent, and nonurgent" (Ignatavicius et al., 2024). Table 4.2 provides examples of client conditions categorized in each tier.

TABLE 4.2 Three-Tiered Triage System and Examples of Clients Triaged in Each Tier	
Tier Level	**Examples of Client Conditions Triaged by Tier**
Emergent (life threatening)	Chest pain Hemorrhage Respiratory distress Stroke Vital sign instability
Urgent (needs quick treatment, but not immediately life threatening)	Abdominal pain (severe) Fractures (compound or multiple) Respiratory infection (especially pneumonia in older adults) Soft-tissue injuries (complex or multiple)
Nonurgent (could wait several hours or longer if needed without fear of clinical deterioration)	Skin rashes Strains and sprains Urinary tract infection

From Ignatavicius, D.D., Rebar, C.R., & Heimgartner, N.M. (2024). *Medical-surgical nursing: Concepts for clinical judgment and collaborative care* (11th Ed.). Elsevier.

Disaster Triage Tag System

Although mass casualty triage practices can vary widely, some concepts are standardized. Most mass casualty response teams at the disaster site and in the acute care setting use a disaster triage tag system that categorizes and ranks clients by their conditions. Priorities for client care are indicated by colored tags and numbers (Ignatavicius et al., 2024):

- *Emergent* (class I) clients are identified with a red tag; these clients have imminent life-threatening conditions.
- Clients who can wait a short time for care (class II) are marked with a yellow tag; these clients have potentially life-threatening *urgent* conditions.
- Nonurgent or "walking wounded" (class III) clients are given a green tag; these clients have *nonurgent* conditions whose care can wait without concern for negative outcomes.
- Clients who are *expected (and allowed) to die or are dead* are issued a black tag (class IV).

Thinking Exercise 4.4 will help you practice what you've learned in this chapter about prioritizing hypotheses. The answer and rationale for the exercise are located at the end of this book.

THINKING EXERCISE 4.4

The nurse is assisting with triaging passengers and crew members who were involved in a small aircraft crash.

History and Physical	Nurses Notes	Orders	Laboratory Results

1730:   Disaster area isolated in desert with large debris field. Six individuals involved in crash with varying degrees of injury:

Client #1: 55-year-old pilot walking around debris field looking dazed and crying. Has superficial laceration on forehead oozing blood slowly. Right wrist feels sore but no other report of pain.

Client #2: 47-year-old adult with large piece of metal through chest and unresponsive; absent pulse and blood pressure.

Client #3: 43-year-old adult with traumatic leg amputation and hemorrhage due to femoral artery laceration; drowsy but oriented and in severe pain.

Client #4: 19-year-old adult with second- and third-degree burns over 45% of body; continuously moaning.

Client #5: 16-year-old adolescent who has small open head wound but is voice responsive; attempting to stand or move to check on other passengers.

Client #6: 13-year-old adolescent who is sitting near Client #1 and screaming to "please wake up"; no apparent injury.

For which of the following clients would the nurse place a red tag for emergent care at the disaster site? **Select all that apply.**
- Client #1
- Client #2
- Client #3
- Client #4
- Client #5
- Client #6

COMMONLY USED MODELS OF PRIORITY SETTING FOR CLIENT CONDITIONS

Many of the prioritization models used today in nursing are aligned with parts of Maslow's hierarchy of needs and the three priority levels. Selecting which model you should use depends on the client situation and the context in which the situation occurs. Six selected priority-setting models appropriate for nursing practice are described in this section. Table 4.3 shows the interrelationships of these models.

Priority Setting Using the ABC Model

The most commonly used priority-setting model in nursing practice is the ABCs, in which A stands for Airway, B stands for Breathing, and C stands for Cardiac/Circulation status. As you probably recognize, client conditions affecting the ABCs are first-level priorities. Assessing for a patent airway is the most important and top priority for any client at any age in any setting. Once an open airway is confirmed or established, evaluating a client's breathing and cardiac/circulation status are the next two essential assessments. To assess the status of the ABCs, ask yourself these questions to help determine the priority of respiratory and cardiovascular client conditions (Thim et al., 2012).

- *Airway: Is the airway patent?* If a client responds in a normal voice, the airway is patent. Signs of a partially obstructed airway include a changed voice, noisy breathing such as stridor or snoring, and labored breathing. With a completely obstructed airway, no respirations are noted. Untreated airway obstruction can rapidly lead to cardiac arrest.
- *Breathing: Is breathing sufficient?* Determine respiratory rate and effort. Inspect movements of the thoracic wall for symmetry and use of secondary respiratory muscles, such as the inter- costals between ribs. Intercostal retraction and labored breathing indicate severe respiratory

TABLE 4.3 Interrelationship of Priority-Setting Models

First-Level Priorities	Second-Level Priorities	Third-Level Priorities
Client conditions that reflect clinical deterioration with critical findings and are life-threatening—these conditions require *emergent or urgent* action	Client conditions that *may lead* to clinical deterioration or become life-threatening without action—these conditions require *prompt* action	Client conditions that are not urgent or acute—actions to meet the client's needs *can wait* without concern for negative outcomes
Selected priority-setting models	**Selected priority-setting models**	**Selected priority-setting models**
• **ABC** (**A**irway, **B**reathing, **C**ardiac function/**C**irculation) • **ABC**VL and **ABC**DE models • **C**URE model (**C**ritical acute client conditions) • Phase 4 mental health crisis	• ABC**VL** model (**V**ital signs and **L**aboratory results) • ABC**DE** model (**D**isability and **E**xposure) • **MAAUAR** model (**M**ental status changes, **A**cute pain, **A**cute impaired urinary elimination, **U**ntreated client conditions, **A**bnormal laboratory and diagnostic test results, **R**isks for safety, skin breakdown, and infection) • C**U**RE model (**U**rgent acute client conditions) • Phase 3 mental health crisis	• **C**U**RE** model (**R**outine maintenance and **E**xtra action or care that is not essential for client safety but important for nurses to provide) • Phases 1 and 2 mental health crisis

distress. Auscultate for normal, adventitious, and abnormal breath sounds; assess peripheral oxygen saturation using pulse oximetry to help determine if breathing is sufficient.

- *Cardiac/Circulation: Are cardiac function and circulation sufficient?* Capillary refill time and heart rate can be assessed in any setting. Skin color changes, diaphoresis, and a decreased level of consciousness are signs of decreased perfusion. Auscultate the heart for normal and abnormal heart tones and measure the client's blood pressure. Hypotension is an important adverse clinical sign. Electrocardiography and continuous cardiac monitoring help determine if cardiac function and circulation are sufficient.

A limitation of using the ABC model is that some clients do not have actual or potential problems related to airway, breathing, and/or cardiac/circulation. For example, a client who has acute kidney impairment or electrolyte imbalance may not have any impairment of the ABCs. This model is also not helpful for clients who are experiencing mental health crises.

CLINICAL JUDGMENT TIP

Remember: The most commonly used priority-setting model in nursing practice is the ABCs, in which A stands for Airway, B stands for Breathing, and C stands for Cardiac/Circulation status. Assessing for a patent airway is the most important and top priority for any client at any age in any setting.

Priority Setting Using the ABCVL Model

After you determine the status of the ABCs, review all of the client's vital signs and laboratory test results. Some clients have abnormal *vital signs* that are not cardiac or circulation related. For example, a very high body temperature (fever) or very low body temperature (hypothermia) can be potentially life-threatening. Clients may also have *laboratory test results* not related to the ABCs, such as abnormal electrolyte values or kidney function studies (e.g., creatinine). These conditions are second-level priorities because they *may lead* to clinical deterioration or become life-threatening without follow-up action. When these conditions are included in a priority-setting approach, the model may be referred to as ABCVL.

Priority Setting Using the ABCDE Model

The Airway, Breathing, Circulation, Disability, Exposure (ABCDE) approach is another expansion of the ABC model. This extended model is a systematic priority-setting approach to the immediate assessment (and treatment) of clients with emergent conditions. Initially developed for medical practice, this model is now the accepted model for clients who require emergent care in any setting (Thim et al., 2012).

Disability (the D in this model) refers to level of consciousness (LOC). Assess the client's LOC using this simple AVPU method (Thim et al., 2012):
- **A**lert
- **V**oice responsive
- **P**ain responsive
- **U**nresponsive

Any client who is not alert or does not respond to a voice command is emergent and a high priority for care.

Exposure (the E in this model) refers to the need to examine the skin for trauma, bleeding, burns, or lesions. These observations often provide clues as to what is causing the client's condition (Thim et al., 2012).

Priority Setting Using the MAAUAR Model

After you determine the status of the ABCs, the MAAUAR model can be used as a second-level priority approach. The MAAUAR model includes:
- **M**ental status changes: A change in mental status, such as acute confusion (delirium), inability to make safe judgments, disorganized thinking, and decreased LOC, could indicate impaired brain function. For example, a client who sustained a traumatic brain injury often experiences a declining LOC due to increased swelling and potential increased intracranial pressure.
- **A**cute pain: Acute pain is a warning sign that the client has an actual health condition that needs to be resolved. For example, severe crushing chest pain may indicate a myocardial infarction.
- **A**cute impaired urinary elimination: Urine output may be inadequate as a result of urinary retention or decreased urine production due to acute kidney injury or chronic kidney disease.
- **U**ntreated client conditions needing immediate attention: Untreated or unaddressed client conditions can lead to medical complications or clinical deterioration. For example, a pregnant client whose gestational hypertension is not managed may develop preeclampsia, a potentially life-threatening condition.
- **A**bnormal laboratory and diagnostic test results: Abnormal laboratory and diagnostic test data can indicate client conditions affecting major organs such as the liver, kidney, and heart.
- **R**isks, including safety, skin breakdown, and infection: Infection (from skin breakdown or other cause) can become systemic and cause sepsis, a potentially life-threatening condition. In older adults, falls can lead to fractures or another major injury.

Priority Setting Using the CURE Model

The CURE model is similar to the client conditions classified by the three priority levels discussed earlier in the chapter, and includes:

C: Critical acute client conditions requiring immediate and emergent action (similar to level-one priorities). Examples of critical acute client conditions include crushing chest pain, labored breathing, and mental health crisis.

U: Urgent acute conditions that place the client at significant safety risk and require prompt action (similar to level-two priorities). Examples of urgent acute client conditions include high fever and decreasing LOC.

R: Routine maintenance care needed for chronic stable client conditions. Examples of chronic client conditions needing routine care include chronic obstructive pulmonary disease and rheumatoid arthritis.

E: Extra action or care that is not essential for client safety but important for nurses to provide (similar to level-three priorities). Examples are emotional support and health teaching regarding stress reduction strategies.

Priority Setting for Mental Health Crises

A mental health crisis may be defined as an acute disruption of psychological homeostasis in which an individual's usual coping mechanisms fail causing distress and functional impairment (Brister, 2018; Wisconsin Technical College System, n.d.). A crisis most often occurs when individuals experience a significant life event, especially if the event was unexpected or unanticipated. Two of the most common types of mental health crises are situational crises (due to personal stressful events) and social crises (due to a natural disaster or man-made event like war).

When a stressful event occurs, individuals progress through one or more crisis phases as outlined in Table 4.4. Be sure to assess clients to determine which phase they are experiencing to help you prioritize their condition.

TABLE 4.4   Crisis Phases (Client Conditions) with Description and Clinical Cues

Crisis Phases (Client Conditions)	Description and Clinical Cues
Phase 1: Normal stress and anxiety	• Exposure to a stressful event causes anxiety as a result of the normal stress response • Individuals are in control of their emotions and behavior
Phase 2: Rising anxiety level	• Use of usual coping mechanisms does not relieve stress • Anxiety levels increase and individuals experience increased discomfort • Feelings of helplessness, confusion, and disorganized thinking may occur • Individuals may experience elevated heart rate and respiration rate
Phase 3: Severe level of stress and anxiety (second-level priority)	• Behaviors become disruptive if new problem-solving methods are unsuccessful • Ability to reason is diminished • Client may yell, swear, become very argumentative, or use threats
Phase 4: Crisis (first-level priority)	• As a result of increased tension that increases to a breaking point level, clients may pace; clench their fists; perspire heavily; and/or demonstrate rapid, shallow, panting breathing • Clients demonstrate emotional lability and possible psychotic thinking • *Clients may be a danger to themselves or others*

Adapted from Wisconsin Technical College System. (n.d.). *3.5. Crisis and crisis intervention.* Retrieved from https://wtcs.pressbooks.pub/nursingmhcc/chapter/3-5-crisis-and-crisis-intervention/

CLINICAL JUDGMENT TIP

Remember: Clients who are in a severe, or Phase 4, mental health crisis need first-level priority care because they could be a danger to themselves or others.

Thinking Exercise 4.5 will help you practice what you've learned in this chapter about prioritizing hypotheses. The answer and rationale for the exercise are located at the end of this book.

THINKING EXERCISE 4.5

The nurse is caring for a 21-year-old client in the college campus health clinic.

History and Physical	Nurses Notes	Orders	Laboratory Results

1805:   Friend brought client to clinic due to superficial bleeding from cutting both arms, including left wrist. Client very distressed, crying, and swearing about the client's ex-partner who "has been having an affair with my best friend for months and I'm the only one who didn't know." Had been in a relationship with ex-partner since high school. Client taking rapid shallow breaths and panting at times. Cut self with razor this afternoon to "help relieve emotional pain." Laughing about plan for revenge by posting mistruths about ex-partner on social media, then screaming and crying about how painful the experience has been. Blames best friend for persuading the client's ex-partner to have an affair. VS: T 98.6°F (37°C); HR 98 beats per minute; RR 36 breaths per minute; BP 118/72 mmHg. Refuses to have pulse oximeter placed. States "that thing can read her thoughts." Medical history includes clinical depression and bulimia nervosa. Attends counseling twice a week using campus resources.

Which of the following conditions is the *priority* for the client at this time? **Select all that apply.**
- Thigh and wrist wounds
- Tachypnea
- Risk for self-harm
- Bulimia nervosa
- Clinical depression
- Psychotic thinking

PRIORITIZING HYPOTHESES TO MAKE SAFE CLINICAL JUDGMENTS

Prioritizing hypotheses requires higher order thinking to determine which client condition is the most important to address or manage in a given clinical situation. A number of factors can affect the ability of nurses to prioritize hypotheses when caring for clients who are experiencing medical complications or clinical deterioration.

Factors that Influence the Ability of Nurses to Prioritize Hypotheses

Nurses make clinical judgments that are affected by many factors in today's multi-layered health care settings. Factors that influence your ability to prioritize hypotheses can be divided into nurse and system or organizational factors.

Nurse Factors

According to a classic study by Hendry and Walker (2004), personal nurse factors that can influence your ability to utilize higher order thinking when prioritizing hypotheses include (Fig. 4.2):
- Level of experience
- Expertise

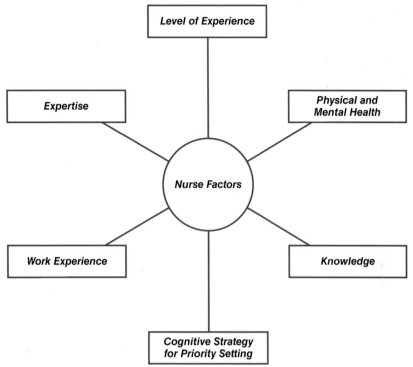

FIG. 4.2 Nurse factors influencing nurses' ability to prioritize hypotheses.

- Work experience
- Cognitive strategy used to set priorities
- Physical and mental health
- Knowledge

Level of experience influences the nurse's ability to accurately prioritize hypotheses. Experienced nurses understand their clients' clinical status by developing relationships and spending time with them. Unlike novice nurses, experienced nurses learn from each client interaction and transfer that learning from one clinical situation to another (Orique et al., 2019).

Experienced nurses often gain *expertise* in a particular specialty such as mental health or obstetrical (OB) nursing. A nurse with clinical expertise in a particular specialty is typically able to prioritize conditions of clients in that specialty. For example, a nurse with expertise in labor and delivery is better able to set priorities for a pregnant client experiencing preeclampsia than a nurse who has had minimal OB experience. An experienced critical care nurse is best able to set priorities for a client admitted to a trauma unit.

Regardless of expertise or level of experience, having *work experience* with clients of any age or condition helps nurses set appropriate priorities for care. For example, a nurse caring for adults should have the ability to apply principles of priority-setting such as the ABCs to care for children who have respiratory distress or compromise.

Cognitive strategies are thought processes used to solve problems. In nursing practice, the priority-setting models described earlier in this chapter are the most common strategies used for prioritizing hypotheses. Selecting which model you should use depends on the client situation and the context in which the situation occurs.

Physical and mental health of nurses can impact the ability to determine client priorities for care. Extreme fatigue and stress can negatively affect the ability to use higher-order thinking to rank client conditions. Fatigue and stress can also promote the development of cognitive biases.

System Factors

System factors can influence your ability to utilize higher order thinking when prioritizing hypotheses. Probably the most important factor is nurses' increasing *workloads* in most health care organizations. Taking care of multiple clients decreases the time you can spend with each client, making it difficult to rank client conditions and potentially jeopardizing client safety. Having inadequate work time leads to missed nursing care which is defined as care left undone, rationed care, or unfinished care (Scott et al., 2018). When care (including assessment) is missed, clinical cues to help generate hypotheses may not be assessed or recognized, which negatively impacts how nurses generate and prioritize client conditions.

Nurses can become overwhelmed with the large amount of complex information received from multiple individuals, technological devices, and clinical systems, causing cognitive overload. As a result of this heavy *workload*, nurses are often overworked, have insufficient time to prioritize client conditions, experience *cognitive overload*, and have minimal opportunity for self-care. As discussed in Chapter 2, cognitive overload can impact the nurse's mental, emotional, and physical well-being, which leads to errors in prioritizing hypotheses. In addition to human resources, nurses need adequate equipment, technology, organizational support, and facility policies and procedures to facilitate their ability to prioritize care when making clinical decisions (Alaseeri et al., 2021).

Role of Nursing Knowledge

Nursing knowledge and knowledge from other disciplines are needed to apply higher order thinking when prioritizing hypotheses. Clinical reasoning requires that nurses integrate that knowledge to make safe, appropriate clinical judgments. A strong knowledge base helps you make (but does not guarantee) sound judgments in each client situation.

In addition to the foundational knowledge outlined in Table 3.3 and in Chapter 3, specific knowledge needed by nurses to accurately prioritize hypotheses includes the following.

Knowledge of Environment where Client Care Is provided

The environment, including the client's home, is part of the context of any clinical situation. Resources, standards of practice, and reimbursement for client care vary depending on the health care environment. For example, a large home health agency in the United States found that the standard practice of scheduling their first home visit after hospital discharge of clients on Medicare was not adequate. As a result, the home care nurses created a decision-making tool to determine which clients were the priority to visit after hospital discharge (Box 4.3).

BOX 4.3   Evidence-Based Practice

How can Clients be Better Prioritized When Transitioned from the Hospital to Home?
Topaz, M., Trifilio, M., Maloney, D., Bar-Bachar, O., & Bowles, K. (2018). Improving patient prioritization during hospital-homecare transition: A pilot study of a clinical-decision support tool. *Research in Nursing and Health Care, 41*(5), 440–447.

Medicare requires that all clients receive a first home visit within 48 hours after the referral is received at the homecare agency. However, for high-risk clients, waiting 48 hours to be assessed by homecare nurses may not be safe practice. In some cases, clients are readmitted to the hospital before the first visit occurs. In this pilot study the researchers tested an innovative clinical-decision support tool called PREVENT to identify clients who may need to be prioritized for earlier homecare visits. During the experimental study phase, high-risk clients received their first homecare nursing visit about one-half a day sooner than required by Medicare (1.8 vs. 2.2 days). As a result, rehospitalizations of newly discharged clients decreased by 9.4%.

Knowledge of Priority-Setting Approaches and Models, Including When and How They Should Be Used

When caring for clients in any environment, you need to determine which priority-setting model is most appropriate and how to use it. For example, the ABC model is appropriate for almost any client in any setting, but determining priorities based on mental crisis phases is only appropriate for clients experiencing a crisis.

Knowledge of Pathophysiology of Client Conditions

Knowledge of the pathophysiology of medical conditions, including common clinical cues, helps you to determine client priorities. The Thinking Exercises in this chapter require you to apply your knowledge of pathophysiology and appropriate priority-setting models to select the correct responses.

CLINICAL JUDGMENT TIP

Remember. Keep in mind that a strong knowledge base of pathophysiology, health care environments, and priority-setting models helps you make (but does not guarantee) sound judgments in each client situation.

Strategies for How to Prioritize Hypotheses

This chapter has explored the process for prioritizing hypotheses and the factors that affect your ability as a nurse to use this clinical judgment cognitive skill. This discussion highlights the strategies you should use to accurately prioritize hypotheses as a client's condition changes or deteriorates (Box 4.4).

BOX 4.4   Strategies for Prioritizing Hypotheses

- Review the list of client conditions (hypotheses) in the clinical situation that were generated from analysis of relevant clinical cues.
- Evaluate hypotheses based on urgency and risk to client safety using the three levels of priority.
- Use an appropriate model of priority setting to rank client hypotheses.
- Remember to consider nurse and system factors that can impact priority setting in the clinical situation.

Review the List of Client Conditions

As defined in Chapter 3, a client condition is a medical disorder or complication that may place the client at risk for clinical deterioration. The first strategy for prioritizing hypotheses is to review the list of client conditions (hypotheses) that were generated from analyzing relevant clinical cues in a given clinical situation. These conditions may be actual or potential and acute or chronic. For example, consider this list of conditions for an 80-year-old alert and oriented client who was living independently in a senior citizen housing apartment before arriving at the ED via 911 for severe crushing chest pain, shortness of breath, and palpitations:

- Severe crushing chest pain with shortness of breath
- New-onset atrial fibrillation with palpitations
- Rheumatoid arthritis and osteoarthritis

- Peripheral vascular disease
- Diabetes mellitus type 2
- Peripheral neuropathy
- Mild depressive disorder
- Transient ischemic attack last year
- Potential for acute ischemic stroke
- Hypertension
- New-onset hyperkalemia
- Sinusitis

Evaluate Hypotheses Based on Urgency and Risk

After reviewing the list of client conditions in a given clinical situation, determine which conditions are acute and which are chronic. The acute conditions for this 80-year-old client include chest pain, atrial fibrillation with palpitations, hyperkalemia, and sinusitis. Then evaluate each acute condition for its urgency and risk to client safety. Ask yourself these questions:

- Which client condition(s) is/are first-level priority?
- Which client condition(s) is/are life-threatening or could become life-threatening, if any?
- Which client condition(s) is/are emergent or urgent, if any?
- Which client condition is the most important to manage first and why?
- What is most important to the client or client's family/guardian?

For the older adult in the example, the first-level priority condition is severe crushing chest pain with shortness of breath because this is a life-threatening clinical situation. This emergent condition, therefore, should be managed first. New-onset atrial fibrillation and hyperkalemia are very serious and *could* become life-threatening; these conditions are urgent and second-level priorities. Sinusitis is nonurgent or a third-level priority condition for care.

Use an Appropriate Model of Priority Setting

Depending on the health care environment and the client, select an appropriate priority-setting model to prioritize hypotheses by ranking client conditions. Using the ABC model, the client is alert and oriented, indicating that the client can communicate and has a patent airway. The client's top priority needs relate to Breathing and Cardiac/Circulation status. Severe crushing chest pain with shortness of breath is a critical finding using the CURE model, again indicating the need for emergent action.

Remember to Consider Nurse and System Factors

As discussed earlier in this chapter, acuity and severity of client conditions are foundational for prioritization. Because acute client conditions can be severe and potentially life-threatening, prioritize these conditions higher than chronic stable conditions. Remember that priority setting should be guided by ethical principles, including justice, fairness, and equity. Although studies show that older adult care is not considered a high priority for bedside nurses, all clients deserve equitable care in any health care environment.

Keep in mind that your ability to prioritize is impacted by your knowledge, experience, health, and cognitive strategy (priority-setting approach). System factors include adequate staffing, equipment, technology, organizational support, and facility policies and procedures.

Thinking Exercise 4.6 will help you practice what you've learned in this chapter about prioritizing hypotheses. The answer and rationale for the exercise are located at the end of this book.

THINKING EXERCISE 4.6

The nurse in NICU is caring for a preterm newborn delivered via C-section at 34 weeks.

History and Physical	Nurses Notes	Orders	Laboratory Results

1525: Preterm neonate admitted to the NICU postdelivery. Apgar score at 1 minute was 5; improved to 9 at five minutes. Baby has noisy breathing, nasal flaring, and periodic intercostal retractions. Slightly bluish-tinged feet and fingers. Moving all extremities and voided ×1. Weak cry at times. Weight 4 lb (1.8 kg); length 16 in (40.6 cm). VS: T 97°F (36.1°C); HR 148 beats per minute; RR 72 breaths per minute; BP 86/52 mmHg; SpO$_2$ 82% on RA. Consult for respiratory therapist and registered dietitian nutritionist.

Complete the following sentence by selecting from the list of word choices below. The nurse determines that the *priority* for the client at this time is managing the neonate's **[Word Choice]**.

Word Choices	
Cyanosis	Respiratory distress
Nutritional status	Hypothermia

END-OF-CHAPTER THINKING EXERCISES

Additional End-of-Chapter Thinking Exercises will help you apply what you've learned in this chapter about prioritizing hypotheses. The answers and rationales for these exercises are located at the end of this chapter.

END-OF-CHAPTER THINKING EXERCISE 4.1

The nurse is caring for a 33-year-old client in the Emergency Department.

History and Physical	Nurses Notes	Orders	Laboratory Results

1410: Admitted to the ED with report of sharp left lower chest pain of 10/10. Client is dyspneic, restless, and has dry, hacking cough. Moaning and grimacing when coughing. Family states client's medical history includes cystic fibrosis, early-stage chronic kidney disease, chronic alcoholism, and major depressive disorder. Drowsy and oriented ×2 (person and place). Bluish-tinged finger tips and lips. Breath sounds markedly diminished in lower left lung; no adventitious or abnormal sounds in right lung. Jugular venous distention present. S$_1$ and S$_2$ present. Bowel sounds present ×4. Able to move all extremities. VS: 100.4°F (38°C); HR 112 beats per minute; RR 30 breaths per minute; BP 90/42 mmHg; SpO$_2$ 89% on O$_2$ at 4 L per minute.

1425: Transported for chest X-ray and possible chest CT scan.

Complete the following sentence by selecting from the list of word choices below. The nurse determines that the *priority* condition for this client is to manage **[Word Choice]**.

Word Choices	
Fever	Tachycardia
Hypotension	Hypoxia

⚡ **END-OF-CHAPTER THINKING EXERCISE 4.2**

The nurse is caring for a 17-year-old client in acute rehabilitation following a cervical spinal cord injury.

History and Physical	Nurses Notes	Orders	Laboratory Results

2035: Client called for nurse with report of new-onset severe, throbbing headache which is worsening to 10/10 acute pain. Alert and oriented ×4. Face flushed and sweaty; client very anxious and restless. Breath sounds clear throughout lung fields. States that abdomen feels distended. Hypoactive bowel sounds ×4. Raised head of bed; urinary catheter draining large amount of clear medium-yellow urine. VS: T 98.6°F (37°C); HR: 56 beats per minute and regular; RR: 24 breaths per minute; BP 206/128 mmHg; SpO$_2$ 97% on RA.

Select **1** client condition that the nurse needs to manage **first** for this client.
- Acute headache pain
- Tachypnea
- Bradycardia
- Anxiety
- Elevated blood pressure
- Abdominal distention

⚡ **END-OF-CHAPTER THINKING EXERCISE 4.3**

The nurse is caring for a 55-year-old client in an acute care unit.

History and Physical	Nurses Notes	Orders	Laboratory Results

1055: Admitted last evening for lower GI bleed. Labs this morning show marked decrease in RBCs, Hgb, and Hct since admission. Two units of packed red blood cells (PRBCs) ordered to begin as soon as possible.

1145: First unit PRBCs started; VS frequently monitored per protocol (VS flowsheet).

1300: Reports feeling "itchy" and having chills at times. Headache started about 10 minutes ago with dyspnea. No urticaria at this time. VS: T 101°F (38.3°C); HR 94 beats per minute; RR 26 breaths per minute; 90/56 mmHg; SpO$_2$ 94% on RA.

History and Physical	Vital Signs				Laboratory Results
Time	Temperature	HR	RR	BP	SpO$_2$ (RA)
1140	98.4°F (36.9°C)	78	18	116/72	98%
1200	98.4°F (36.9°C)	80	20	114/70	98%
1215	99.2°F (37.3°C)	86	20	106/68	97%
1230	100°F (37.8°C)	88	22	102/60	96%
1300	101°F (38.3°C)	94	26	90/56	94%

Complete the following sentence by selecting from the list of word choices below. The *priority* for this client is to manage the client's **[Word Choice]**.

Word Choices
Allergy
Headache pain
Transfusion reaction

END-OF-CHAPTER THINKING EXERCISE 4.4

The nurse is caring for a 60-year-old client admitted yesterday to a long-term care facility for rehabilitation after bilateral total knee arthroplasties.

History and Physical	Nurses Notes	Orders	Laboratory Results

0300:   Client scheduled to have PT and OT after breakfast in the morning. History of osteoarthritis, obesity, hypertension, and ulcerative colitis. Nursing assistant supervised client ×2 tonight to ambulate independently with walker to bathroom. Had diarrhea ×2 in past hour with abdominal cramping. Client now back in bed. Given acetaminophen for postsurgical pain of 4/10.

0350:   Called nurse with new-onset chest pain of 8/10 and shortness of breath. States feeling like "my heart is racing and beating out of my chest." Diaphoretic and lightheaded. Alert and oriented ×4 but very anxious about new signs and symptoms. Continues to have intermittent abdominal cramping. VS: 98.6°F (37°C); HR 102 beats per minute, irregular; RR 24 breaths per minute; BP 92/46 mmHg; SpO$_2$ 90% on RA.

Which of the following client conditions is the **priority** for client care at this time? **Select all that apply.**
- Diarrhea
- Abdominal cramping
- Impaired gas exchange
- Postoperative knee pain
- Anxiety

Answers and Rationales for Thinking Exercises

CHAPTER THINKING EXERCISES

THINKING EXERCISE 4.1

Answer:
The client's *priority* for care at this time is to manage the client's **chest pain**.

Rationale: This client presented to the ED with chest pain, nausea and vomiting, shortness of breath, left jaw pain, tachycardia, and lightheadedness. The client also has an elevated heart and respiratory rate. All of these findings are serious and acute because they occurred abruptly. Chest pain could indicate a possible myocardial infarction which could be life-threatening and is an emergent condition. Nausea and vomiting, an elevated blood pressure of 168/100, and hyperglycemia are not life-threatening unless they worsen. Therefore, the correct response to this Thinking Exercise for the client's priority for care is chest pain.

THINKING EXERCISE 4.2

Answer:
The *priority* for nursing care is to manage the client's **internal bleeding** as evidenced by **tachycardia** and **hypotension**.

Rationale: The priority for client care is the condition that is life-threatening and would require emergent action. The client has abdominal trauma caused by multiple gunshot wounds (GSWs) which show old blood on the dressings. One bullet penetrated through the client's entire body causing perforation of the right ileum with probable active bleed. Although the bleeding is not visible, the client has clinical cues that support the client's loss of blood and resulting hypovolemia—tachycardia and hypotension. Severe pain and anxiety are not first-level priorities because they are not life-threatening. The leg fracture requires prompt action but is not life-threatening at this time.

THINKING EXERCISE 4.3

Answer:
Select **2 priority** client conditions that require nursing action.
- ○ Urinary tract infection
- **X** Dehydration
- ○ Malnutrition
- **X** Hyperglycemia
- ○ Osteoarthritis pain
- ○ Fluid overload
- ○ Decreased peristalsis

Rationale: The client is an older adult who has a history of diabetes mellitus (DM) type 2 and other chronic disorders. The client's FSBG level has been high for at least 3 days (metformin dose was increased) indicating hyperglycemia. The client lost 9 lb (4.1 kg) in the last 3 days, has dry skin, and dry mucous membranes. These findings plus an elevated body temperature, hypotension, and tachycardia indicate dehydration. An elevated blood urea nitrogen (BUN) supports this client condition. BUN increases due to kidney impairment, dehydration, or increased metabolic activity. The client's kidneys are not impaired as evidenced by a normal serum creatinine. The client is likely experiencing hyperglycemic hyperosmolar syndrome as a diabetic emergency which can occur in clients who have DM type 2. This complication requires emergent action to prevent hypovolemic shock and possible death. Fluid has shifted from the client's vascular system into the interstitial tissues (dependent edema) most likely due to low protein from a poor appetite. Therefore, the client does not have fluid overload. While the client's nutritional status is somewhat compromised as evidenced by a low prealbumin, malnutrition is not the client's priority condition. A prealbumin below 10 mg/dL (100 mg/L) is indicative of malnutrition. While the client may have decreased GI motility (decreased peristalsis) as demonstrated by hypoactive bowel sounds, this condition is not a priority problem requiring emergent action. The client does not have a urinary tract infection because the urine culture is not positive. Osteoarthritis is a chronic health problem which causes persistent pain. This condition is not life threatening and, therefore, not urgent or emergent.

THINKING EXERCISE 4.4

Answer:

For which of the following clients would the nurse place a red tag for emergent care at the disaster site? **Select all that apply.**

- ○ Client #1
- ○ Client #2
- **X** Client #3
- **X** Client #4
- ○ Client #5
- ○ Client #6

Rationale: In a mass casualty event, clients are given colored tags to identify their priority for care status. Clients requiring emergent care are assigned red tags; these clients have imminent life-threatening conditions. Client #3 is experiencing hemorrhage due to a traumatic leg amputation. Hemorrhage is a life-threatening condition and therefore the client would need a red tag. Client #4 has massive second and third degree burns over almost half of the body and requires a red tag. Burns involving more than 30% of the body are life-threatening and require emergent care due to the likelihood of severe fluid and electrolyte imbalances and infection. Client #2 would be evaluated as needing a black tag because the client is impaled with large metal debris and has no vital signs. Clients #1 and #6 would likely need a green tag because their care can wait without concern for negative outcomes. Client #5 likely would receive a yellow tag due to a decreased level of consciousness (voice responsive) with a small open head wound and the client trying to help others.

THINKING EXERCISE 4.5

Answer:

Which of the following conditions is the **priority** for the client at this time? **Select all that apply.**

- ○ Thigh and wrist wounds
- ○ Tachypnea
- **X** Risk for self-harm
- ○ Bulimia nervosa
- ○ Clinical depression
- ○ Psychotic thinking

Rationale: The client is experiencing Phase 4 of a mental health crisis after discovering that the client's partner was having an affair. As a result of this significant and stressful life event, the client cut one wrist and both thighs. This need for self-harm is the priority client condition. However, the wounds are superficial and oozing blood. The bleeding is not an arterial bleed or hemorrhage and the wounds are therefore not the priority for care. Tachypnea and panting can occur in a crisis but are not life-threatening at this time. The client has psychotic thinking as evidenced by the delusion that the pulse oximeter could read the client's thoughts. However, this thinking is not life-threatening at this time. The client's history of depression and bulimia nervosa is also not life-threatening and therefore not the priority for the client's care.

> ## THINKING EXERCISE 4.6
>
> **Answer**:
> The nurse determines that the ***priority*** for the client at this time is managing the neonate's **respiratory distress**.
>
> **Rationale**: A 34-week preterm neonate's lungs are not completely developed and contain excess fluid. Therefore, the newborn usually has signs and symptoms of respiratory compromise, such as nasal flaring, intercostal retractions, tachypnea (more than 60 breaths per minute), and an SpO_2 less than 90%. The digital cyanosis is expected for a newly delivered neonate. A temperature of less than 97°F (36.1°C) would be considered hypothermia. The neonate will be placed in a heated isolette to control body temperature. The nutritional status is not known at this time but the neonate will likely be fed through an NGT because the baby likely does not have the strength to drink an adequate amount of formula from a bottle or breast. Using the ABC model for priority setting, respiratory distress is the priority for the client at this time.

END-OF-CHAPTER THINKING EXERCISES

> ## END-OF-CHAPTER THINKING EXERCISE 4.1
>
> **Answer**:
> The nurse determines that the ***priority*** condition for this client is to manage **hypoxia**.
>
> **Rationale**: The client has localized chest pain, diminished breath sounds, dyspnea, and tachypnea (increased respiratory rate). These clinical cues suggest that the client has respiratory distress. The client's SpO_2 is below normal, indicating that the client's respiratory distress is causing hypoxia. The client's drowsiness (decreased LOC) and disorientation may be due to a lack of oxygen to the client's brain. Using the ABC priority model, hypoxia as a result of respiratory distress (breathing) is potentially life-threatening and is, therefore, the priority client condition. Hypotension, fever, and tachycardia could become life-threatening if any of these vital signs worsen. However, if the cause of the client's hypoxia is identified and managed, these vital signs would likely return to a usual level for the client. Given the client's history of cystic fibrosis and the clinical cues in the situation, the client likely has a left pneumothorax.

> ## END-OF-CHAPTER THINKING EXERCISE 4.2
>
> **Answer:**
> Select **1** client condition that the nurse needs to manage **first** for this client.
> - Acute headache pain
> - Tachypnea
> - Bradycardia
> - Anxiety
> - **X** Elevated blood pressure
> - Abdominal distention
>
> **Rationale:** The client likely has autonomic dysreflexia (AD), which is an abnormal involuntary autonomic nervous system response to stimulation in clients who experience a high-level spinal cord injury. This sympathetic response causes severe, life-threatening hypertension, reflex bradycardia, severe headache, diaphoresis above the level of injury, and facial and neck flushing. The nurse would raise the head of the bed (which was done) and check for causes of the AD, such as a kinked urinary catheter, which was also done. The nurse would then contact the health care provider or Rapid Response Team to manage the elevated blood pressure to prevent the client from having a stroke, a potentially life-threatening complication. When the severe hypertension is treated, the client's headache and other signs and symptoms should also improve, especially if the cause of the AD is resolved.

⚡ END-OF-CHAPTER THINKING EXERCISE 4.3

Answer:
The *priority* for this client is to manage the client's **transfusion reaction**.

Rationale: The client developed clinical cues consistent with a reaction to receiving the first blood transfusion, including fever, chills, itching, headache, and hypotension. Itching may indicate an allergic response to the transfusion, but the new-onset signs and symptoms indicate that the client has a different type of reaction. The transfusion would need to be stopped to prevent life-threatening problems such as respiratory distress. The client's headache is not life-threatening.

⚡ END-OF-CHAPTER THINKING EXERCISE 4.4

Answer:
Which of the following client conditions is the **priority** for client care at this time? **Select all that apply.**
- ○ Diarrhea
- ○ Abdominal cramping
- **X** Impaired gas exchange
- ○ Postoperative knee pain
- ○ Anxiety

Rationale: The client's surgery increases the risk for postoperative pulmonary complications, especially venous thromboembolism (deep vein thrombosis/pulmonary embolus). This complication is very common after lower extremity total joint arthroplasty. The client's clinical cues, including new-onset chest pain, shortness of breath, palpitations, diaphoresis, tachycardia, hypotension, and anxiety, are consistent with pulmonary embolism. This condition impairs gas exchange and is potentially life-threatening. The client's abdominal cramping and diarrhea are consistent with the chronic condition in the client history of ulcerative colitis. The client's knee pain is not severe and is being managed with acetaminophen. Therefore, it is not the priority client condition.

REFERENCES

Alaseeri, R., Rajab, A., & Banakhar, M. (2021). Do personal differences and organizational factors influence nurses' decision making? A qualitative study. *Nursing Reports, 11*(3), 714–727.

American Association of Colleges of Nursing. (2021). *The Essentials: Core competencies for professional nursing education.* Author.

Brister, T. (2018). *Navigating a mental health crisis: A NAMI resource guide for those experiencing a mental health emergency.* National Alliance on Mental Illness. https://www.nami.org/Support-Education/Publications-Reports/Guides/Navigating-a-Mental-Health-Crisis/Navigating-A-Mental-Health-Crisis?utm_source=website&utm_medium=cta&utm_campaign=crisisguide.

*Hendry, C., & Walker, C. (2004). Priority setting in clinical nursing practice: Literature review. *Journal of Advanced Nursing, 47*(4), 427–436.

Hossain, F., & Clatty, A. (2021). Self-care strategies in response to nurses' moral injury during COVID-19 pandemic. *Nursing Ethics, 28*(1), 23–32.

Ignatavicius, D. D., Rebar, C. R., & Heimgartner, N. M. (2024). *Medical-surgical nursing: Concepts for clinical judgment and collaborative care* (11th ed.). Elsevier.

Ingram, A., & Powell, J. (2018). *Patient acuity tool on a medical-surgical unit.* American Nurse. https://www.myamericannurse.com/patient-acuity-medical-surgical-unit/.

*Maslow, A. H. (1943). *A theory of human motivation.* Martino Publishing, Mansfield Centre. [reprinted 2013].

Orique, S. B., Despins, L., Wakefield, B. J., Erdelez, S., & Vogelsmeier, A. (2019). Perception of clinical deterioration cues among medical-surgical nurses. *Journal of Advanced Nursing, 75*(11), 2627–2637.

Potter, P. A., Perry, A. G., Stockert, P. A., & Hall, A. M. (2023). *Fundamentals of Nursing* (11th ed.). Elsevier.

Scott, P. A., Harvey, C., & Papastavrou, E. (2018). Resource allocation and rationing in nursing care: A discussion paper. *Nursing Ethics, 26*(5). https://doi.org/10.1177/0969733018759831

Suhonen, R., Stolt, M., Habermann, M., Hjaltadottir, I., Vryonides, S., et al. (2018). Ethical elements in priority setting in nursing care: A scoping review. *International Journal of Nursing Studies, 88,* 25–42.

*Thim, T., Krarup, N. H. V., Grove, E. L., Rohde, C. V., & Lofgren, B. (2012). Initial assessment and treatment with the airway, breathing, circulation, disability, and exposure (ABCDE) approach. *International Journal of General Medicine, 5,* 117–121.

Topaz, M., Trifilio, M., Maloney, D., Bar-Bachar, O., & Bowles, K. (2018). Improving patient prioritization during hospital-homecare transition: A pilot study of a clinical-decision support tool. *Research in Nursing and Health Care, 41*(5), 440–447.

Wisconsin Technical College System. (n.d.). *3.5 Crisis and crisis intervention.* https://wtcs.pressbooks. pub/nursingmhcc/chapter/3-5-crisis-and-crisis-intervention/.

*Denotes classic reference

How to Generate Solutions

LEARNING OUTCOMES

1. Describe the types of thinking needed to generate solutions to improve clinical outcomes.
2. Differentiate common solutions to consider and potential solutions to avoid to generate solutions that address priorities for providing client care.
3. Identify solutions that are client centered, focused on determinants of health, and evidence-based.
4. Identify nurse and system factors that can affect the ability to generate solutions.
5. Discuss strategies for generating solutions to make safe, appropriate clinical judgments.

KEY TERMS

Analytical thinking: Using a logical process to eliminate ideas to narrow possibilities to the most likely specific solution/s.

Clinical outcomes: Measurable changes in clinical cues, health, ability to function, quality of life, or survival that result from client care.

Creative thinking: Thinking in nursing care that is used to generate solutions for client care that are simple, useful, effective, cost-effective, and safe.

Cultural competency: The ability to engage effectively with people across cultures.

Cultural humility: Dynamic process using self-reflection to acknowledge one's own biases to provide client-centered, individualized care that honors the beliefs, customs, and values of the individual.

Evidence-based practice (EBP): The deliberate use of current best evidence when planning and providing nursing care for clients.

Implicit bias: Automatic attitudes, behaviors, and actions (either positive or negative) which involve unintentional assumptions about individuals or groups that occur involuntarily without a person's awareness; also called unconscious or hidden bias.

Innovative thinking: The ability to generate new and original ideas.

Negligence: Failing to provide the expected standard of care for the client's condition that results in injury or harm to the client. This can also include: failure to assess, insufficient monitoring, failure to communicate important information, failure to notify provider, and failure to follow protocols.

Nonmaleficence: The avoidance or minimization of harm to the client.

Risk reduction: Preventing and reducing threats and harm to clients, staff, and the organization.

Scientific method: The process of scientific thinking that also reflects the National Council of State Boards of Nursing Clinical Judgment Measurement Model (NCSBN CJMM) and includes: defining the problem (recognizing cues), making observations (recognizing cues), forming a hypothesis (analyzing and prioritizing hypotheses), creating a prediction and testing the prediction (generating solutions and taking action), and drawing conclusions (evaluating outcomes).

Scientific thinking: Knowledge seeking that is intentional and uses inductive and deductive reasoning to make observations, see patterns, and make inferences.

Social determinants of health: Environmental conditions that affect a wide range of health, functioning, and quality-of-life outcomes and risks.

Solution generation: Identifying expected outcomes and using hypotheses to determine interventions to move the client toward the desired outcomes.

GENERATING SOLUTIONS

As described in Chapter 1, solution generation is an essential cognitive clinical judgment skill that requires multiple types of thinking and must consider multiple aspects of client needs and priorities. Effective use of this cognitive skill results in solutions (actions) that are safe, effective, client-centered, cost-effective, and promote progress toward desired client outcomes. This chapter explores how to generate solutions that result in safe, appropriate clinical judgments.

Definitions

Nurses generate solutions with the goal of improving client clinical outcomes. Clinical outcomes are measurable changes in clinical cues, health, ability to function, quality of life, or survival that result from client care. Clinical outcomes do not always result in "curing" or resolving a client condition. For example, a decrease in blood pressure for a client who has hypertension is an improvement in the clinical situation. Through use of blood pressure readings, it is possible to show measurable progress (or deterioration of) the client's condition or clinical outcome.

The highest priority for all nurses is to prevent harm from occurring to clients while in our care. Risk reduction is the process of anticipating events or situations that might result in harm to clients or even staff. When generating solutions, consider risk-reducing solutions that prevent potential harm. It is much easier to prevent events from occurring than to treat consequences after they occur. Evidence-based practice is the deliberate use of current best evidence when planning and providing nursing care for clients. Be sure to consult the evidence to generate solutions that are most effective, current, and effectively reduce the risk for deterioration of the client's condition.

Solutions should be client-centered (also referred to as person-centered). To generate client-centered solutions nurses need to demonstrate cultural competence and humility and be aware of the potential for implicit bias. Implicit bias includes automatic attitudes, behaviors, and actions (either positive or negative) and involves unintentional assumptions about individuals or groups that occur involuntarily without a person's awareness (Narayan, 2019; Sabin, 2022; Thirsk et al., 2022). Cultural competency is the ability to engage effectively with people across cultures. Cultural humility is broader and is defined as a "dynamic and lifelong process focusing on self-reflection and personal critique, acknowledging one's own biases" (Khan, 2021). Cultural humility is more client-centered in that it recognizes the uniqueness of individuals who might share a cultural background and requires that the provider seek to understand the person as an individual with individual preferences all the while incorporating cultural competency during the process. Cultural humility involves creating a professional relationship with the client that intends to honor their beliefs, values, and customs (Stubb, 2020). With education, self-reflection, self-awareness, and cultural humility, you can be proactive in removing implicit bias from clinical judgment decisions and solutions generated. See Chapter 3 for more discussion on implicit bias.

Types of Thinking Needed to Generate Solutions

The one constant in health care is change. Nurses encounter new clients each day, with varying clinical situations which require continual use of multiple types of thinking to generate solutions to best meet the needs of each individual client. Chapter 1 discusses different types of thinking that nurses use. These methods of thinking are especially important when generating solutions to meet clinical outcomes. Thinking like a nurse develops over time and is enhanced through knowledge gained and nursing care experiences. The ability to generate solutions also improves over time as the nurse encounters multiple client situations and is able to gain experience with generating solutions for a variety of client care issues.

Creative and innovative thinking are both needed for generating solutions. Creative thinking in nursing care is used to generate solutions for client care that are simple, useful, effective, cost-effective, and safe (Cheraghi et al., 2021). Creative thinking is needed to develop solutions that are also client centered. For example, a nurse may need to promote a nutritious diet for a client who has specific religious dietary preferences. The solutions to promote the client's nutrition should incorporate the client's dietary preferences. Innovative thinking involves generating solutions that are new and being implemented for the first time. One solution can be as simple as attempting to decrease agitation in a client by calling the family and/or by playing the client's favorite soft music. Or innovation can be as complex as becoming a nurse entrepreneur who designs a new product or technology that improves client care or client care processes. For example, the crash cart was developed by nurse Anita Dorr who wanted to improve the response time and interventions for clients experiencing cardiac or emergency events (University of Illinois-Chicago, n.d.). Not only did Dorr create a new product, she also created an improved process for response to emergency situations in the health care environment.

Analytical thinking (as defined in Chapter 1) is using a logical process to eliminate ideas to narrow possibilities to the most likely specific solution/s. When a nurse faces a client care challenge and begins to generate solutions, it is important to determine which solutions might be *most* effective in helping the client achieve the desired outcomes. Additionally, the nurse must use analytical thinking to determine which solutions may be harmful to the client or contraindicated for a particular client situation. These types of solutions need to be avoided. Using creative and innovative thinking, the nurse may develop 10 solutions that may improve the client's outcomes in a given clinical situation. Then, using analytical thinking, the nurse may determine that two of the solutions being considered are contraindicated for the client. The nurse may also decide that five of the solutions would be helpful but would not address the client's condition quickly enough, which could result in deterioration of the client's condition. The nurse then concludes that the remaining three solutions would be most effective and client-centered, and would meet the outcomes in the most efficient way.

Generating solutions also requires scientific thinking. Scientific thinking utilizes an established process for thinking called the scientific method, which also aligns with Layer 3 of the NCSBN Clinical Judgment Measurement Model (CJMM). This intentional process is described as:

- Defining the problem (recognizing cues)
- Making observations (recognizing cues)

- Forming a hypothesis (analyzing and prioritizing hypotheses)
- Creating a prediction and testing the prediction (generating solutions and taking action)
- Drawing conclusions (evaluating outcomes)

Fig. 5.1 shows the relationship between the Scientific Method of Thinking with the NCSBN clinical judgment cognitive skills. Scientific thinking is described as knowledge seeking that is intentional and uses inductive and deductive reasoning to make observations, see patterns, and make inferences. Nurses generate solutions based on the client data obtained and patterns determined from clustering data. These data are used to make inferences about what client outcomes are desired. Nurses examine the research and other sources of evidence to find solutions recommended for the particular client condition. Scientific thinking can help you generate solutions based on client data and evidence-based standards of care to address the priority actual or potential client condition.

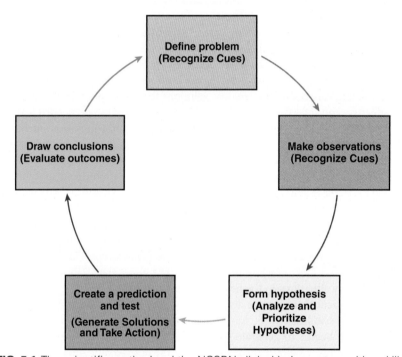

FIG. 5.1 The scientific method and the NCSBN clinical judgment cognitive skills.

Chapter 1 also discusses the importance of thinking ahead, thinking in action, and thinking back. These types of thinking are relevant when generating solutions to help clients achieve desired outcomes. The nurse must anticipate reducing client risk at all times to keep clients safe and promote optimal outcomes. In other words, nurses need to think ahead to generate solutions that can prevent client conditions or prevent worsening of the client's conditions. Nurses are thinking ahead and reducing risk when solutions are generated to prevent a venous thromboembolism (VTE) in a postsurgical client by promoting ambulation, applying sequential compression devices (SCDs), and administering prescribed, prophylactic low-dose anticoagulant medication.

Chapter 3 discusses the use of predictive models (PPMP) and predictive thinking to identify potential client conditions that help direct thinking in generating solutions. Use of predictive models and predictive thinking are evidence-based methods for thinking ahead to generate effective solutions that predict and manage risk. Thinking in action is required when nurses are in a crisis or emergency situation and solutions must be generated quickly to make clinical judgments that improve client outcomes. Thinking back requires nurses to look back on solutions generated and evaluate their effectiveness to determine if these are solutions that would be helpful in future client situations.

CLINICAL JUDGMENT TIP

Remember: Experienced nurses must incorporate creative, innovative, analytical, and scientific thinking when generating solutions to achieve desired client outcomes. These types of thinking anticipate what the client may be experiencing now (thinking in action) or in the future (thinking ahead). The nurse must use analytical thinking when reflecting on solutions generated (thinking back) to determine if these solutions would be appropriate for future client situations.

Thinking Exercise 5.1 will help you practice what you've learned in this chapter about generating solutions. The answer and rationale for the exercise are located at the end of this book.

THINKING EXERCISE 5.1

The nurse is caring for an 85-year-old client in a long-term care unit.

History and Physical	Nurses Notes	Orders	Laboratory Results

1500:   Client found on floor in room. Walker beside client, tipped over on floor. States "I don't know what happened. My hip hurts and I can't get up." In supine position, left leg externally rotated. Client rubbing left hip area. Skin tear noted left elbow, 1.5 in (4 cm) × 2.3 in (6 cm), 0.2 in (0.5 cm) deep with moderate amount of bleeding. Client alert and oriented × 4, PERRLA. Hand grips 3+ and equal in strength. Able to move three extremities with full ROM; denies pain. Unable to move left leg. Respirations nonlabored and without distress; lung sounds clear throughout. VS: T 98.6°F (37°C); HR 100 beats per minute and regular; RR 20 breaths per minute; B/P 150/88 mmHg; SpO$_2$ 95% on RA. Pain in left hip reported at 10/10.

Select **2** appropriate actions that the nurse could take at this time.
- Notify the health care provider.
- Assist client to stand to determine if weight bearing is tolerable.
- Monitor client overnight and report findings.
- Position the client on the affected side.
- Monitor for signs of shock.
- Provide oral fluids.

PROCESS OF GENERATING SOLUTIONS

The process of generating solutions begins with a review of priorities for an individual client's care. These priorities are developed with input from the client and client's guardian/family and are used to develop desired or expected clinical outcomes. As mentioned in Chapter 4, developing clinical outcomes should involve the client and client's guardian/family so that the solutions are in alignment with the client's priorities for health.

Review of Priorities for Client Care

The process of generating solutions should be focused on client priority conditions. Chapter 4 discusses how to prioritize hypotheses and rank them according to the level of priority. Models for priority setting including the ABCDE and the MAAUAR models are discussed in Chapter 4 as evidence-based methods that can be used to help the nurse set priorities for client conditions and rank them based on urgency, likelihood, risk, client preference, or time. The nurse then uses these client priority conditions to determine what outcomes are most desired. Chapter 4 provides a detailed discussion on setting priorities for care based on client condition.

Developing Clinical Outcomes to Address Priorities for Client Care

Clinical outcomes are used to measure how effective the care was. Client priorities are determined, clinical outcomes are defined, and solutions can then be generated to positively address the client priorities. All care provided needs to focus on achieving desired clinical outcomes and be driven by the best available evidence. Outcomes may be developed for client conditions or for interventions. Client condition-focused outcomes describe what will be observed in the client when the condition no longer exists or is managed at an acceptable level. Intervention-focused outcomes describe the achievement of the desired response to the intervention. Fig. 5.2 provides examples of client condition and intervention-focused clinical outcomes.

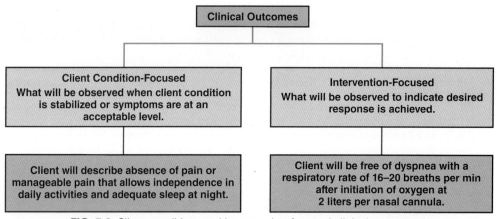

FIG. 5.2 Client condition- and intervention-focused clinical outcomes.

Outcomes should be developed in partnership with the client and/or family. The CMS (Center for Medicare and Medicaid Services) focuses on continual improvement and measurement of care to ensure quality of care. One high-priority requirement for the CMS is that facilities must assess and report data on patient-reported outcomes (PROs). PROs are the status of a person's health condition or health behavior that comes directly from the client without interpretation of anyone else such as a nurse or a physician (CMS, 2022). The key areas that must be assessed include health-related quality of life, symptoms and symptom burden, and health behaviors. All of these outcomes are assessed through data gathered directly from the client through self-report. PROs are measured using indicators called patient-related outcome measures (PROMs). PROMs demonstrate whether a nurse or clinician is actually improving care from the client's perspective. Reporting PROMs creates a feedback loop to measure quality of care that is actually determined by the client (Hostetter & Klein, n.d.). Client-centered care is a priority for the CMS to ensure clients and families are engaged as partners in their care; this process results in higher quality care and better outcomes for clients.

Effectively developed outcomes are not only condition/intervention based and client centered, but are also specific, measurable, achievable, agreed upon by all parties, realistic, and time bound (SMART). To be specific, the client condition, for example, should be clearly identified and not blended with other client conditions. Each outcome is focused on one client priority. Outcomes need to be measurable so that progress or the lack of progress can be determined. Outcomes should be agreed to (client centered), achievable, and realistic. For example, it may not be reasonable for someone with persistent pain to be pain free. A more achievable and realistic goal would be for the client to have decreased pain to an acceptable level for the client. Finally, outcomes should be time-bound and identify a time frame for achieving desired results.

CLINICAL JUDGMENT TIP

Remember. Clients and families must be included when developing clinical outcomes. Outcomes should include measurement by both the nurse and by the client's report of achievement or lack of achievement of the desired outcome, if possible.

Determining Solutions for Attaining Clinical Outcomes

Once the desired outcomes are determined, the nurse next generates solutions that could be helpful in attaining these outcomes. As discussed earlier, you would want to involve the client and family when selecting interventions, if possible. When a client is in rapid decline or the client is experiencing an urgent or emergent health condition, the nurse needs to intervene quickly and specifically. If the client is experiencing an urgent health condition or rapid decline in condition, the client might not be able to make health decisions. In urgent situations, there may not be time to consult the family prior to taking action. But whenever possible, it is best to include the client in the decision-making for their care as long as it does not delay care that would cause a worsening of the condition.

Two types of solutions are considered to meet clinical outcomes: independent and collaborative. An independent solution allows the nurse to perform the solution without assistance or "permission" from other members of the health care team. A collaborative solution involves team members across health care professions and may require instruction or "permission" from a physician or other health care prescriber. These categories of interventions are discussed further in Chapter 6.

Solutions should be generated that manage both client conditions and contributing factors. The nurse should give high priority to designing interventions aimed at managing the factors that are contributing to the condition. For example, if a client is experiencing dehydration due to excessive vomiting, administer antiemetic medication in addition to replacing fluids with IV therapy. This will help reduce the cause of the fluid volume loss.

Assessments and monitoring parameters are also appropriate solutions (nursing actions) needed to make safe clinical judgments. Solutions should be selected that define parameters for monitoring the client so that the nurse can determine whether progress or lack of progress toward the outcome is being made. Determine how each outcome will be assessed. For example, for a client who has dehydration, assessments should include daily weights so that progress toward achieving adequate fluid balance can be monitored closely. Recall that weight is the most reliable indicator of fluid balance.

Assessments should also be performed to measure the achievement of outcomes for potential client conditions that could possibly occur. For example, a client with a severe traumatic brain injury (TBI) needs to have vital signs, pupil size/shape and reaction, and level of consciousness frequently monitored to assess for potential increased intracranial pressure. The data obtained from frequent monitoring can indicate whether new or different actions may be needed. If the assessment data for the client with a TBI show a widening pulse pressure, bradycardia, and restlessness, the nurse would then suspect increased intracranial pressure and generate different solutions, including notifying the primary care provider and initiating a rapid response. In addition to direct client assessment, the nurse should identify laboratory and diagnostic imaging results that are important to monitor for achieving desired outcomes. For a client with dehydration, for instance, it would be important for the nurse to monitor serum electrolytes and urine specific gravity to determine progress or lack of progress toward achieving fluid and electrolyte balance. Solutions must be consistent with facility or agency policy, and the most recent and best evidence. Each facility has slight variations of established solutions for selected client care situations. For example, a hospital may have pregenerated actions for hospitalized clients who are oversedated due to opioid therapy. These interventions must be grounded in the most current evidence. Health care is rapidly changing, and new and better ways of improving client outcomes are emerging daily. The nurse continually reviews new evidence and practice guidelines as they become available. It is important for nurses to participate in the development of facility policies and procedures supported by any new or relevant evidence-based practice updates.

Common Solutions to Consider

Many common solutions to consider are generated from the nurse's prior experience, knowledge, review of facility policy, and current evidence. Even novice nurses start at the bedside with a background of basic nursing solutions that can be considered. Begin by selecting assessment and monitoring parameters that would be key in determining improvement or lack of improvement in client conditions. These assessment solutions should include assessments of vital signs, relevant body systems (e.g., use of assessment techniques to monitor heart sounds, lung sounds, appearance of skin), subjective data from client and/or family, and monitoring of trends in laboratory or other diagnostic tests.

Solutions must first and foremost protect client safety and anticipate safety risks. These solutions must be implemented early when risks for injury are present. For example, clients at risk for falls should be placed on fall risk protocols. Clients at risk for venous thromboembolism (VTE) need sequential compression devices. Clients who state that they might be a danger to themselves due to mental health disorders should be placed on suicide precautions and receive frequent and/or constant monitoring. Clients at high risk for seizures should have oxygen and suction available at the bedside.

Nurses need to protect the safety of the client and the safety of the family, staff, and other clients on the unit. Solutions should promote safety in the health care or home care environment. For example, for clients with infectious disease, the nurse needs to generate solutions for infection transmission prevention, such as isolation protocols, personal protective equipment (PPE), and hand hygiene so that others are protected from the spread of any infection or infectious disease. Additionally, nurses may need to generate solutions that protect vulnerable clients from infection, such as those that are immunocompromised. In this case, the nurse might need to place the client in a negative airflow room or ask that all visitors wear protective isolation PPE when visiting. For the immunocompromised client, the nurse needs to monitor the client for early signs of infection by assessing vital signs (especially temperature), performing routine physical assessment, and monitoring lab results (especially WBC count in the CBC).

Other common solutions include providing basic care and comfort, many of which nurses learn about in their early Foundations courses. Solutions can be generated for proper positioning of the client for increased comfort and respiratory function with a schedule for repositioning to promote skin health and improved circulation. Elevation of injured, swollen limbs on pillows can assist to ease the client's discomfort and tissue swelling. Administration of breathing treatments and oxygen therapy can ease the discomfort related to dyspnea. In the hectic environment of modern health care, it is sometimes easy to overlook basic comfort and care solutions that can improve client conditions in any setting. Table 5.1 describes some common solutions for a wide range of physiologic client conditions that may be or become urgent or emergent and require making clinical judgments.

TABLE 5.1   Common Solutions for Urgent or Emergent Physiologic Client Conditions

Actual or Potential Client Conditions	Common Solutions
Dehydration/fluid loss	• Administer IV fluids • Encourage oral fluids as tolerated • Monitor intake and output • Monitor vital signs frequently (especially pulse and blood pressure) • Monitor urine specific gravity • Monitor weight
Difficulty breathing/ respiratory distress	• Elevate head of bed • Administer oxygen therapy • Monitor vital signs frequently including SpO_2 • Assess lung sounds frequently; observe for signs of distress or retractions • Consult respiratory therapy • Monitor diagnostic test results such as chest X-rays for concerns (e.g., pneumonia) • Monitor lab results for complete blood count (CBC) for concerns (e.g., infection)
Impaired mobility	• Encourage cough and use of incentive spirometer to prevent respiratory complications • Assess client's strength in each extremity each shift • Assess casted extremity every hour for capillary refill, skin color, skin temperature, movement, and pain • Administer pain medications as needed,. • Monitor urinary output, bladder/abdominal distention, intake and output, bowel movement pattern, and vital signs in client with spinal cord injury • Apply sequential compression devices to prevent venous thromboembolism in the client with limited mobility and high risk (e.g., client with fracture)
Impaired skin integrity/risk for impairment	• Reposition client routinely in bed to promote circulation and prevent skin breakdown • Assess skin every shift and with repositioning for signs of nonblanching erythema in light-skinned persons; palpate skin to assess for changes in temperature, pain, discomfort, and induration (thickening, hardening of tissue) for dark-skinned persons • Maintain toileting schedule to prevent incontinence • Provide perineal cleansing and use protective barrier cream when incontinent to protect skin from moisture • Monitor medical equipment device sites frequently for potential skin breakdown and apply protective devices when available (i.e., for nasal cannulas, assess ears, and provide protective padding) • Consult wound therapy nurse
Ineffective perfusion	• Monitor vital signs frequently, especially pulse, blood pressure, and SpO_2 • Assess cardiac sounds for adventitious sounds, rate, and rhythm • Assess peripheral pulses frequently with bilateral comparison • Assess neurological status frequently (i.e., level of consciousness, orientation ×4, grip and extremity strength, pupil size and reactivity, behavior) • Initiate and monitor continuous telemetry • Monitor diagnostic tests including EKG, echocardiogram, and stress testing • Monitor cardiac enzymes lab results • Monitor CBC for Hgb and Hct

Continued

TABLE 5.1   Common Solutions for Urgent or Emergent Physiologic Client Conditions—cont'd

Actual or Potential Client Conditions	Common Solutions
Infection/risk for infection	• Offer oral fluids frequently to maintain hydration • Administer IV fluids • Administer antibiotics • Monitor vital signs often, especially temperature and pulse • Monitor CBC results • Monitor diagnostic results • Monitor wounds for signs of infection (i.e., redness, discharge, swelling) • Implement isolation protocols for infectious disease • Wear required PPE (personal protective equipment; i.e., gloves, mask, gown) when caring for clients with infectious disease • Maintain aseptic technique during procedures • Monitor urinary output for amount, color, clarity, and particulates
Neurologic impairment	• Monitor vital signs frequently, especially pulse, blood pressure, respirations, and SpO$_2$ • Assess neurological status frequently (i.e., level of consciousness, orientation ×4, grip and extremity strength, pupil size and reactivity, behavior) • Reorient client to person, place, time, and situation frequently • Monitor intracranial pressure • Initiate seizure precautions (i.e., oxygen and suction at the bedside) • Administer antiseizure medication as needed for seizures • Restrict fluid intake if indicated
Pain	• Assess client frequently through self-report on pain scale to determine level of pain • Use pediatric faces pain scale to assess pain in children 3–8 years old • Monitor behavior and facial expressions for clients under 3 and for those who are unable to verbalize level of pain • Provide parenteral or oral pain medication as needed • Apply ice packs as needed • Elevate affected extremity using pillows • Maintain a quiet and dark environment to promote sleep

CLINICAL JUDGMENT TIP

Remember: Oftentimes, the solutions that can provide improvement in client conditions are ones that nurses learn early in their nursing education, such as those listed in Table 5.1.

Nurses need to use their knowledge, experience, and review of the evidence to generate solutions for a wide range of specific client conditions. Examples of condition-specific solutions include:

• Cardiac monitoring for a client with a dysrhythmia.
• Monitoring vital signs and surgical site for a postoperative client.
• Regular blood glucose monitoring for a client with diabetes mellitus; interventions for extreme high or low glucose levels.

The nurse must be familiar with each specific client condition, determine effective solutions for improving the condition, determine what to avoid that might make the condition worse, and determine what to monitor to fully understand the status of the condition.

In addition to creating solutions, nurses need to use their knowledge and expertise to *anticipate* solutions as well. Anticipating solutions that might be needed for the client can aid in saving time and improve client outcomes. For example, if a client presents to the emergency department with severe vomiting and diarrhea lasting several days, anticipate solutions for probable dehydration. Recall that older adults and infants can become dehydrated within hours rather than days. The nurse knows to obtain laboratory results as soon as possible because electrolytes might be depleted and replacements may be needed. The nurse is not diagnosing the client with dehydration or electrolyte imbalance, but is anticipating possible client conditions. Once prescribed, the nurse can initiate IV access, initiate appropriate fluids and electrolytes, and continue to monitor electrolyte lab values.

The nurse can also generate possible collaborative solutions which involve the health care team. Examples of collaborative solutions include:

- The nurse, the medical provider, and the respiratory therapist creating solutions for maintaining appropriate gas exchange levels and a patent airway with oxygen therapy, breathing treatments, and medications for a client with respiratory distress. In some cases, continuous positive airway pressure (CPAP) therapy or mechanical ventilation may be required.
- The nurse, the radiology staff member, and the medical provider creating solutions for diagnostic examination and stabilization of a fracture, and pain management for a client presenting with a suspected fracture of the tibia.
- The nurse, the medical provider, and the respiratory therapist responding to a client in cardiac arrest by implementing emergency protocols and resuscitation measures.

Not only do condition-specific solutions need to be designed, but preventive solutions may need to be generated. For example, common preventive solutions for the postsurgical client may include monitoring lung sounds, temperature, and oxygen saturation for any potential indication of respiratory complications so that early interventions can be implemented. Encouraging coughing and deep breathing or the use of an incentive spirometer regularly can also prevent respiratory complications from occurring in the postsurgical client. These types of nursing actions prevent complications and client deterioration.

Potential Solutions to Avoid

When determining potential solutions to achieve targeted outcomes, nurses must select solutions that will not result in worsening of the client condition or cause an additional condition. An important ethical priority for nurses is nonmaleficence, which means do no harm. A client with chronic heart failure who becomes dehydrated and needs IV fluids may need to receive these fluids at a slower rate than other clients because the heart failure can be worsened by a rapid fluid infusion. This example also stresses the importance of creating solutions that are individualized for each client. There is no "one size fits all" when generating solutions.

Another important priority when generating solutions is to avoid negligence. Negligence is failing to notice or use reasonable care which results in harm for the client. In the client with heart failure, it would be negligent for the nurse to fail to frequently assess the client for worsening heart failure including monitoring vital signs, auscultating heart and lung sounds, documenting daily weights, monitoring edema, and monitoring the client for dyspnea. If new-onset edema and/or dyspnea occur and the nurse did not notice these changes for some time, the nurse would demonstrate a failure to notice.

Negligence also can occur if the nurse deviates from the traditional standard of care for a particular condition. For instance, a traditional standard of care is to determine blood return prior to administering an IV medication. Administering IV medication through an IV catheter without obtaining blood return for confirmation of placement would be deviating from the standard of care and could result in client harm. Any solutions generated should prevent failure to notice potential client conditions and should follow the traditional, but evidence-based, standard of care. Box 5.1 provides an example of the importance of selecting parameters to monitor, determining solutions that anticipate potential client conditions, and the consequences for failure to create solutions for assessment that result in harm to the client.

BOX 5.1   Evidence-Based Practice

Prevalence and Analysis of Medical Device-Related Pressure Injuries: Results from the International Pressure Ulcer Prevalence Survey

Kayser, S. A., VanGilder, C. A., Ayello, E. A., & Lachenbruch, C. (2018). Prevalence and analysis of medical device-related pressure injuries: Results from the International Pressure Ulcer Prevalence Survey. *Advances in Skin & Wound Care, 31*(6), 276–285. https://doi.org/10.1097/01.ASW.0000532475.11971.aa

The authors used data from a large, international survey of acute care hospitals, long-term acute care hospitals, long-term care facilities, and rehabilitation facilities to determine the prevalence and analysis of medical device-related pressure injuries (MDR-PIs). This survey included reports from over 1000 facilities who surveyed over 100,000 clients per year. The list of devices that the survey responder had available to choose from included: endotracheal tubes, nasogastric tubes, casts/splints, nasal oxygen devices (nose and ears), CPAP/BiPAP masks, halos, sequential compression devices, and cervical collars.

Results of the study showed that:
- Most MDR PIs were facility acquired (75%)
- Most were located on the ears (29%) and the feet (12%)
- Most were associated with nasal oxygen tubes (32%), cast/splints (12%), and CPAP/BiPAP masks (9%)

This study also concluded that MDR PIs form faster than non-MDR PIs. Timely proactive assessment and prevention are critical. Assessment and prevention are especially important for those with oxygen tubing/masks and casts/splints as these are the most common types of devices for causing MDR PIs.

The most important method for determining solutions to avoid is to review and be fully informed of the most recent evidence and care standards. Review of the evidence can help nurses understand the prevalence of a condition and the likelihood of occurrence to generate solutions to prevent potential harm. For example, when caring for clients who have oxygen therapy or a cast or splint, the nurse would incorporate solutions such as:
- Circulation assessments on the casted extremity
- Application of protective devices or padding such as padded wraps to protect ears from a nasal cannula
- Monitoring for reports of pain or sudden increase in pain, especially burning pain (indicates pressure)
- Promoting nutrition and hydration
- Reporting and documenting any skin changes immediately.

CLINICAL JUDGMENT TIP

Remember: Nurses must not only know which solutions to select but also know which solutions to avoid that might make the client condition worsen. There is no "one size fits all" when determining solutions. Be sure to individualize solutions to meet specific client outcomes.

Thinking Exercise 5.2 will help you practice what you've learned in this chapter about generating solutions. The answer and rationale for the exercise are located at the end of this book.

THINKING EXERCISE 5.2

The nurse is caring for a 12-year-old client in the Emergency Department.

History and Physical	Nurses Notes	Orders	Laboratory Results

1300: Client presents to ED accompanied by parent. Client states "It's really hard for me to catch my breath. My asthma is flared up. I haven't taken my allergy medicine this week. I always have allergies in the spring." Parent states client has had asthma since early childhood which is usually well-controlled by daily cetirizine and occasional use of albuterol rescue inhaler. States that the family has had financial challenges recently and has had difficulty affording medications. Client well-nourished and well-groomed. Client dyspneic with labored breathing; audible wheezes noted. Skin warm, moist; fingernail beds have bluish tinge with sluggish capillary return >3 seconds, and dark skin tones appear ash gray. Wheezes on expiration throughout all lung fields. Chest symmetric; no injuries noted; no retractions noted. Apical pulse steady and regular. VS: T 98.6° F (37° C); HR 110 beats per minute; RR 30 breaths per minute; B/P 125/78 mmHg; SpO$_2$ 92% on RA. Pain reported at 0/10. Wt. 110 lbs. (50 kg).

Determine whether the following potential orders are anticipated or not anticipated by the nurse at this time.

Potential Orders	Anticipated	Not Anticipated
Start oxygen at 2 L via nasal cannula		
Initiate IV access		
Give oral prednisone now for airway inflammation		
Administer acetaminophen orally now for discomfort		
Administer albuterol via nebulizer now and repeat every 20 minutes for 1 hour if needed		
Obtain chest X-ray		
Consult social services		
Teach family how to develop asthma action plan		

GENERATING CLIENT-CENTERED SOLUTIONS

Developing effective solutions that adequately address client health care priorities requires the nurse to create solutions that are client centered, address relevant determinants of health, and based on sound and current evidence.

Considering Client and Family Preferences

Client and family preferences must be considered when generating outcomes. The statement "nothing about me without me" is an important reminder for nurses working to create clinical outcomes and interventions that are focused on client and family preferences. Generating outcomes that incorporate client and family preferences actually results in higher quality care. Research has shown that when clients are engaged in their care, it can lead to measurable improvements in safety and quality of care.

While client preferences should always be considered, nurses must provide care that is family-centered as well. The Institute for Client and Family-Centered Care (IPFCC, n.d.) defines client- and family-centered care as an approach to the planning, delivery, and evaluation of health care grounded in a collaboration between health care providers, clients, and their families. Clients define who their family is and determine how family members may participate in care and decision-making. For example, a client may be a fall risk due to acute confusion while hospitalized. Providing education to a client's family on preventing falls such as calling for assistance with ambulating the client or reminding the client to avoid climbing out of bed involves family members in promoting the overall safety of the client.

Nurses must generate solutions for the most important client priorities. Yet these priorities may or may not be in alignment with what the client or family determines to be a priority. For example, a client may present to the Emergency Department experiencing a hypertensive crisis but may have concerns about being admitted to the hospital. The client may be the sole care provider for an aging parent with dementia. The client's priority is the need to ensure that someone is caring for their parent while the nurse is focused on addressing the hypertensive crisis to prevent a stroke. Both priorities are important but have differing impacts. If the client's parent is unsupervised, the impact will be immediate in that the parent will not be supervised and may become injured. The client may feel that the risk for stroke is not as immediate a need as seeing that the parent is supervised and cared for. The nurse may need to consult a social worker to obtain resources for providing for the immediate care of the parent so that the client can receive prompt medical care for the hypertensive crisis.

CLINICAL JUDGMENT TIP

Remember. When generating solutions, it is important to communicate and collaborate with your client and their family to determine what the client perceives as the priority condition for their care.

Identifying Social Determinants of Health

The Healthy People 2030 initiative defines social determinants of health as the environmental conditions that affect a wide range of health, functioning, and quality-of-life outcomes and risks. People are impacted by environmental conditions where they are born, live, work, play, and age (US Department of Health and Human Services [USDHHS], 2020). The social determinants of health consist of five major categories outlined in Table 5.2.

According to the World Health Organization (WHO), achieving quality outcomes requires taking a broad view of client circumstances and paying attention to social determinants of health. Social determinants of health can have an even larger impact on clients' health conditions than coexisting health conditions or lifestyle choices (WHO, n.d.). Generating client-centered solutions requires that the nurse consider the context of where the client lives, works, and plays to generate solutions that have the greatest positive impact on health. The nurse must examine how the client may be impacted by their race and/or ethnicity, income, education, housing, environment and whether or not the client experiences a violent or unsafe environment. Then the nurse must generate solutions that attempt to positively impact the client's environment that may ultimately positively impact their health (Table 5.3).

TABLE 5.2 Social Determinants of Health Categories and Impact

Categories	Impact on Health
Economic stability	• People with steady income and employment are more likely to be healthy • People with disabilities, injuries, or chronic conditions may be limited in their ability to work. This results in being unable to afford healthy food, health care, adequate housing, and education
Education access and quality	• People with higher levels of education tend to be healthier and live longer • Children who routinely experience forms of social discrimination, who are from low-income families, attend poorly performing schools, or have disabilities are more likely to struggle with school and less likely to obtain higher education. This means these children are less likely to get safe, high-paying jobs and are at increased risk for chronic health conditions
Health care access and quality	• Many people in the United States have limited access to health care or insurance Those without insurance are less likely to have a primary care provider and may not be able to afford health care services • Some people live too far away from health providers to receive routine services. Lack of access to health care or resources negatively impacts health and increases risk for negative health outcomes due to unmanaged chronic conditions or failure to identify and treat critical health conditions in a timely manner
Neighborhood and built environment	• Neighborhoods and residences have a major impact on health and include the places where people live, work, learn, and play • People who live in neighborhoods with high rates of violence, or unsafe air or water are at increased risk for illness or injury • Racial/ethnic minorities and those who are of low income are more likely to live in places with these health risks • Workplaces can also contribute to increased health risks such as places with loud noise or repetitive motion
Social and community context	• Relationships with family, friends, coworkers, and community members can impact health and well-being • Unsafe neighborhoods, discrimination, or lack of financial stability can have a negative impact on safety and health

US Department of Health and Human Services. (2020). *Healthy people 2030*. Retrieved from https://health.gov/healthype ople/priority-areas/social-determinants-health

TABLE 5.3 Examples of Solutions to Positively Impact Social Determinants of Health

Category	Potential Solutions
Economic stability	• Assist those with disabilities or limited income in linking with available community health or economic resources • Provide information on community resources such as meals for the elderly, veterans' benefits for those eligible, government assistance such as TANF (Temporary Assistance for Needy Families), homeless shelter information, food assistance such as SNAP (Supplemental Nutrition Assistance) or WIC food support for families

Continued

TABLE 5.3   Examples of Solutions to Positively Impact Social Determinants of Health—cont'd

Category	Potential Solutions
Education access and quality	• Refer families to area educational resources • Identify relevant assessments needed for children for potential health care risks that can impact educational performance including, but not limited to: lead levels, hemoglobin, vision screenings, hearing screenings, dental screenings, nutrition screenings, immunization status, signs of being bullied, or signs of abuse • Generate solutions to address any concerns such as resources for eyeglasses, low-cost dental care, free lead/hemoglobin screenings, or referrals to social services for any signs of abuse • Refer families to organizations like Head Start, which provides high-quality early childhood education and nutrition at no cost for those who meet income guidelines
Health care access and quality	• Educate clients and families on any available resources for insurance such as HealthCare.gov or Medicare where low-income persons can qualify for insurance benefits • Refer clients to any area health care resources that are offered at no or reduced cost such as area health departments • Assist clients with applying for prescription discounts • Educate clients on how to obtain or navigate services such as telehealth. Telehealth may help those in rural locations access needed providers
Neighborhood and built environment	• Conduct environmental assessments for the client • Obtain subjective data regarding the conditions where the client works, lives, and plays • Provide area resources for any concerns identified
Social and community context	• Obtain subjective data on the relationships and social support that the client may have • Identify any risk factors to health or safety such as lack of nearby family or friends, social isolation, lack of financial stability, or unsafe neighborhood • Connect client with area groups for support • Provide resources on any free or low-cost mental health services • Provide assistance with obtaining low-cost prescription medication for chronic conditions such as depression or anxiety • Refer clients to support groups such as Alcoholics Anonymous for addiction support at no cost or area NAMI (National Alliance on Mental Illness) organizations which provide support groups and free online resources for mental health conditions

US Department of Health and Human Services. (2020). *Healthy people 2030*. Retrieved from https://health.gov/healthype ople/priority-areas/social-determinants-health

Children are at greatest risk for negative health risks due to an unsafe or unhealthy environment. The early impact of unsafe environments can cause lifelong health conditions. For example, children exposed to the following common environmental conditions may suffer the following negative health impacts:
• Chronic exposure to secondhand smoke can result in developing asthma and chronic upper respiratory conditions.
• Exposure to lead in paint or water can result in development of permanent developmental delays.

- Living within 0.2–0.3 miles of a major highway can result in a high risk for developing asthma, asthma attacks, impaired lung function, premature death, and death from cardiovascular diseases (American Lung Association, 2022).

It is especially important when determining solutions for children that the nurse carefully consider the environment where the child lives, attends school, and plays when generating solutions to improve client conditions.

Additionally, the nurse needs to work within the environment of the client and family preferences and available resources when generating solutions. Any solution should be practical and easily implemented. Solutions should be developed in cooperation with the client and family and demonstrate not only cultural competence, but cultural humility as well. Clients and families must be provided support so any solution can be sustainable. Nurses are important sources of information to families about available resources that can help with health care needs.

CLINICAL JUDGMENT TIP

Remember: When generating solutions, it is important to consider any social determinants of health that may be negatively impacting a client's condition and generate solutions that demonstrate cultural humility.

Using Best Current Evidence

Generating solutions must be focused on desired clinical outcomes and be driven by the best available evidence. To give care that is based on the best available evidence, you might question current practices. Health care has shifted from practices based in tradition ("We do it this way because that's the way it's always been done") to evidence-based practice (EBP) ("We do it this way because the most current research shows we achieve the best outcomes when we do it this way"). Through experience, nurses generate a wealth of knowledge about various solutions. But nurses should also be continually questioning if this is the best way of providing care. Is there new research that provides solutions that are better at improving client outcomes? Do the policies and procedures at my organization reflect current practice? Question what you do, why you do it, what your clients' experiences are, and how client care and nurses' jobs can be improved.

Nurses and nursing students need to understand their responsibilities related to EBP. Box 5.2 describes these responsibilities for participating in research and EBP.

Nurses may be overwhelmed with knowing how to review research articles or understanding which articles are high-quality studies. Box 5.3 summarizes some tips for effectively reviewing the literature to determine effective solutions for client care.

Incorporating best current evidence is particularly useful when caring for clients who experience clinical deterioration or medical complications. As defined in Chapter 2, clinical deterioration is a dynamic state in which the client progresses to a worsened clinical condition increasing morbidity, body organ dysfunction, prolonged hospital or agency length of stay, and/or death. Box 5.4 summarizes best practice standards developed by nurses to improve clinical outcomes for clients experiencing clinical deterioration.

Clinical practice guidelines (CPGs) are an excellent source of well-established standards for providing care that reflects the most current evidence. CPGs can be found on infection control practices, infectious disease management, and vaccination recommendations on the Center for Disease Control and Prevention (CDC) Website. Clinical practice guidelines are also specific to specialty areas through national nursing organizations such as the Emergency Nurses Association

---

BOX 5.2   Responsibilities for EBP for Nurses and Nursing Students

*Reflect on your daily practices, thinking analytically about the clients and situations you encounter—seek out evidence of findings that might improve nursing care. For example, if you're caring for someone with leg edema after heart surgery, you should be asking, "I wonder if there are any new studies explaining why this happens and what can be done about it?"

   *Know the rationale behind your actions and the level of evidence that supports it. For example, are the rationales behind your actions supported by clinical practice guidelines? A textbook? Your instructor or another clinical expert?

   *Raise questions that might prompt researchers to formulate questions to guide a study. For example, you could ask your manager, "Because we seem to be having an increase in infections again, should we revisit our hand-sanitizing procedures?"

   *Help researchers collect data. If you're asked to complete a questionnaire or to document specific data for research purposes, it is your professional responsibility to do so, diligently and accurately, as long as it doesn't interfere with nursing care.

   *Acquire and share knowledge related to research and EBP. We must constantly ask ourselves questions like, "Am I making time to become familiar with EBP related to the clinical situations in which I'm involved?" and "Do I interact with others (peers, educators) to learn more about research and EBP?"

BOX 5.3   How to Review Research Articles

*Ask your leaders and educators for help with finding and using research articles. However, be sure that you understand the following basic facts about choosing useful research articles and information:

a. Choose refereed or peer-reviewed publications (articles are reviewed for accuracy).

b. Read the abstract first. If it seems applicable, skip to the end of the article and review the summary/conclusion and discussion. If the article seems relevant, read the entire study.

c. Always ask, "How valid and reliable are these results?" "How sure am I that this study was conducted in a way that I can trust that the results are accurate?" and "How does this information compare with what other publications say about this topic?" Consider whether there is vested interest by the researchers or publishers. Think independently, and ask questions. How will this article inform your future practice when making clinical judgments?

d. Larger studies such as systematic or scoping reviews, meta-analysis, and clinical practice guidelines provide the strongest evidence; expert opinion is the lowest level of evidence. Generally, the larger the study sample size, the more reliable the results.

e. Look for evidence from the last 5 years for the most recent results.

f. Look for EBP alerts or newsletters which are often provided which provide the latest updates in client care trends and solutions.

(ENA) or the American Association of Critical Care Nurses (AACCN). Additionally, web-based subscriptions such as UptoDate can provide recommendations for care practices.

CLINICAL JUDGMENT TIP

Remember. To generate solutions to make safe and appropriate clinical judgments, nurses need to utilize evidence that supports the most effective practice standards.

   Thinking Exercise 5.3 will help you practice what you've learned in this chapter about generating solutions. The answer and rationale for the exercise are located at the end of this book.

BOX 5.4 Evidence-Based Practice

What are the Best Practices for Managing Clients Experiencing Clinical Deterioration?

Park, S., & Kellerman, T. (2022). *Acute nursing care: Recognition and response to deteriorating clients.* Retrieved March 19, 2023 from https://anmj.org.au/acute-nursing-care-recognition-and-response-to-deteriorating-clients/.

Failing to notice and respond to client deterioration is widely known to be associated with increased risk of an adverse event and increased risk of mortality. The solutions developed below provide nurses with an easy-to-remember ABCDEF guideline for noticing and intervening early when client deterioration occurs.

A. **Call for help**
   - Using the emergency call button or alerting a Rapid Response; do not leave the client unattended
B. **Collect more information/data**
   - History of present complaint, recently administered medications, recent vital signs and observations, fluid balance, nurse's and provider's notes
   - Look for trends
C. **Position the client**
   - Depending on how the client presents will depend on the position that you put your client in. You will generally be guided by your client's vital signs and symptoms and overall condition.
     - Unconscious/breathing: recovery position (as long as no spinal injury is suspected)
     - Hypotensive: flat with legs elevated
     - Not breathing: Fowler's or semi-Fowler's
     - Acute coronary syndrome: semi-upright
D. **Oxygen therapy**
   - Oxygen may be need for rapid deterioration, use high-flow oxygen therapy only for short term
   - For stroke and cardiac episodes without evidence of shock, guide oxygen therapy with pulse oximetry readings. Do not exceed an oxygen saturation of >92% on room air
   - If the client does not appear critically ill, titrate the flow of oxygen to maintain saturations of >94%
   - For clients with chronic obstructive pulmonary disease (COPD), monitor for signs of respiratory distress and make sure that this is communicated when the Rapid Response Team (RRT) arrives
E. **Prepare equipment for the RRT teams**
   - Think about what the medical teams may need, e.g., IV access, fluids, blood tests, medications, etc. and prepare accordingly
F. **Handover to applicable health care professionals**
   - When the medical teams arrive to help, it is extremely important that a concise, accurate, and efficient handoff is given using an evidence-based method of handoff communication such as ISBAR

Nurses are the most likely health care professionals to positively impact the outcomes for the clinically deteriorating client by promptly generating solutions. Being familiar with evidence-based guidelines aids the nurse in being prepared.

⚡ THINKING EXERCISE 5.3

The nurse is caring for a 68-year-old client who is being admitted to the acute care telemetry unit.

History and Physical	Nurses Notes	Orders	Laboratory Results

0900:   Client states "I feel really weak. I've had an ulcer I think for some time now; I usually use antacids for the pain. Yesterday the pain became worse and I even got sick. It looked really weird like coffee grounds. Today it feels like my heart is skipping a beat." Client grimacing and holding hand over upper abdomen while providing recent history. BS present × 4 quadrants, abdomen soft, flat. Reports tenderness to light palpation LUQ. S_1 and S_2 present; tachycardia and irregular HR. Client has history of atrial fibrillation managed with daily apixaban and metoprolol. Twelve-lead ECG shows atrial fibrillation with HR 108. Radial and pedal pulses 2+ and slightly irregular bilateral. States last bowel movement yesterday morning; normal in consistency. Client voided 100 mL clear, straw-colored urine without pain or difficulty. Respirations unlabored; lungs clear to auscultation over all fields. Alert and oriented ×4. Moves all extremities with full ROM. Walks unassisted; gait steady. VS: T 98.6°F (37°C); HR 108 beats per minute; RR 16 breaths per minute; B/P 90/54 mmHg; SpO_2 95% on RA. PERRLA. Pain reported at 6/10 on a 0–10 pain scale and indicates pain is in upper left quadrant.

Continued

> ↘ **THINKING EXERCISE 5.3—cont'd**
>
> For each body system below, specify the potential nursing actions that would be appropriate for the care of the client. Each body system may support more than one nursing action.

Body Systems	Potential Nursing Actions
Gastrointestinal	☐ Place nasogastric tube to low continuous suction
	☐ Monitor results of esophagogastroduodenoscopy (EGD)
	☐ Massage abdomen every 2 hours or as needed for pain
	☐ Start regular diet
Cardiac	☐ Initiate continuous telemetry monitoring
	☐ Administer apixaban orally
	☐ Give diltiazem IV
	☐ Administer nitroglycerin sublingual prn chest pain; repeat as needed every 5 minutes for up to 15 minutes
Vascular	☐ Monitor CBC for trends
	☐ Initiate IV access
	☐ Start IV fluids
	☐ Type and cross for 2 units of PRBCs (packed red blood cells)

GENERATING SOLUTIONS TO MAKE SAFE CLINICAL JUDGMENTS

As discussed in this chapter, being able to generate effective solutions for improving client outcomes is an essential cognitive skill needed to make safe and appropriate clinical judgments. Having an understanding of factors that influence the ability to generate solutions, a strong knowledge base in nursing, and an understanding of the role of the client condition (mental health and physical) is essential when making clinical judgments, especially when generating solutions.

Factors that Influence the Ability of Nurses to Generate Solutions

There are several factors that both negatively and positively influence the ability of nurses to critically think to generate solutions. The ability to generate solutions is influenced by both nurse factors and situational circumstances similar to those discussed in Chapter 3. Nurses can also develop habits that can actually improve the ability to generate solutions. Awareness of these nurse factors, situational (system) factors and strategies to improve thinking can be the first step toward improving generation of solutions. Improving thinking results in creative, comprehensive, client-centered solutions that improve clinical outcomes.

Nurse Factors

Many personal factors can influence the ability of nurses to generate creative solutions. Clinical judgments are often more influenced by what the nurse brings to the situation (knowledge and experience) than the objective data in the situation. Nurses need to first understand their own thinking characteristics (or lack of) and work to continually develop behaviors and habits to improve generating solutions. Table 5.4 summarizes key personal characteristics and behaviors often exhibited by expert thinkers who are most skilled at generating solutions.

TABLE 5.4 Personal Thinking Factors for Generating Solutions

Thinking Factors	Behaviors and Characteristics
Autonomous/responsible	Self-directed in thinking, accountable for own actions
Confident, courageous, persistent, resilient	Has faith in ability to think and learn; overcomes challenges and learns from failed attempts to improve
Creative	Continually looking for new and better way solutions; offers alternate approaches
Curious and inquisitive	Continually questioning; researching evidence for best practices; seeking broader understanding; looking for new and better ways of providing care
Effective communicator	Speaks and writes clearly, communicating thoughts clearly to others. Listens well and has empathy for others' thoughts, feelings, and ideas
Fair-mindedness and moral development; honest	Aware of own values, has a good sense of right and wrong, and approaches situations with an attitude of "I must consider all viewpoints and make decisions in the key players' best interests"
Health-oriented	Manages stress, personal health, and well-being; this creates a better frame of mind to creatively generate solutions
Proactive and improvement-oriented for self, clients, and systems	Self-identifies learning needs and continually seeks out new knowledge; learns from prior experience/mistakes
	Clients: Generates solutions that continually promotes health to maximize function and comfort
	Systems: Identifies risks and problems with health care systems; promotes safety quality, satisfaction, and cost efficiency
Reflective and self-corrective	Continually reflects on nursing care provided with the idea of continually improving. Asks for feedback; corrects own thinking; finds ways to avoid future mistakes
Self-aware	Aware of own learning, personality, and communication style preferences; self-aware when emotions or self-interest may be influencing thinking
Skilled in creating an inclusive environment for working with diverse individuals	Avoids implicit bias in thinking; demonstrates cultural humility when generating solutions

From Alfaro-LeFevre, R. (2019). *Evidence-based critical thinking indicators.* All rights reserved. Available at http://www. AlfaroTeachSmart.com.

System Factors

System or situational factors can also affect nurse thinking for generating effective solutions. Clinical judgments can be impacted by the context in which the situation occurs and the culture of the nursing unit. It is important to examine any factors that may be influencing thinking so these factors may be targeted for improvement when needed. Table 5.5 summarizes key system and situational factors that can affect nurse thinking for generating solutions.

Like any skill, generating solutions improves with practice and establishing new or improving current thinking habits. Current habits can also be a barrier to thinking, such as resistance to change, stereotyping, needing to be right, making assumptions, jumping to conclusions, and "one size fits all." The nurse must continually self-reflect on current habits to avoid any of these types of behaviors, identify if these habits might be negatively impacting thinking to generate solutions,

TABLE 5.5 System and Situational Factors Affecting Generating Solutions	
System/Situational Factors	**Potential Impacts**
Awareness of risks	Awareness of potential risks can help you generate proactive solutions such as placing a client on fall precautions. Hyper-awareness of risks can potentially impede thinking as it can cause the fear of failure which may overwhelm one's courage to develop solutions
Awareness of available resources	Knowing about available resources is key in generating solutions. This knowledge helps a nurse find needed resources for clients. It is also helpful to know what resources are available to help the nurse
Culture of nursing unit	The culture of the nursing unit can make a huge impact on generating solutions. A collaborative, team-oriented unit focused on continual improvement results in solutions that are comprehensive. The staff of a unit that openly discusses "near misses" or "missed nursing care" often promotes creative solutions. A negative unit that is punitive when mistakes occur and opposed to change negatively impacts the creation of new solutions
Distractions and interruptions	Distractions and interruptions impede thinking—the more distractions, the more difficult it is to stay focused. The more distracting an environment is, the more likely errors can occur. Creativity is impeded by continual interruption in thinking
Knowledge and experience	Having knowledge and experience with a situation is very helpful in generating solutions. The more knowledge and/or experience a nurse has with a particular condition or procedure, the easier it is for the nurse to recall or generate effective solutions for implementation
Negative talk	Focusing too much on what could go wrong can impede creativity for solutions. Positive thinking and reinforcement are essential for building confidence in thinking by focusing on what is being done right
Presence of motivating factors	The presence of motivational factors helps the nurse to engage in thinking and creating solutions. These could be the motivation to improve client outcomes or system processes, the motivation to continually improve, or the motivation to continually learn
Time	Time can be an enhancing or impeding factor. Time limitations can be motivating factors—deadlines stimulate us to get things done. If there's too little time, however, you may generate solutions more quickly than you'd like and come up with less-than-satisfactory solutions

and identify methods for improvement. Table 5.6 describes habits that promote thinking when generating effective solutions.

Through awareness of factors that both promote and inhibit the generation of solutions, nurses can work toward improving abilities and avoid potential barriers. The habits of thinking for generating solutions are continually developed throughout the career of the nurse and improve over time with practice and gained experiences. Much self-reflection is needed on current practices to determine areas needing improvement. Practicing self-reflection for improvement results in improvement in:

- The nurse's thinking abilities
- Client outcomes
- Processes and procedures of the system

Role of Nursing Knowledge Base

Effective clinical judgment requires recall of nursing knowledge to be applied to a client situation or care process to generate solutions to meet desired clinical outcomes. A nurse's knowledge base contains not only knowledge of disease processes but also is composed of the nurse's experience with skills, specialty, and prior client care experiences. The knowledge base of nurses is reflective

TABLE 5.6   Habits to Promote Nurse Thinking

Nurse Thinking Habits	Nurse Thinking Behaviors
Be a systems thinker	Look for relationships among key pieces of the whole rather than simply "one client at a time." Look for ways to not only improve client outcomes but also to improve outcomes by improving overall processes and procedures. In this way, a much larger positive impact can be had
Begin with the end in mind	Start with the desired client or process outcome in mind. Then work toward generating solutions for the outcome
Communicate effectively	Work to understand others' points of view before sharing yours; be open to ideas and information
Emotional intelligence	Develop the capacity to be aware of, control, and express one's emotions; handle interpersonal relations fairly and empathetically when generating solutions
Know your priorities	Determine priorities for solutions and maintain focus accordingly. Don't be distracted to put last things first
Lifelong learning	Commit to lifelong learning; continually research evidence; seek new and improved solutions for intervention
Mutual benefit	Create solutions that aim to benefit all
Practice cultural humility and avoid implicit bias	Continually self-reflect to avoid any implicit bias being demonstrated in solutions. Continually gain awareness and experience in caring for diverse clients while demonstrating cultural humility and generating client-centered solutions
Proactive and responsible for self	Anticipate what might occur and create solutions in advance to prevent or reduce risk whenever possible; maintain accountability for self in all communications and solutions

Adapted from Dolansky, M., & Moore, S. (2013). Quality and safety education for nurses (QSEN): The Key is systems thinking. *OJIN: The Online Journal of Issues in Nursing, 18*(3); Senge, P., Fritz, R., & Wheattly, M. (2018). *Learning organizations: The promise and the possibilities*. The Systems Thinker. Retrieved from https://thesystemsthinker.com/learning-organizations-the-promise-and-the-possibilities/

of their level of experience and the individual characteristics of each nurse. This means that nurses who have had more practice caring for a particular group of clients within their specialty have had a wide range of client care experiences. For example, they have performed a large number of skills, and have an enhanced ability to generate creative solutions for improving client outcomes. These experienced nurses work at the expert level and are able to generate a wide range of diverse solutions based on previous client care experiences. While this knowledge base builds and improves over time, new nurses need to be able to demonstrate safe clinical judgments, including generating effective client care solutions based on nursing knowledge and informed by evidence.

The American Association of Colleges of Nursing (AACN) (2021) Core Competencies for Professional Nursing require that nursing graduates demonstrate the ability to clinically reason and integrate nursing knowledge, evidence, and knowledge from other disciplines to inform and support clinical judgments. Development of nursing knowledge is composed of three facets: knowledge, skills, and attitudes. A nurse gains knowledge over time through participation in a wide range of care experiences and by lifelong learning. Additionally, over time the nurse has the opportunity to develop professional attitudes. These attitudes become more sophisticated and informed throughout the career of a nurse through enhanced ability to critically think. Skills are enhanced and refined over time through the ability to practice these in a variety of client care situations. Skills are not only psychomotor, such as taking vital signs and inserting IVs, but can include professional skills such as communication, incorporating cultural humility, client assessment, providing referrals, delegation, and collaboration with the team.

Quality and Safety Education for Nurses (QSEN, 2020) established competencies for new nurses with the goal of continuously improving the quality and safety of health care systems. QSEN established proposed targets for the knowledge, skills, and attitudes that must be developed in prelicensure programs for graduates to be able to generate safe, client-centered care solutions that are focused on improving client outcomes. QSEN expectations for new graduates include having knowledge, skills, and abilities in the following six areas: client-centered care, teamwork and collaboration, EBP, QI, safety, and informatics. Table 5.7 provides some examples of the expectations for each area that provide a knowledge base for nurses to generate effective solutions. These competencies are now integrated into the AACN *Essentials* because the QSEN initiative was completed.

TABLE 5.7   QSEN Competencies for Generating Solutions

Competency	Knowledge	Skills	Attitudes
Client-centered care	• Integrate, communicate, and demonstrate understanding of multiple dimensions of client-centered care	• Provide client-centered care with sensitivity and respect for this diversity	• Value seeing health care situations "through the client's eyes"
Teamwork and collaboration	• Understand scopes of practice/roles of health care team members and demonstrate effective collaboration to improve client outcomes	• Function and communicate competently within own scope of practice as a member of the health care team	• Value the perspectives and expertise of all health team members
EBP	• Understand how the strength and relevance of available evidence influences the choice of interventions in provision of client-centered care	• Locate and read original research and evidence reports	• Value EBP and the need for continuous improvement in clinical practice based on new knowledge
QI	• Understand the desired outcomes of care in the setting where one is in clinical practice	• Seek information about outcomes of care for populations served; use quality measures to understand performance	• Understand that continuous QI is an essential part of daily work; value measurement and its role in good client care
Safety	• Recognize human factors that contribute to an unsafe environment; incorporate basic safety design principles; avoid common unsafe practices; promote factors that create a culture of safety	• Demonstrate effective strategies to reduce risk of harm to self or others	• Value own role in preventing errors; value vigilance and monitoring by clients/families/members of the health care team
Informatics	• Utilize information and technology to create safe client solutions	• Document and plan client care in an electronic health record; navigate the electronic health record	• Value technologies that support creation of solutions that incorporate error prevention and care coordination

Adapted from QSEN. (n.d.). QSEN Competencies. Retrieved from https://www.qsen.org/competencies-pre-licensure-ksas

Role of Client Condition

Effective solutions are client-centered, grounded in current evidence, considerate of relevant determinants of health, and the result of nursing knowledge. But the type of client condition you manage is a key driving force behind all solutions created. In addition to generating solutions for physiologic client conditions such as hypertensive crisis or hemorrhage, you will likely encounter clients who have acute mental/behavioral health conditions such as suicidal ideation or violence toward others.

As discussed in Chapter 4, potential mental health crises may be the priority client condition. Common mental/behavioral health conditions include:

- Suicide attempt
- Intentional harm to others
- Acute psychotic episode with violence
- Alcohol and drug withdrawal
- Delirium tremens

If a client is threatening or being violent toward others, deescalation interventions are typically used. In the hospital setting, you may need to call a Code Gray or other agency-specific code for an expert response team, including security personnel. Examples of these evidence-based deescalation solutions are listed in Box 5.5.

BOX 5.5   Examples of Commonly Used Deescalation Solutions

- Be empathetic, calm, and nonjudgmental
- Respect the client's personal space
- Maintain neutral nonverbal facial expressions and gestures
- Listen to the client carefully
- Allow client to verbalize
- Allow time for client to work through their feelings and calm down

---

Strategies for How to Generate Solutions

The process of generating solutions involves understanding strategies to promote creative and innovative thinking. Often it is a matter of generating new ideas or reconstructing old ones to better fit a particular situation (Cheraghi et al., 2021). This chapter has explored the process for generating solutions and the factors that affect your ability as a nurse to use this clinical judgment cognitive skill. This discussion highlights the strategies you should use to effectively generate solutions to positively impact a client's condition changes or deterioration (Box 5.6).

BOX 5.6   Strategies for Generating Solutions

- Develop expected clinical outcomes for the priority client condition
- Create a list of possible solutions for the priority client condition based on your knowledge and experience
- Remember to use the strategy for thinking in action and thinking ahead when generating solutions
- Collaborate with relevant health care team members, client, and family
- Analyze solutions for potential implementation

Develop Expected Clinical Outcomes for the Priority Client Condition

After determining the client's priority physiologic or mental/behavioral health condition, decide on one or more expected clinical outcomes to manage or resolve the condition. Be sure the desired outcomes are specific, measurable, and realistic. For example, if the client is experiencing hypotension and tachycardia as a result of GI bleeding, you would expect that as a result of appropriate and timely interventions, the client's blood pressure and pulse would return to baseline or a normal range. Vital signs are specific, measurable, and realistic results that indicate whether the client's blood volume increased to adequately perfuse major body organs.

Create a List of Possible Solutions for the Priority Client Condition

When the expected outcome(s) for the client are established, think of all the possible solutions that *could* help achieve that outcome. For the example of the client who has GI bleeding, some solutions could be directed toward increasing the client's body fluids, including oral and IV fluids. Other solutions could be directed toward determining and treating the cause of the bleeding. For example, a client with advanced cirrhosis and bleeding esophageal varices would likely need vasopressors or an invasive procedure to locate and stop the bleeding. In some cases, the cause of GI bleeding is unknown and the client requires diagnostic testing.

Remember to Use Thinking in Action and Thinking Ahead

Remember to use the strategy for thinking in action and thinking ahead when generating solutions. Determine what solutions are needed now (thinking in action) and what solutions would help this condition in the future (thinking ahead). Not only do nurses need to solve current client care conditions, but they also need to always be working to prevent any potential conditions that could occur.

Collaborate with Relevant Health Care Team Members

One of the most common methods for generating solutions is to consult with relevant interprofessional health team members. Consulting expert team members, such as the medical provider, respiratory therapist, or pharmacist, may result in a more rapid generation of solutions. Collaboration can help create a wider range of potential solutions that may be better targeted for improving the condition in a more expedient manner.

The team huddle is an evidence-based method for working with the care team to develop solutions or identify potential safety concerns for the client. The team gathers on a daily basis to discuss the client's progress, identify concerns, and present potential solutions for improving the client's outcomes (Shaikh, 2020). Huddles have been shown to improve client safety in areas such as medication errors, serious safety events, wrong-site surgery, and poor hand hygiene. Huddles have also been shown to have secondary benefits such as facilitating immediate clarification of issues, having fewer interruptions during the workday, and creating a culture of empowerment and collaboration in health care teams.

Remember that, when generating solutions, the client and client's family are also part of the relevant health care team. One strategy for incorporating client input is through the Bedside Shift Report (BSR). The BSR involves handing off care from one nurse to the next at the bedside in a face-to-face interaction that involves the client and family members so that the client is aware of and participates in the plan for care, if possible. The BSR has been shown to improve client and nurse satisfaction (Dorvil, 2018).

Analyze Solutions for Potential Implementation

After the list of potential solutions has been developed, begin to analyze these potential solutions for possible implementation. Ask yourself, which solutions are indicated for this particular client condition? If orders are needed, determine which orders you would anticipate for this particular client situation. Consider summarizing solutions so that you can examine the situation comprehensively. Cluster related solutions to see if any relationships exist that provide insight about which solutions are the most appropriate. Evaluate each proposed solution to decide if it is the best for this particular client condition to prevent or manage clinical deterioration or mental/behavioral health crisis.

Thinking Exercise 5.4 will help you practice what you've learned in this chapter about generating solutions. The answer and rationale for the exercise are located at the end of this book.

THINKING EXERCISE 5.4

The nurse is caring for an 81-year-old client in an acute care unit.

History and Physical	Nurses Notes	Orders	Laboratory Results

1700: Client has history of uncontrolled diabetes mellitus type 2, hypertension, TIAs, and family history of cardiovascular disease. States, "I wish I could have a few minutes for a cigarette break. It is very stressful being in the hospital. I have a pretty bad headache tonight too." Admitted for surgical and wound care therapy for large open wound to left heel area. Client alert and oriented × 4, PERRLA. Full ROM × 4 extremities, grips =, 3+, leg strength, = bilaterally. States "not feeling the best tonight. Not sure what is wrong." Client ate 25% of evening meal. Dressing to left heel dry and intact. Respirations easy and without distress, lung sounds clear to auscultation throughout. S_1 and S_2 present, apical pulse rate regular. VS: T 99°F (37°C); HR 110 beats per minute; RR 24 breaths per minute; B/P 178/108 mmHg; SpO_2 94% on RA. Headache pain reported at 8/10.

1900: Client difficult to arouse, confused, unable to follow commands, disoriented to place, time, and situation. Speech somewhat slurred. States "My head hurts so bad. My leg feels numb. The light is hurting my eyes." Face asymmetric in appearance, drooping of left eye and left side of mouth. Grips 3+ on right, 1+ left. Leg strength 3+ right, 1+ left. Respirations slightly increased from previous assessment; lung sounds clear to auscultation throughout. S_1 and S_2 heard throughout, apical pulse rate regular. VS: T 100.6° F (38.1° C); HR 120 beats per minute; RR 28 breaths per minute; B/P 200/125 mmHg; SpO_2 89% on RA. Headache pain reported at 10/10.

The nurse begins to plan care for the client. For each potential order, specify whether the order is indicated or not indicated for the client.

Potential Orders	Indicated	Not Indicated
Lower head of bed		
Perform stroke scale assessment		
Suction client's oropharynx		
Start oxygen at 2 L via nasal cannula		
Monitor vital signs and neurologic assessments frequently		
Obtain blood for glucose testing		
Anticipate fibrinolytic therapy		
Administer antiseizure medication		
Teach client how to use assistive devices for ambulation		
Initiate Rapid Response Team		

END-OF-CHAPTER THINKING EXERCISES

Additional End-of-Chapter Exercises will help you apply what you've learned in this chapter about generating solutions. The answers and rationales for these exercises are located at the end of this chapter.

⚡ END-OF-CHAPTER THINKING EXERCISE 5.1

The nurse is caring for a 52-year-old in an urgent care setting.

History and Physical	Nurses Notes	Orders	Laboratory Results

2100: Client states "I have been sick for 4 days. I can't stop coughing, and ache all over. I've had a fever of 100 this week. I'm having a lot of nasal congestion, too." Alert and oriented × 4. Respirations unlabored; lungs clear to auscultation over all fields, denies shortness of breath. Slightly loose cough noted, client states nonproductive. Clear nasal discharge noted. BS present × 4 quadrants, abdomen soft, flat. S_1 and S_2 present, regular HR. Walks unassisted; gait steady. VS: T 100.4°F (38°C); HR 88 beats per minute; RR 18 breaths per minute; B/P 128/84 mmHg; SpO_2 95% on RA. Pain described as overall body aches, reported at 4/10 on a 0–10 pain scale.

Complete the following sentence by selecting from the lists below. The nurse would anticipate that _____ **1 [Select]** _____ and _____ **2 [Select]** _____ would be indicated for the client at this time.

Options for 1	Options for 2
Nasal swabs for RSV, influenza, and COVID-19	Azithromycin
Oxygen therapy	Oral fluids
Oseltamivir	Chest X-ray

⚡ END-OF-CHAPTER THINKING EXERCISE 5.2

The nurse is caring for a 16-year-old pregnant client in a community health clinic.

History and Physical	Nurses Notes	Orders	Laboratory Results

2100: Client states "I haven't been feeling the greatest, especially the last month or so. I did a pregnancy test at home awhile back and was surprised to learn that I am pregnant. My parents are upset about the pregnancy, but they are supportive. My last period was around early November. My parents do not have insurance at their jobs; they are undocumented workers. I haven't been to a doctor or dentist for anything in at least 2 years. I have been feeling tired and having occasional headaches. I have a headache today. I had a little spotting of blood yesterday." Client alert and oriented × 4, PERRLA. Lungs clear to auscultation over all fields. BS present × 4; abdomen protuberant consistent with pregnancy. Estimated date of delivery (EDD) 8/16; client 35 weeks pregnant. S_1 and S_2 present, regular HR. 1+ nonpitting edema bilateral lower extremities. Client has not had prenatal care. No history of chronic health conditions. Urinalysis today shows 2+ protein in urine, otherwise negative. VS: T 98.6° F (38° C); HR 88 beats per minute; RR 20 breaths per minute; B/P 188/98 mmHg; SpO_2 99% on RA. Denies pain. Wt. 180 lbs. (81.6 kg).

Complete the following sentence by selecting from the lists of options below. The nurse should anticipate _____ **1 [Select]** _____ and obtaining _____ **2 [Select]** _____

Options for 1	Options for 2
Referring the client for immediate evaluation	Blood sugar, Hgb A_1C, and glucose tolerance test
Allowing the client to return home for daily blood pressure monitoring	Serum creatinine, platelet count, and liver enzymes
Scheduling an appointment within 1 week with obstetric care provider for evaluation	CBC, serum electrolytes, and BUN

END-OF-CHAPTER THINKING EXERCISE 5.3

The nurse is caring for an 8-month-old client in the acute pediatric unit.

History and Physical	Nurses Notes	Orders	Laboratory Results

2000:   Admitted to the acute care unit accompanied by parent. Parent states "My baby has been so congested; the congestion makes it difficult to eat." Parent states baby has been healthy until current illness. States that child is breastfed and receives some rice cereal and baby fruits. States that child has had some vaccines but prefers the child receive these on a slower schedule than what the CDC recommends. Child has had 2-month and 4-month vaccines, but not 6-month vaccines. Baby dyspneic with rapid breathing; no stridor or audible wheeze. Large amount of clear nasal secretions and crusting bilateral nares. Skin warm, moist, pale pink in color, no cyanosis. Expiratory wheezing noted throughout lung fields upon auscultation, anterior and posterior. Loose, frequent cough present. Chest symmetric, no injuries noted, moderate intercostal retractions noted. Apical pulse steady and regular. Baby well-nourished and well groomed. VS: T 100.6°F (38.7°C); HR 150 beats per minute; RR 40 breaths per minute; B/P 110/78 mmHg; SpO$_2$ 90% on RA. Baby quiet in parent's arms. Wt. 18 lbs. (8.2 kg).

The nurse has reviewed the nurse's notes and is planning care. For each potential order, specify whether the order is indicated or not indicated for the care of the client.

Potential Orders	Indicated	Not Indicated
Start IV fluids		
Suction frequently		
Start oxygen at 4–6 L per minute via nasal cannula		
Give albuterol via nebulizer		
Obtain blood for glucose testing		
Administer acetaminophen orally now		
Obtain chest X-ray		
Initiate droplet precautions		
Place baby in negative-airflow pressure room		

The nurse is caring for a 28-year-old client admitted to the acute care unit.

History and Physical	Nurses Notes	Orders	Laboratory Results

1330:   Client states, "I live on the streets; I don't have an address. My leg is really killing me." Client has history of ongoing methamphetamine use for 5 years. Right lower leg red, hot swollen, shiny. Diameter of left calf 12.2 in (31 cm), right calf 25.6 in (65 cm). Client states leg is painful and tender to touch. Rates pain 9/10. Track marks noted between toes bilaterally. Wound on right ankle, 1.2 in (3 cm) in diameter with some purulent drainage; erythema surrounding wound. Rest of skin warm, moist, pale pink. Pedal pulses 2+, regular. Lungs clear throughout; respirations nonlabored. S_1 and S_2 present, regular HR. Abdomen soft and concave. Client states has "limited access to food and gets by the best I can." Teeth in poor condition; numerous caries noted with two teeth missing left lower side. Leg strength 4/4, equal bilaterally. Client has slight limp when walking due to leg tenderness. Thin and poorly groomed. States "I don't have regular access to bathing or clothing." Allergies: Penicillin, peanuts. VS: T 102.6°F (38.7°C); HR 110 beats per minute; RR 20 breaths per minute; B/P 128/88 mmHg; SpO$_2$ 96% on RA. Wt. 145 lbs. (65.9 kg).

2100:   Client reports leg pain 9/10. Right lower leg red, hot, shiny, elevated on two pillows. Dressing to right ankle has quarter sized blood-tinged purulence. Client states "I really don't feel well. Feels like my heart is racing and I'm so hot." Client alert and oriented × 4. Has not voided since 1430. VS: T 103.2°F (39.6°C); HR 130 beats per minute; RR 28 breaths per minute; B/P 90/68 mmHg; SpO$_2$ 92% on RA.

Which of the following actions would the nurse plan to implement based on the client's condition? **Select all that apply**.
- Administer ketorolac IV.
- Administer vancomycin IV.
- Administer piperacillin tazobacter IV.
- Monitor serum lactate.
- Initiate oxygen therapy.
- Obtain blood cultures.
- Obtain chest X-ray.
- Start IV fluids.
- Type and cross for 2 units of PRBCs (packed red blood cells).
- Obtain urinalysis.

The nurse is caring for a 72-year-old client in the Emergency Department (ED).

History and Physical	Nurses Notes	Orders	Laboratory Results

1400:   Client states "My chest is hurting; I've had this cough for over a week now and it just doesn't get better." Productive cough, short of breath, taking a breath every 3–4 words, maintaining tripod position. Lungs have crackles left lower lobe; lung sounds diminished bilateral lower lobes anterior and posterior. Client reports pain 7/10 over left lower chest. Skin warm, moist, dark skin tones ash gray. Pedal pulses 2+, regular, bilateral 1+ edema noted. S_1 and S_2 present, HR regular. Abdomen soft, mild ascites. Bowel sounds present × 4. Client states "I usually drink about a 12-pack of beer per day but I haven't been up to drinking the last 2 days." Leg strength 4/4, equal bilateral. Grips strong, equal bilaterally. Alert and oriented × 4, PERRLA. VS: T 103.4° F (39.7° C); HR 115 beats per minute; RR 32 breaths per minute; B/P 168/94 mmHg; SpO$_2$ 88% on RA. Wt. 155 lbs. (70.3 kg).

Which of the following nursing actions would the nurse plan to implement? **Select all that apply**.
- Perform CIWA-Ar (Clinical Institute Withdrawal Assessment for Alcohol) assessment.
- Draw arterial blood gases.
- Place on seizure precautions.
- Prepare for paracentesis.
- Initiate oxygen therapy.
- Draw blood for cardiac enzymes.
- Obtain chest X-ray.
- Start regular diet.

END-OF-CHAPTER THINKING EXERCISE 5.6

The nurse is caring for a 54-year-old admitted to the acute care unit with diverticulitis and bloody diarrhea.

History and Physical	Nursing Flowsheet	Orders	Laboratory Results

Parameters	Results Today 0700	Results Yesterday (1400) (Admission)
Temperature	102.8°F (39.3°C)	100.4°F (38°C)
Pulse rate	HR 115 beats per minute	HR 85 beats per minute
Respiratory rate	RR 24 breaths per minute	RR 12 breaths per minute
Blood pressure	B/P 185/96 mmHg	B/P 140/74 mmHg
Nausea and vomiting	Present; emesis ×3 since 0400, clear, green	Absent
Light palpation of abdomen	Abdomen rigid	Abdomen soft, states tender in LLQ
Pain	10/10, generalized throughout abdomen	4/10 LLQ

Based on the client's recent assessment findings and medical history, the nurse will need to **1 [Select]** and **2 [Select]**.

Options for 1	Options for 2
Provide a quiet environment for client to rest	Administer antidiarrheal medications
Teach the client how to splint the abdomen for pain	Administer ondansetron orally
Remain with the client	Type and cross for 2 units of PRBCs
Apply ice packs as needed for pain	Initiate the Rapid Response Team

Answers and Rationales for Thinking Exercises

CHAPTER THINKING EXERCISES

⚡ THINKING EXERCISE 5.1

Answer:
Select **2** appropriate actions that the nurse could take at this time.
X Notify the health care provider.
○ Assist client to stand to determine if weight bearing is tolerable.
○ Monitor client overnight and report findings.
○ Position the client on the affected side.
X Monitor for signs of shock.
○ Provide oral fluids.

Rationale: The client has evidence of a possible hip fracture (history of recent fall, pain in the left hip, inability to move left leg, and external rotation of the left leg). This is a condition that requires immediate attention and possibly surgical treatment if a hip fracture has occurred. It would be most important for the nurse to notify the provider so that the client can be transferred for evaluation, X-rays, and potential surgery. This type of injury can be quite severe and result in shock; it will be important for the nurse to stay with the client and monitor for any signs that shock may be occurring (increased thready pulse, decreased blood pressure, narrowed pulse pressure, increased respiratory rate, and anxiety can be early signs of shock). It is not appropriate for the nurse to help the client to bear weight on the affected limb as this is contraindicated for a potential hip fracture and may cause further injury. Monitoring the client overnight is contraindicated and will delay needed treatment. Positioning the client on the affected side is also contraindicated and could cause further injury. Finally, it is possible the client may require surgery later that day to repair the fracture and should remain NPO (nothing by mouth) until further instructions have been received from the provider.

⚡ THINKING EXERCISE 5.2

Answer:

Order	Anticipated	Not Anticipated
Start oxygen at 2 L via nasal cannula	X	
Initiate IV access	X	
Give oral prednisone now for airway inflammation		X
Administer acetaminophen now for discomfort		X
Administer albuterol via nebulizer now and repeat every 20 minutes for 1 hour if needed	X	
Obtain chest X-ray	X	
Consult Social Services	X	
Teach family how to develop asthma action plan	X	

THINKING EXERCISE 5.2—cont'd

Rationale: The nurse would anticipate that orders would be directed toward immediate correction of impaired gas exchange and airway impairment due to the constriction of the bronchioles caused by irritation resulting from exposure to allergic triggers. Usually, this is controlled by daily antihistamines (cetirizine), but the client has been financially unable to obtain this medication on a regular basis. Lack of regular maintenance medication due to limited financial resources resulted in the exacerbation of asthma causing extreme dyspnea and wheezing. To improve the client's outcome of improved gas exchange, the nurse could anticipate that the provider will order oxygen via nasal cannula to correct the low SpO$_2$ of 92%. Also, intravenous access will likely be needed to administer medications that can act in a rapid manner because this is an emergent situation. While steroids will likely be needed, oral prednisone will have a much slower effect than intravenous; it is more likely that intravenous steroids such as methylprednisolone will be ordered. The client has no reports of pain so acetaminophen is not indicated at this time. The albuterol nebulizer treatment is indicated and should be initiated as soon as possible to dilate the bronchioles and provide immediate breathing relief. The chest X-ray would likely be ordered to ensure there are no other causes for the wheezing such as a foreign body or pneumonia. Consulting social service is an excellent idea to work with the family in finding resources for medications. Finally, it will be very important to provide client education about an asthma action plan so that the family is aware of how to monitor and treat the child's asthma at home and know when to seek medical attention.

THINKING EXERCISE 5.3

Answer:

Body System	Potential Nursing Interventions
Gastrointestinal	☒ Place nasogastric tube to low continuous suction
	☒ Monitor results of esophagogastroduodenoscopy (EGD)
	☐ Massage abdomen every 2 hours or as needed for pain
	☐ Start regular diet
Cardiac	☒ Initiate continuous telemetry monitoring
	☐ Administer apixaban orally
	☒ Give diltiazem IV
	☐ Administer nitroglycerin sublingual prn chest pain; repeat as needed every 5 minutes for up to 15 minutes
Hematologic/vascular	☒ Monitor CBC for trends
	☒ Initiate IV access
	☒ Start IV fluids
	☒ Type and cross for 2 units of PRBCs (packed red blood cells)

Rationale: Because the client has evidence of upper gastrointestinal bleeding (pain, history of ulcer, and coffee ground emesis, rapid pulse, low blood pressure, weakness) and atrial fibrillation (history of atrial fibrillation with ECG showing atrial fibrillation), interventions are needed to address the blood loss, the source of the bleeding, and returning the heart to normal sinus rhythm.

Continued

Potential nursing actions to help manage the client's GI bleeding include insertion of a nasogastric (NG) tube which is connected to low continuous suction to decrease secretions in stomach. An EGD would be ordered; it would be important to review the results and report these to the provider as soon as they become available so that the source of the bleeding can be identified. Since the client has an NG tube, the client would be NPO and a regular diet would be contraindicated. Abdominal massage is not indicated and could even be harmful if the source of bleeding is continually irritated. Nursing actions related to the client's atrial fibrillation would include telemetry monitoring to monitor heart rhythm continually. Diltiazem would be a drug of choice to return the heart rate to normal sinus rhythm. Apixaban would be contraindicated in a client with an active bleeding condition because it is an anticoagulant and would not be appropriate or safe. Nitroglycerin is not indicated because the client does not have a history of angina or chest pain. Other appropriate nursing actions include monitoring the CBC for trends in the hemoglobin (Hgb) and hematocrit (Hct) which indicate improvement or lack of improvement related to blood loss. Intravenous access would be anticipated along with fluid replacement to replace volume lost. Additionally, typing and crossmatching for possible administration of PRBCs would be appropriate as blood transfusions may be needed if the Hgb or Hct are critically low.

⚡ **THINKING EXERCISE 5.4**

Answer:

Potential Orders	Indicated	Not Indicated
Lower head of bed		X
Perform stroke scale assessment	X	
Suction client's oropharynx		X
Start oxygen at 2 L via nasal cannula	X	
Monitor vital signs and neuro assessments frequently	X	
Obtain blood for glucose testing	X	
Anticipate fibrinolytic therapy		X
Administer antiseizure medication		X
Teach client how to use assistive devices for ambulation		X
Initiate Rapid Response Team	X	

Rationale: The client is exhibiting signs of a hemorrhagic stroke caused by bleeding into the brain tissue resulting from severe hypertension. The client has a sudden excruciating headache along with photophobia, extreme elevated blood pressure/temperature/heart rate/respirations. The client also exhibits facial drooping and left-sided weakness. There is a noticeable deterioration in mental status and presence of confusion/disorientation. Initiating a rapid response is indicated as the client has significant deterioration and stroke requires rapid intervention. Completing the stroke scale as soon as possible would be very helpful in determining client status. It would be appropriate to initiate oxygen therapy due to the low SpO$_2$ and monitor vital signs and neuro status frequently to assess for improvement or worsening of client condition. It would also be important to obtain a blood glucose result as soon as possible as the client has a history of DM type 2 and hypoglycemia can mimic emergent neurologic disorders. Because the client has evidence of a potential hemorrhagic stroke, lowering the head of the bed is not indicated as this may increase intracranial pressure. Fibrinolytic therapy would not be indicated as this is for ischemic stroke rather than hemorrhagic. It is likely this client will need a CT scan to confirm stroke type before fibrinolytics can be administered. Suctioning the client, administering seizure medication, and teaching about assistive devices are not indicated at this time. There is no evidence of excessive oral secretions or seizure activity at this time. Teaching the client about assistive devices is not indicated at this time as this is an emergent situation and the client would not be able to comprehend teaching while in severe pain and distress.

END-OF-CHAPTER THINKING EXERCISES

END-OF-CHAPTER THINKING EXERCISE 5.1

Answer:
The nurse would anticipate that **nasal swabs for RSV, influenza, and COVID-19** and **oral fluids** would be indicated for the client at this time.

Rationale: The client is exhibiting symptoms of a viral respiratory infection. The provider would order nasal swabs to determine whether the symptoms are due to influenza, RSV, or COVID-19. Oxygen therapy is not indicated at this time as the SpO_2 is 95% on RA. Oseltamivir is not indicated at this time as this therapy needs to be initiated within the first 48 hours of the start of symptoms and the client has been ill for 4 days. Azithromycin is an antibiotic and is not effective in treating viral infections. The lungs are clear to auscultation, the cough is nonproductive, and the temperature is low-grade so there is no indication for a chest X-ray at this time. Encouraging oral fluids is appropriate and helpful to maintain hydration of the client and decrease viscosity of secretions.

END-OF-CHAPTER THINKING EXERCISE 5.2

Answer:
The nurse should anticipate **referring the client for immediate evaluation** and obtaining **serum creatinine, platelet count, and liver enzymes**.

Rationale: It will be important to refer the client immediately for evaluation by a health care provider as the client has had no prenatal care and has extremely high blood pressure (188/98), headaches, proteinuria, and spotting. This client likely has preeclampsia, which can cause extremely dangerous complications such as cerebral edema and hemorrhage. It would be important for this client to be evaluated as soon as possible so that preventive measures can be taken. Additionally, clients with preeclampsia are at risk for thrombocytopenia, renal insufficiency, and impaired liver function, so the nurse would anticipate laboratory testing to include serum creatinine, platelet count, and liver enzyme studies.

END-OF-CHAPTER THINKING EXERCISE 5.3

Answer:

Potential Orders	Indicated	Not Indicated
Start IV fluids	X	
Suction frequently	X	
Start oxygen at 4–6 L per minute via nasal cannula		X
Give albuterol via nebulizer		X
Obtain blood for glucose testing		X
Administer acetaminophen orally now		X
Obtain chest X-ray	X	
Initiate droplet precautions		X
Place baby in negative airflow pressure room		X

Continued

END-OF-CHAPTER THINKING EXERCISE 5.3—cont'd

Rationale: For the baby with bronchiolitis secondary to RSV, IV fluids would be indicated to maintain hydration. The baby is at risk for dehydration due to the decreased ability to feed due to copious nasal secretions. For this reason, frequent nasopharyngeal suctioning is needed. A chest X-ray would be indicated due to the severity of the baby's symptoms and the need to rule out pneumonia. At this time there is no need to obtain a blood glucose result. The baby would not need a negative-airflow pressure room with a diagnosis of RSV. Clients with RSV are placed on contact precautions rather than droplet precautions as the virus is spread through contact with infected materials. Oxygen would be more appropriate at 1–3 L for an infant; 4–6 L is too high. Albuterol is not indicated as RSV is caused by mucus in the airways rather than bronchospasm. Acetaminophen is not indicated at this time; the client is not experiencing pain and there is only a low-grade temperature. Administering acetaminophen for a low-grade temperature will suppress the baby's own immune response to the disease.

END-OF-CHAPTER THINKING EXERCISE 5.4

Answer:
Which of the following actions would the nurse plan to implement? **Select all that apply.**
X   Administer ketorolac IV
X   Administer vancomycin IV
o   Administer piperacillin tazobacter IV
X   Monitor serum lactate
X   Initiate oxygen therapy
X   Obtain blood cultures
o   Obtain chest X-ray
o   Start IV fluids
o   Type and cross for 2 units of PRBCs (packed red blood cells)
o   Obtain urinalysis

Rationale: This client is exhibiting symptoms of cellulitis of the leg, possibly secondary to the wound on the ankle. The client has some symptoms of a deep vein thrombosis, but the ankle wound combined with the generalized edema, erythema, and inflammation of the lower leg is more characteristic of cellulitis. The client is also beginning to show possible signs of sepsis. Signs of sepsis exhibited include increasing temperature, respirations, and heart rate with decreasing blood pressure and SpO_2. The client is experiencing severe pain and rates pain at 9/10. The client has a history of methamphetamine abuse so tolerance for pain medication is likely to be high. The nurse should plan to administer the ketorolac for the high pain level. The client is allergic to penicillin so piperacillin/tazobactam would be contraindicated. Vancomycin would be appropriate to treat cellulitis, although a broad spectrum may be needed if it is determined the client has sepsis. The serum lactate should be monitored as increased levels can indicate sepsis. Oxygen therapy should be initiated due to the decreased SpO_2. Blood cultures would be obtained to determine if sepsis is present. There is no indication for a chest X-ray (no respiratory distress or symptoms). IV fluids are needed for hydration and medication administration, but there is no indication for a blood transfusion. A urinalysis would not provide useful information as to whether the client has sepsis.

END-OF-CHAPTER THINKING EXERCISE 5.5

Answer:
Which of the following nursing actions would the nurse plant to implement? **Select all that apply.**

X Perform CIWA-Ar (Clinical Institute Withdrawal Assessment for Alcohol) assessment
X Draw arterial blood gases
X Place on seizure precautions
○ Prepare for paracentesis
X Initiate oxygen therapy
X Draw blood for cardiac enzymes
X Obtain chest X-ray
○ Start regular diet

Rationale: This client has a history of recent alcoholism (12 pack of beer per day) and is exhibiting a mild amount of ascites and edema in the lower extremities. The client is exhibiting extreme fever, tachycardia, tachypnea, elevated blood pressure, SpO_2 of 88% on RA, severe dyspnea (tripod position, can only say three to four words at a time), chest pain, crackles in the left lower lobe, and a productive cough. These findings would indicate the client may have pneumonia. This client is at risk for potential seizure activity and alcohol withdrawal symptoms that could be very severe. It would be important for the nurse to initiate a CIWA assessment to monitor withdrawal symptoms and intervene if needed. It would be important to place the client on seizure precautions to prevent injury should a seizure occur. The ascites is mild and a paracentesis would not be indicated at this time. A regular diet is contraindicated as the client is experiencing edema and would require a low-salt diet to prevent further fluid retention. The nurse should anticipate an arterial blood gas test to confirm the SpO_2 as the SpO_2 can be unreliable in clients who have darker skin tones. A chest X-ray would be indicated to determine if the client has pneumonia or other lung conditions. Oxygen therapy is indicated due to the low SpO_2. Cardiac enzyme testing is also indicated to determine if the chest pain is cardiac- or respiratory-related.

END-OF-CHAPTER THINKING EXERCISE 5.6

Answer:
Based on recent assessment findings and medical history, the nurse will need to **remain with the client** and **initiate the Rapid Response Team.**

Rationale: This client is experiencing an exacerbation of diverticulitis which is resulting in bloody diarrhea. The client likely has developed an abscess in the abdominal area secondary to the diverticulitis. The client's symptoms have progressed over time and reflect a sudden increase in temperature, pulse rate, respiratory rate, and blood pressure; the client also has nausea and vomiting. There has been a significant increase in pain and it is no longer localized. The abdomen has progressed from soft and tender to boardlike and rigid. The nurse should recognize the client may be experiencing peritonitis and should not leave the client unattended. The nurse should also initiate a Rapid Response Team call as the client's condition is likely to rapidly deteriorate. Peritonitis is a potentially fatal condition requiring immediate intervention.

REFERENCES

Alfaro-LeFevre, R. (2019). *Evidence-based critical thinking indicators*. Retrieved from http://www.AlfaroTeachS mart.com.

American Association of Colleges of Nursing. (2021). *The Essentials: Core competencies for professional nursing education*. Retrieved from https://www.aacnnursin g.org/Portals/42/AcademicNursing/pdf/Essentials-2021.pdf.

American Lung Association. (2022). *Living near highways and air pollution*. Retrieved from https://www.lung.org/clean-air/outdoors/who-is-at-risk/highways.

Centers for Medicare and Medicaid Services (CMS). (2022). *Client-reported outcome measures*. Retrieved from https://mmshub.cms.gov/sites/default/files/Clie nt-Reported-Outcome-Measures.pdf.

Cheraghi, M. A., Pashaeypoor, S., Dehkordi, L. M., & Khoshkest, S. (2021). Creativity in nursing care: A concept analysis. *Florence Nightingale Journal Nursing, 29*(3), 389–396. https://doi.org/10.5152/FNJN.2021.21027

Dolansky, M., & Moore, S. (2013). Quality and safety education for nurses (QSEN): The Key is systems thinking. *OJIN: Online Journal of Issues in Nursing, 18*(3).

Dorvil, B. (2018). The secrets to successful nurse bedside shift report implementation and sustainability. *Nursing Management, 49*(6), 20–25.

Hostetter, M., & Klein, S. (n.d.). *Using client-reported outcomes to improve health care quality.* The Commonwealth Fund. Retrieved from https://www.commonwealthfund.org/publications/newsletter-article/using-client-reported-outcomes-improve-health-care-quality.

Institute for Client and Family-Centered Care. (n.d.). *Client and family centered care.* Retrieved from https://www.ipfcc.org/about/pfcc.html.

Kayser, S. A., VanGilder, C. A., Ayello, E. A., & Lachenbruch, C. (2018). Prevalence and analysis of medical device-related pressure injuries: Results from the international pressure ulcer prevalence survey. *Advances in Skin & Wound Care, 31*(6), 276–285.

Khan, S. (2021). *Cultural humility vs cultural competence-and why providers need both.* Health City. Retrieved from https://healthcity.bmc.org/policy-and-industry/cultural-humility-vs-cultural-competence-providers-need both#:~:text=The%20term%20%22cultural%20humility%22%20was,curiosity%20rather%20than%20an%20endpoint.

Narayan, M. C. (2019). Addressing implicit bias in nursing: A review. *AJN, 119*(7), 36–43.

Park, S., & Kellerman, T. (2022). *Acute nursing care: Recognition and response to deteriorating clients.*
Retrieved from https://anmj.org.au/acute-nursing-care-recognition-and-response-to-deteriorating-clients/.

QSEN. (2020). QSEN competencies. Retrieved from https://www.qsen.org/competencies-pre-licensure-ksas.

Sabin, J. A. (2022). Tackling implicit bias in health care. *New England Journal of Medicine, 387,* 105–107.

Senge, P., Fritz, R., & Wheattly, M. (2018). *Learning organizations: The Promise and the possibilities.* The systems thinker. Retrieved from https://thesystemsthinker.com/learning-organizations-the-promise-and-the-possibilities/.

Shaikh, U. (2020). *Improving client safety and team communication through daily huddles.* Agency for Healthcare Research and Quality (AHRQ). Retrieved from https://psnet.ahrq.gov/primer/improving-client-safety-and-team-communication-through-daily-huddles.

Stubbe, D. (2020). Practicing cultural competence and cultural humility in the care of diverse clients. *Focus, 18*(1), 49–51.

Thirsk, L. M., Panchuk, J. T., Stahlke, S., & Hagtvedt, R. (2022). Cognitive and implicit bias in nurses' judgment and decision-making: A scoping review. *International Journal of International Studies, 133.*

University of Illinois-Chicago. (n.d.) Emergency nurses association collection. Retrieved from https://nursing.uic.edu/nursing-research/centers-labs-interest-groups/midwest-nursing-history-research-center/collections/organizations/emergency-nurses-association-collection/.

US Department of Health and Human Services. (2020). *Healthy people 2030.* Retrieved from https://health.gov/healthypeople/priority-areas/social-determinants-health.

World Health Organization (WHO). (n.d.). *Social determinants of health.* Retrieved from https://www.who.int/health-topics/social-determinants-of-health#tab=tab_1.

6

How to Take Actions

THIS CHAPTER AT A GLANCE...

Taking Actions
- Definitions
- Need for Immediate Actions When Making Clinical Judgments

Categories of Nursing Actions
- Independent Nursing Actions
- Collaborative Nursing Actions

Direct Versus Indirect Nursing Actions
- Direct Nursing Actions

- Indirect Nursing Actions

Taking Actions to Make Safe Clinical Judgments
- Factors that Influence the Ability of Nurses to Take Actions
- Role of Nursing Knowledge Base
- Role of Client Condition and Context
- Strategies for How to Take Actions

End-of-Chapter Exercises

LEARNING OUTCOMES

1. Explain the importance for taking immediate actions when making clinical judgments.
2. Differentiate independent and collaborative nursing actions.
3. Describe direct and indirect nursing actions for improving client outcomes.

4. Discuss factors that influence the ability of nurses to take actions for making safe clinical judgments including the role of nursing knowledge base and the role of the client condition.

KEY TERMS

Actions: Nursing interventions and assessments that are implemented to assist the client in improving health and attaining desired clinical outcomes.

Behavioral actions: Actions that are designed to help a client improve or manage behaviors such as decreasing anxiety or managing agitation.

Bullying: Bullying is the "repeated, unwanted, harmful actions intended to humiliate, offend and cause distress" (American Nurses Association, n.d., b).

Client- and family-centered actions: Actions that focus on what the client and/or family perceives as a priority clinical condition for improving their health conditions.

Collaborative actions: Actions that require instructions from or participation by the interdisciplinary health care team.

Direct actions: Interventions that are directly implemented by the nurse interacting with the client.

Independent actions: Nursing interventions that are nurse-initiated and performed without supervision or direction from others.

Indirect actions: Interventions the nurse takes that do not involve interacting with the client, but are on behalf of the client.

Physiologic actions: Actions designed to improve the client's physiologic symptoms and/or condition.

Safety actions: Actions that promote the safety of the client.

Workplace violence: An actual act or threat of physical violence, harassment, or intimidation.

TAKING ACTIONS

As described in Chapter 1, taking actions is an essential cognitive skill that requires the nurse to examine the list of potential solutions identified for each desired clinical outcome and determine which actions should be implemented to meet the client's priority needs. Taking actions requires understanding of the client needs and priorities. The nurse must also determine how and in what order each action will need to be implemented to adequately address priorities. Nurses recognize cues, analyze and prioritize cues, generate solutions to address priorities, and then take actions toward the client conditions and clinical outcomes that are the highest priority.

Taking actions is an essential cognitive skill that results in assisting the client toward desired clinical outcomes in the most efficient and expedient manner. Effective use of this cognitive skill results in actions that are safe, effective, client centered, cost-effective, and promote progress toward desired client outcomes. This chapter explores how to take actions that result in safe, appropriate clinical judgments.

Definitions

Chapter 5 discussed the cognitive skill of generating solutions where the nurse develops a wide range of potential solutions to address the priorities for the client condition. Once solutions have been developed, the nurse must then decide which action/s to take and in what order. The nurse selects from a wide range of possible independent or collaborative actions. Independent actions are nursing interventions that are nurse-initiated and performed without supervision or direction from others. Collaborative actions are interventions that require instructions from or participation by the interprofessional health care team. Collaborative actions may be prescribed by a health care provider, registered dietitian nutritionist, pharmacist, respiratory therapist, or rehabilitation therapist. Consulting a team member to collaborate on providing client's treatment or administering a prescribed medication is also a collaborative action.

The nurse utilizes both direct and indirect actions when providing client care. Direct actions are interventions that are directly implemented by the nurse interacting with the client, such as obtaining vital signs or administering medication. Indirect actions are interventions the nurse takes that do not involve interacting with the client, but are on behalf of the client. Examples of indirect actions include monitoring lab values or initiating isolation precautions. Each of these types of actions is discussed in further detail later in this chapter. The nurse relies on nursing knowledge and experience when selecting appropriate actions and action types.

Need for Immediate Actions When Making Clinical Judgments

Chapter 1 discusses a model by Levett-Jones et al. (2010) which outlines the five rights of clinical reasoning that help nurses manage clients at high risk for medical complications or clinical deterioration. These rights include recognizing the right cues and taking the right action at the right time for the right reason for the right client. When clients are experiencing or have the potential to experience rapid deterioration, recognizing what interventions are needed and implementing immediate nursing actions can help prevent any deterioration from occurring or can result in reversing deterioration. When nurses fail to take actions to recognize deterioration, implement relevant assessments, quickly consult relevant health care team members, or rapidly implement urgently needed interventions, client harm and even death can occur. Chapter 5 discusses that this failure to notice or to act is defined as negligence, and violates an important ethical principle of nursing.

To be prepared for taking immediate actions, nurses must anticipate which client condition has high potential for clinical deterioration. Chapter 2 reminds nurses to be intensely monitoring clients who (Padilla & Mayo, 2018):

- Are emergency admissions
- Have acute or preexisting health conditions
- Have had recent surgeries
- Are experiencing critical illnesses

Clients with these conditions likely have the most need for taking immediate action for any deterioration of their condition.

Chapter 4 describes the differences between emergent, urgent, and nonurgent client conditions. Emergent client conditions are described as *life-threatening situations* in which the client could suffer significant harm without taking immediate therapeutic and/or diagnostic action. Clients have multiple, complex health conditions that require the nurse to be prepared to perform comprehensive assessments, prioritize health care needs, and quickly address any emergent conditions that arise. Chapter 4 also discusses the levels of priority for client conditions and describes emergent conditions as Level 1 which are conditions that reflect clinical deterioration with critical findings and could even result in death. Examples of physiologic emergent, Level 1 priority conditions are described in Table 4.1 and can include symptoms of severe cardiac or respiratory distress. Mental health conditions can also be determined to be Level 1 priorities, such as when clients are exhibiting thoughts of suicide or harming others. When taking actions, the nurse needs to be prepared to monitor the client for emergent needs and be able to intervene rapidly to prevent negative clinical outcomes and prevent client harm.

Deterioration of a clinical condition can happen very quickly. One example of rapid deterioration is a postoperative client who has respiratory depression as a result of opioid drug therapy. You should be aware that for any client on opioid therapy, potential deterioration can occur at any time. The risk is increased for opioid-naïve clients who do not routinely use these types of medications. Monitor all postoperative clients being treated with opioids continually for potential deterioration in respiratory status. If deterioration occurs, take immediate actions. In the case of respiratory depression, you should.:

- Initiate a rapid response.
- Immediately assess relevant vital signs, respiratory status, neurologic status, pupil size and reaction, orientation, and level of consciousness.
- Administer naloxone hydrochloride to reverse the effects of the opioids.
- Support the client's respiratory status with oxygen and suction at the bedside in case it should be needed.
- Monitor the client's level of pain because the reversal agent also reverses the analgesic effects of the opioid and pain will recur.

All of these assessments and nursing interventions should occur instantly and without delay to prevent further deterioration of the client's respiratory status. Failing to notice the client's deterioration or failing to take immediate actions could result in client death in this situation and would demonstrate negligence by the nurse. Table 6.1 provides additional examples of emergent deterioration of client conditions and examples of immediate nursing actions that would be indicated.

CLINICAL JUDGMENT TIP

Remember: Nurses must be prepared at all times to use their clinical judgment skills to take immediate actions when a client's condition deteriorates. This process requires that the nurse be able to recognize relevant cues, evaluate hypotheses based on urgency, prioritize what is needed, and take actions on client conditions to prevent or reverse clinical deterioration.

TABLE 6.1 **Examples of Client Conditions that Require Immediate Actions**	
Client Condition	**Immediate Actions Needed**

Autonomic dysreflexia	• Place client in sitting position
	• Assess for and remove/manage the cause
	  • Check for urinary retention or catheter blockage
	  • Check urinary catheter tubing for kinks/obstruction
	  • If no urinary catheter, check for bladder distention and catheterize immediately if indicated
	  • Check for fecal impaction and remove if needed
	  • Monitor blood pressure
	• Give medications as ordered to lower blood pressure

Ischemic stroke	• Initiate rapid response • Anticipate order for intravenous antihypertensive medications • Monitor the client's blood pressure and mean arterial pressure
Status epilepticus	• Protect client from injury • Establish an airway; consult an anesthesia provider or respiratory therapist in the event intubation is needed • Initiate a rapid response • Administer oxygen • Initiate intravenous access and fluids • Administer lorazepam or diazepam via intravenous push
Surgical wound evisceration	• Initiate rapid response and notify surgeon • Place client supine with hips and knees bent • Elevate head of bed 15–20° • Place moistened sterile dressings over exposed viscera using aseptic technique • Assess for shock

Adapted from Ignatavicius, D.D., Rebar, C.R., & Heimgartner, N.M. (2024). *Medical-surgical nursing: Concepts for interprofessional collaborative care* (11th ed.). Elsevier.

Thinking Exercise 6.1 will help you practice what you've learned in this chapter about taking actions. The answer and rationale for the exercise are located at the end of this book.

THINKING EXERCISE 6.1

The nurse is caring for a 35-year-old client in the Emergency Department (ED).

History and Physical	**Nurses Notes**	**Orders**	**Laboratory Results**

1630:   Client is 1-month post-kidney transplantation. States "I don't know what it is but I really don't feel well. I haven't been urinating as much and I feel wiped out." Breath sounds clear throughout all fields. S_1 and S_2 present and regular. Abdomen soft, slightly distended, tenderness to flank at surgical site. Surgical wound dry, no redness or drainage, well approximated. Last bowel movement was yesterday and soft. Bowel sounds present × 4 quadrants. States slightly nauseated; denies vomiting. Skin hot and dry with usual pigmentation. Client voided 25 cc dark yellow urine. VS: T 102.4°F (39.1°C); HR 98 beats per minute; RR 16 breaths per minute; B/P 178/102 mmHg; SpO_2 98% on RA. Wt. 150 lbs. (68.2 kg).

THINKING EXERCISE 6.1—cont'd

Select whether the following anticipated orders are indicated or not indicated for the client at this time.

Anticipated Orders	Indicated	Not Indicated
Obtain serum creatinine, BUN, and potassium		
Insert indwelling urinary catheter		
Obtain abdominal/renal CT scan		
Prepare client for renal biopsy		
Administer increased doses of immunosuppressive drugs		
Initiate intravenous steroids		
Prepare client for emergency surgery to remove kidney		
Prepare client for dialysis		

CATEGORIES OF NURSING ACTIONS

Chapter 5 discusses two types of solutions for taking actions that can be used to meet desired clinical outcomes: independent and collaborative. Remember that independent solutions are potential actions the nurse can perform without assistance or "permission" from other members of the health care team. Collaborative solutions are actions that involve team members across health care professions and may require instruction or "permission" from a physician or other health care prescriber. Although some textbooks state that some nursing actions are *dependent*, nurses always need to think about every action to determine if it is appropriate and safe for the client. Therefore, this book does not include this category. When taking actions, nurses use both independent and collaborative actions to provide a comprehensive approach which will best result in improving the client condition.

Chapter 5 discusses priorities to consider when generating independent and collaborative solutions for taking action which include:
- Considering client and family preferences
- Identifying relevant social determinants of health
- Using best current evidence

These priorities are also important when considering which action/s to take. Keep in mind that it is very important to consider client and family preferences whenever possible. For example, a client who is experiencing blood loss and does not wish to receive blood products will need an alternative solution for taking actions that may be different than the first-line standard of care. Nurses need to be aware of and consider any potential social determinants of health that might impact the client when determining actions. In some cases, the nurse's actions include assisting the client to obtain needed resources. The nurse must take actions using solutions that are based on the most recent evidence and reflect current practice. All actions, both independent and collaborative, must be evidence-based to provide optimal care for the client.

Nurses use a wide range of independent and collaborative actions that address a variety of client needs when making clinical judgments to improve clinical outcomes, including:

- Client and family actions
- Physiologic actions
- Behavioral actions
- Safety actions

Family actions are actions that address the needs and priorities of the client and/or family. Chapter 5 introduced PROMs (patient-/client-related outcome measures) which are health outcomes determined in conjunction with or by the client. **Client- and family-centered actions** are actions that focus on what the client and/or family perceives as a priority clinical condition for improving their health conditions. **Physiologic actions** are actions designed to improve the client's physiologic symptoms and/or condition. **Safety actions** are actions that promote the safety of the client. Clients with health care conditions (especially those that are hospitalized) are at increased risk for a wide range of safety concerns which may include but are not limited to:

- Falls
- Pressure injuries
- Secondary infections
- Medical errors
- Venous thromboembolism (VTE)
- Sepsis

Behavioral actions are actions that are designed to help a client improve or manage behaviors such as decreasing anxiety or managing agitation. The nurse must utilize clinical judgment to implement effective independent and collaborative family, physiologic, behavioral, and safety actions to provide care that addresses the comprehensive health care needs of the client.

Independent Nursing Actions

Independent actions are nursing interventions that are nurse-initiated and performed without supervision or direction from others. When taking action, nurses must be aware of the scope of practice for the state in which they live and only perform independent actions that are within their legal scope to provide independently. Many actions require an advanced practice provider license for prescribing medication, performing procedures, or ordering diagnostic testing. These actions would be outside the scope of practice for generalist registered or licensed practical nurses. It is important for nurses to be very familiar with the scope of practice for the state where they practice when determining which independent actions to take.

Knowing the correct evidence-based procedure or method of performing any action is critical. A nurse who has not learned how to use a specific type of piece of equipment should not utilize the device until properly educated. Nurses must know what types of precautions are needed when taking actions and what types of observations may be needed following the action. Nurses are responsible for not only performing the intervention, but also knowing potential side or adverse effects that might occur and be prepared to intervene as necessary (Potter et al., 2021). For example, a nurse monitoring a cardiac monitor needs to be familiar with cardiac rhythms and be prepared to properly intervene when a dysrhythmia occurs.

The nurse uses the cognitive skills of recognizing cues, analyzing cues, prioritizing hypotheses, and generating solutions to determine which independent actions to take depending on the client's condition. Be sure to take actions that focus on the client and family, physiologic, behavioral, and safety needs. Table 6.2 provides examples of independent client and family, physiologic, behavioral, and safety actions.

TABLE 6.2 Independent Client and Family, Physiologic, Behavioral, and Safety Actions

Type of Action	Independent Nursing Action

Client and family actions	• Provide education on client condition
	• Support client and/or family preferences which may include:
	  • Desire for or against resuscitation (DNR)
	  • Beliefs regarding blood transfusions or medical treatments
	  • Dietary preferences
	  • Spiritual support or preferences
	  • Nontraditional health practices
	  • Organ donation
	• Inform health care team of client preferences
	• Provide emotional support through therapeutic communication to client/family

Physiologic needs	• Assess vital signs • Monitor laboratory results • Administer CPR if indicated and preferred by client • Monitor intake and output • Assess level of pain • Perform neurovascular assessments on casted extremity • Monitor fetal heart tones • Elevate head of bed for client with respiratory distress.
Behavioral actions	• Reorient client with confusion to person, place, time, and/or situation • Use therapeutic communication to decrease anxiety • Provide calm, soothing environment for client who is agitated or distressed • Perform mini-mental status exam or other mental status assessment • Implement suicide precautions for those at risk for self-harm (this is also a safety action) • Implement deescalation techniques for client with agitation (this is also a safety action)
Safety actions	• Implement fall risk precautions • Maintain suction at the bedside for clients at risk of aspiration • Reposition clients frequently to prevent skin breakdown • Monitor temperature and CBC for clients at risk for infections • Ambulate clients when indicated to prevent VTE or other health complications • Monitor wounds for signs of infection or bleeding • Implement isolation protocols for infectious disease • Monitor medical equipment device sites frequently for potential skin breakdown and apply protective devices when available.

Data from Ignatavicius, D.D., Rebar, C.R., & Heimgartner, N.M. (2024). *Medical-surgical nursing: Concepts for clinical judgment and collaborative care* (11th ed.). Elsevier.

Collaborative Nursing Actions

Collaborative nursing actions are interventions that require instructions from or participation by the interdisciplinary health care team. As stated earlier, be sure you fully understand the scope of practice for the state in which you work to know which actions are independent and which require collaboration with another health care provider. Be sure to only perform those collaborative actions for which you are prepared or educated.

Collaborative actions that require instructions from another member of the health care team include actions that must be prescribed. Examples of prescribed actions include administering medications, infusion fluids, oxygen therapy, respiratory treatments, or diet selection. The nurse needs to know when a collaborative action may be needed, even though it should not be performed without obtaining permission. For example, the nurse needs to recognize that a client with an SpO$_2$ of 88% likely needs supplemental oxygen. Depending on agency policy, the nurse *may* need to contact the provider to obtain the order for administering this therapy.

The nurse needs to be familiar with which providers have prescriptive authority and for what interventions. For example, a physical therapist can prescribe therapy and methods for ambulation for a client. A physician, nurse practitioner, resident physician, or physician assistant is able to prescribe medication, diet, or treatments. A respiratory therapist can order supplemental oxygen therapy and breathing treatments. The nurse also must be familiar with which type of provider to contact for each client care situation. For example, a nurse would contact the client's surgeon when a postoperative client is having increased pain at the surgical site. But when this same client is having a hypertensive crisis, the surgeon may prefer that the nurse notify the hospitalist physician who is managing the unit and has more experience treating this type of complication. Collaborative actions take expert coordination and communication by the nurse to effectively involve the correct team member for the correct action at the correct time.

Other types of collaborative actions include nurse-driven protocols and standing orders. Nurse-driven protocols are formal, agreed-upon policies that allow nurses to make certain decisions based on their scope of nursing practice without consulting a health care provider for intervention orders. These protocols are evidence-based policies developed by and agreed upon by the health care team and include input from physicians, pharmacists, nurses, and any other relevant team stakeholder such as respiratory or physical therapy (Barto, 2019). The purpose of nursing protocols is to improve client outcomes, promote client safety in a timely manner, and improve quality of care. Hospitals use protocols that are developed to address core CMS (Center for Medicaid and Medicare Services) guidelines. CMS reduces payment to hospitals when clients develop certain health care-associated complications during hospitalizations (Center for Medicaid and Medicare Services, 2022). For example, CMS reviews hospital data and may reduce payment for any hospitalized client who develops the following secondary infections:

- Central line-associated bloodstream infection (CLABSI)
- Catheter-associated urinary tract infection (CAUTI)
- Surgical site infection (SSI)
- Methicillin-resistant *Staphylococcus aureus* (MRSA) bacteremia
- *Clostridium difficile* infection (CDI)

The aim of this fee reduction is to encourage hospitals to provide optimal care in a timely manner to prevent these complications from occurring.

A hospital might elect to use a nurse-driven protocol for removal of urinary catheters to prevent urinary tract infections in order to prevent CAUTI. Protocols usually begin with algorithms for assessment to determine if the client meets the criteria for the protocol. One sample protocol provided by Agency for Healthcare and Research Quality (AHRQ, 2020) states that the nurse should assess a client each morning for presence of a urinary catheter and if so, evaluate the need for continued use. Then the nurse would review if the client demonstrates or meets any of the following criteria for maintaining the catheter with the algorithm listed in Table 6.3.

TABLE 6.3 Sample Protocol for Urinary Catheter Removal to Prevent CAUTI

CATHETER DISCONTINUATION PROTOCOL FOR INDWELLING URINARY CATHETERS

DAILY MORNING ASSESSMENT: DOES THE CLIENT MEET ANY OF THE CRITERIA BELOW?

Criteria	Yes	No
Client has urinary retention or neurogenic bladder	☐	☐
Catheter for short perioperative use and/or for urologic study	☐	☐
Client requires highly accurate output measurements in ICU	☐	☐
Catheter placed by urology service	☐	☐
Needs assistance with healing severe perineal wounds in incontinent clients	☐	☐
Requires strict immobilization for trauma	☐	☐
Is undergoing hospice or comfort care and catheter was requested by client	☐	☐
If answer to any of the above criteria is no, discontinue urinary catheter.	Date discontinued	Time

Observation of client after discontinuing catheter:

6 hours post catheter removal: Client voids with no symptoms	No action needed	
Client voids within 6 hours but has symptoms of abdominal fullness or discomfort, complete bladder scan	<300 mL: Observe and repeat post-void bladder scan within 2 hours. If symptoms persist, contact provider	>300–500 mL, intermittent catheterization. Repeat post-void bladder scan once every 6 hours and if symptoms persist, contact provider
Client unable to void within 6 hours, complete bladder scan	<300 mL: Repeat scan within 2 hours if symptoms persist and contact provider	>300–500 mL; intermittent catheterization. Repeat bladder scan once every 6 hours if symptoms persist and contact provider

Adapted from the Agency for Healthcare and Research Quality (AHRQ). (2020). Toolkit for reducing catheter-associated urinary tract infections in hospital units: Implementation Guide, Appendix M. Example of a nurse-driven protocol for catheter removal. Retrieved from https://www.ahrq.gov/hai/cauti-tools/impl-guide/implementation-guide-appendix-m.html

This protocol is designed to prevent ongoing urinary catheter use in hospitalized clients. Unnecessary catheterization can result in urinary tract infections and complications such as sepsis, which can be life-threatening. This protocol provides nurses the authority to remove a catheter when the client no longer meets the criteria. Protocols are an effective, evidence-based method for preventing any delay of care; they provide nurses the autonomy and authority to take actions in certain circumstances.

CLINICAL JUDGMENT TIP

Remember: Be sure to check your agency's policies and protocols for taking actions. Protocols are an effective, evidence-based method for preventing any delay of care; they provide nurses the autonomy and authority to take actions in certain circumstances.

Standing orders are collaborative actions that are preapproved evidence-based orders developed by relevant health care team stakeholders. They may be implemented in a variety of settings including the emergency department, critical care unit, acute care unit, and ambulatory care clinic setting. Standing orders allow for more timely action by giving preapproval from the prescriber for a nurse to implement needed interventions using specific assessment criteria. The standing order describes the parameter of the situation where the nurse may act to carry out specific orders for a client experiencing symptoms or health care needs. Situations that may utilize standing orders include but are not limited to:

- Administering immunizations
- Health screenings
- Telephone triage and advice
- Obtaining lab tests or implementing treatments for certain conditions that are time-sensitive
- Enhancing client comfort (e.g., acetaminophen for fever)

Standing orders can provide the nurse autonomy in certain situations to act quickly and independently in improving a client's condition and preventing deterioration. For example, for clients having a myocardial infarction, the nurse can obtain electrocardiogram (ECG) results and administer aspirin while waiting for a provider to arrive and provide further orders. Rapid administration of aspirin prevents or slows clotting of platelets in the blood supply that supplies the heart (Ignatavicius et al., 2024). Standing orders and nurse-driven protocols are effective, evidence-based collaborative actions for improving client clinical outcomes.

CLINICAL JUDGMENT TIP

Remember: Nurses utilize both independent and collaborative actions within the scope of their practice when taking actions to improve the client's clinical condition. Collaborative actions require participation and possibly prescriptions or instructions from other team members prior to implementation. The nurse needs to be familiar with which collaborative action may be needed to request these actions from the appropriate health care professional.

Research is emerging demonstrating the effectiveness of nurse-led interventions. Kelly et al. (2022) conducted a systematic review and meta-analysis to determine the effectiveness of nurse-led interventions for cancer-related symptoms (Box 6.1).

BOX 6.1   Evidence-Based Practice

How effective are nurse-led interventions?
Kelly, D., Campbell, P., Torrens, C., Caralambous, A. Ostlund, U., Eicher, M., Larsson, M., Nohavova, I., Olsson, C., Simpson, M., Patiraki, E., Sarp, L., Wiseman, T., Oldenmenger, W., & Wells, M. (2022). The effectiveness of nurse-led interventions for cancer symptom management 2000–2018: A Systematic review and meta-analysis. *Health Sciences Review, 4,* 1–11.

The authors conducted a scoping review of current research articles to identify the effectiveness of nurse-led interventions for cancer symptom management. The review of the selected 149 studies revealed that nurse-led interventions were effective in relieving the discomfort associated with cancer and cancer therapies. More specific results of this study included that nurse-led interventions were effective in improving:

- Nausea and vomiting
- Constipation
- Fatigue
- Psychological morbidity (anxiety, depression, mood)

Interestingly enough, the researchers did not find clear evidence that nurse-led interventions were effective in managing pain, although it is reported that other studies have found that nurse-led, nonpharmacological interventions for pain are effective. This research provides evidence that supports the importance of the nurse to be able to determine and implement interventions for clients to alleviate symptoms of discomfort.

Although the study did not address which types of interventions are more or less effective, the study did demonstrate that when nurses provide interventions for relieving symptoms associated with cancer, clients experience relief from discomfort or potentially life-threatening symptoms, such as nausea and vomiting.

The study by Kelly et al. (2022) supports the importance of effective clinical judgment for taking actions and the use of independent and collaborative nurse-led actions for improving client conditions. Use of protocols, standing orders, and evidence-based independent and collaborative nursing actions result in care that can be provided in a timely manner without delay by repeatedly obtaining permissions from other health care professionals. These tools result in the nurse being able to more rapidly take actions to prevent further clinical deterioration or increased discomfort.

Thinking Exercise 6.2 will help you practice what you've learned in this chapter about taking action. The answer and rationale for this exercise are located at the end of this book.

THINKING EXERCISE 6.2

The nurse is caring for a 17-year-old client in the Emergency Department (ED).

History and Physical	Nurses Notes	Orders	Laboratory Results

2100:   Client identifies self as transgender person and reports history of type 1 diabetes mellitus. States "I feel so shaky and thirsty. My head is killing me. I vomited twice this afternoon. I feel like I have to urinate all the time." Client reports being unhoused and has irregular access to needed supplies to manage diabetes. Client's skin feels warm and dry, face flushed. Fruity scent to breath; client breathing rapidly, respirations deep. Breath sounds clear throughout lung fields. S_1 and S_2 present and regular. Abdomen soft and flat, bowel sounds present ×4 quadrants. Last bowel movement was yesterday and soft. States slightly nauseated. Appears drowsy, oriented × 4. VS: T 98.4°F (36.9°C); HR 80 beats per minute; RR 32 breaths per minute, deep; B/P 88/60 mmHg; SpO_2 98% on RA. Wt. 140 lbs. (63.5 kg).

Select whether the following potential nursing actions are indicated or not indicated for the client at this time.

Potential Nursing Actions	Indicated	Not Indicated
Initiate intravenous fluids		
Administer oral glucose		
Initiate intravenous regular insulin		
Initiate intravenous long-acting insulin		
Initiate cardiac monitoring		
Obtain bedside glucose and ketone samples		
Obtain glucose, electrolytes, and blood gases		
Obtain BUN, creatinine, and liver enzymes		
Administer oral carbohydrates (e.g., orange juice)		

DIRECT VERSUS INDIRECT NURSING ACTIONS

The nurse considers a variety of solutions before taking actions to improve a client's clinical condition. As discussed previously, the nurse can select independent or collaborative actions to meet the client's needs. These action types can be further divided into two categories: direct and indirect nursing actions. The nurse must select the appropriate direct and/or indirect actions to meet the client's needs. Direct actions involve providing care directly to the client through interaction with the client. Indirect actions involve providing care that directly benefits the client, but does not require interaction with the client. You need to be familiar with both types of actions to select the best action for improving the client condition in the most efficient way.

Direct Nursing Actions

Direct nursing actions are interventions that are directly implemented by the nurse interacting with the client. Direct actions can be nurse-initiated, such as when a nurse changes a client's position to improve the client's comfort. Direct actions can also be provider-initiated (collaborative), such as when a provider orders a medication that the nurse administers. Regardless of who initiates the action, a direct action involves a nurse performing an action that directly involves interaction with a client.

Nurses perform a wide range of direct actions daily which comprise the majority of client care. Direct actions include not only nursing interventions but also client assessments. Table 6.4 provides examples of independent and collaborative direct care actions to manage client conditions affecting various body systems.

TABLE 6.4   Examples of Direct Actions for Client Conditions Affecting Various Body Systems

Body Systems	Direct Nursing Actions
Cardiovascular	• Administering CPR • Assessing peripheral pulses • Obtaining pulse and blood pressures • Applying compression stockings to decrease edema and prevent VTE • Administering antihypertensive medication
Gastrointestinal	• Assessing bowel sounds • Palpating the abdomen • Administering enteral feedings • Inserting a nasogastric (NG) tube • Administering proton pump inhibitor medications (PPI) • Removing sutures or surgical staples
Integumentary	• Repositioning clients frequently to prevent skin breakdown • Assessing skin frequently to monitor for potential areas of breakdown • Providing wound care and utilizing prescribed dressings • Inspection of skin for lesions using ABCDE method (**A**symmetry, **B**order [irregular], **C**olor [consistency], **D**iameter [<6mm], and/or **E**levation)
Neurologic	• Assessing level of consciousness and alertness • Reorienting client with confusion to person, place, time, and/or situation • Assessing strength, gait, and symmetry of movement • Obtaining vital signs • Assessing pupils • Administering antiseizure medications • Assisting with lumbar puncture procedure • Managing pain

TABLE 6.4   Examples of Direct Actions for Client Conditions Affecting Various Body Systems—cont'd

Body Systems	Direct Nursing Actions
Respiratory	• Administering a nebulizer treatment • Assessing lung sounds • Assisting the client with incentive spirometer • Initiating and titrating oxygen therapy • Providing oral care for client on ventilator • Assessing respirations for rate, quality, and effort • Assessing chest for retractions • Assisting with insertion of chest tubes • Administering oxygen therapy
Urinary	• Administering intravenous fluids • Administering diuretic medications • Managing and discontinuing urinary catheters • Implementing dialysis procedures • Obtaining temperature to determine presence of infection

Data from Ignatavicius, D.D., Rebar, C.R., & Heimgartner, N.M. (2024). *Medical-surgical nursing: Concepts for clinical judgment and collaborative care* (11th ed.). Elsevier.

Indirect Nursing Actions

Indirect nursing actions support client care and work to improve the client condition, but do not require interaction directly with the client. These actions are performed on behalf of the client and may occur away from the client's bedside. Using indirect actions, the nurse utilizes resources to enhance client care or more deeply evaluate the client's condition. The nurse may use indirect measures to manage the client's environment or equipment to promote safety, such as using aseptic technique for preparing parenteral medications. Indirect measures can also be used to evaluate the client's condition by reviewing or monitoring lab values, history of present illness, or diagnostic reports.

An indirect nursing action that nurses use frequently is communication with the health care team on behalf of the client to improve the client's condition. The nurse participates in or coordinates the care of the client with other members of the team through effective communication. Research has shown that the use of evidence-based methods for communicating in the health care environment results in improved clarity of communication, decreased medical errors, and improved client safety. The Joint Commission (TJC, 2017) reports that the potential for client harm is increased when a health care team member receives information that is inaccurate, incomplete, not timely, or is otherwise not what is needed. TJC (2017) recommends that communication be standardized using tools, templates, checklists, or mnemonics to communicate needed information in a consistent manner. This standardization ensures that communication will be comprehensive and help team members perform more consistently. One evidence-based tool used as an indirect care action for communication is the SBAR communication tool. SBAR communication requires that the nurse communicate the situation, background, assessment, and make a recommendation for the client.

- **S**ituation: Describe what is happening with the client.
- **B**ackground: Explain any background information that may be relevant to the current situation.
- **A**ssessment: Describe assessment data and analysis of the client's problem or need.
- **R**ecommendation/**R**equest: State what is needed or what outcome is desired.

The SBAR tool is described as a tool that is appropriate to communicate to the health care team when a client's situation changes and/or deteriorates. As part of the SBAR communication, nurses must take indirect action by making recommendations or requests for what the client may need. The nurse is often the first person to be aware when client conditions change or the client experiences clinical deterioration. The nurse must report this change to the appropriate provider using the SBAR format and make a request or recommendation for what the client may need. Examples of nurse-driven recommendations or requests include:

- Request the provider prescribe an increased dose of pain medication or an alternative pain medication when the current dose is not effective
- Request the provider prescribe acetaminophen for fever or discomfort
- Recommend to a respiratory therapist that a client have regimen or PRN nebulizer treatments for increased wheezing
- Request the provider order a urinalysis for the older client experiencing painful urination, fever, and delirium
- Recommend to the provider that a client at a long-term care unit be transported to an emergency department for evaluation after a fall and report of wrist pain

Nurses frequently are required to hand-off a client to another member of the health care team. For example, when a client clinically deteriorates on an acute care unit, the nurse may need to hand-off the client to another care provider in a critical care unit or operating suite. Handing-off a client requires that the nurse take actions to communicate to the receiver the client condition and what the plan is for care. Inadequate hand-off communication results in a wide range of adverse events including wrong-site surgery, delay in treatment, falls, and medication errors (TJC, 2017).

The I-PASS communication tool is an evidence-based communication tool for effective client hand-offs from one provider to another which results in comprehensive and consistent communication across levels of care (I-PASS Safety Institute, 2022). I-PASS communication requires the nurse to report:

- **I**llness severity: Describe how acute the illness is at this time: stable or unstable.
- **P**atient summary: Events leading up to admission, hospital course so far, ongoing assessment plan.
- **A**ction List: What needs to be done, when, by whom?
- **S**ituation awareness and contingency plans: What's going on now; what might happen and what is the plan for this?
- **S**ynthesis by receiver: The receiver summarizes the information learned about the client and has a chance to ask further questions. This closes the feedback loop and ensures understanding.

Using standardized tools for communicating to other health care providers is an evidence-based, indirect action for ensuring consistent, comprehensive communication and results in improved clinical outcomes.

Perhaps the most important indirect communication method a nurse uses is documentation of the client's condition, assessment data/client findings, nursing actions, and evaluation of the effectiveness of those actions. Clear documentation informs other team members of the exact status of the client and provides data that are useful when the health care team makes decisions about care. Data that are incomplete or inaccurate can result in the wrong care being prescribed or wrong actions taken. The nurse must take actions to ensure that documentation for the client is clear, comprehensive, effective, and completed in a timely manner.

Fig. 6.1 provides examples of independent and collaborative indirect care actions in each of the action types discussed previously in this chapter (Client and Family, Physiologic, Behavioral, and Safety categories).

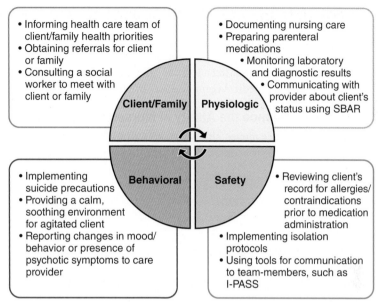

FIG. 6.1 Examples of indirect client/family, physiologic, behavioral, and safety nursing actions.

Thinking Exercise 6.3 will help you practice what you've learned in this chapter about taking action. The answer and rationale for the exercise are located at the end of this book.

THINKING EXERCISE 6.3

The nurse is caring for a 32-year-old client in an acute care obstetrics suite.

History and Physical	Nurses Notes	Orders	Laboratory Results

0500:   Client in active labor, G2, P1. Client at 40W2D gestation by LMP/sonogram. Ultrasound showed no fetal abnormalities at 20 wks. Received appropriate prenatal care. States previous pregnancy uncomplicated; delivered at 38 weeks by SVD. States "I think my water broke." S_1 and S_2 present with regular rate. Breath sounds clear throughout lung fields; respirations slightly increased due to progress of labor. Minimal edema in lower legs and feet. Gravid uterus, fundal height at 40 cm, fetus appears vertex, contractions every 2 minutes + fetal movement although client states movements have been somewhat decreased the last few minutes. Fetal heart rate baseline 150 and variably decreases to 120; fetal monitor shows variable deceleration during uterine contractions. Vaginal exam reveals cervix dilated to 7 cm, fully effaced, fetus station +1, umbilical cord is present in vaginal canal with clear amniotic fluid drainage present. VS: T 99.0°F (37.2°C); HR 98 beats per minute; RR 24 breaths per minute; B/P 140/88 mmHg; SpO_2 98% on RA. Wt. 175 lbs. (79.6 kg).

Select **3** actions the nurse should take **immediately**.
○ Ask another nurse team member to initiate rapid response and notify provider
○ Insert gloved fingers into vaginal canal to manually relieve compression of the cord
○ Place client into side-lying position
○ Ask a nurse team member to administer oxygen 2 L by nasal cannula
○ Ask a nurse team member to start or increase intravenous fluids
○ Ask a nurse team member to prepare for forceps delivery

TAKING ACTIONS TO MAKE SAFE CLINICAL JUDGMENTS

Taking actions to make safe clinical judgments requires higher order thinking to determine the most efficient and expedient method for improving clinical deterioration and attaining desired clinical outcomes. A number of factors can affect the ability to take actions when caring for clients who are experiencing medical complications or clinical deterioration.

Factors that Influence the Ability of Nurses to Take Actions

Many factors influence nurses' ability to take actions. Similar to other cognitive skills described in this book, taking actions is influenced by both nurse factors and system (organizational) factors.

Nurse Factors

Some of the same nurse factors described in Chapter 4 also impact the ability of the nurse to take actions in a timely manner. Nurse factors influencing the ability to take actions include:
- Level of experience
- Expertise and knowledge
- Work experience
- Knowledge of potential nursing actions
- Physical and mental health

The nurse's *level of experience* can greatly impact the ability to take actions. When compared to experienced nurses, novice nurses have had limited opportunity to practice clinical judgment skills, including taking actions. Novices also have limited experience evaluating the effectiveness of nursing care provided for continual improvement. By contrast, experienced nurses have had multiple opportunities to take actions and evaluate outcomes of that action. Professional nursing experience results in continually building a knowledge base and improving clinical judgment skills, including taking actions.

Novice nurses have a basic entry-level understanding about client conditions and their management, and have not worked in many different health care settings. By contrast, nurses who have several years of experience have had much more opportunity to work with different types of:
- Clients, families, cultures
- Health conditions
- Health complications
- Technology and equipment
- Health care settings or units

A nurse who has *work experience* with different types of clients, conditions, technologies, and settings is able to respond and take actions much more quickly than a novice nurse. With work experience, the nurse becomes increasingly skilled at recognizing the need to take actions by rapidly recognizing and analyzing cues, and prioritizing hypotheses.

> **CLINICAL JUDGMENT TIP**
>
> *Remember:* Professional nursing experience results in continually building a knowledge base and improving clinical judgment skills, including taking actions.

With an extensive level of experience in caring for particular types of clients in certain types of settings, the nurse gains *expertise* in certain areas of nursing practice. For example, a nurse who consistently cares for clients in the critical care setting becomes very familiar with the actions needed for these types of complex-care clients. In this setting, the nurse typically encounters the same types of client conditions and utilizes the same technology repeatedly, gaining increased ability to effectively take actions when caring for their clients. The expert nurse is also skilled at quickly determining whether a client condition is nonurgent, urgent, or emergent. This skill enables the expert to determine how quickly a necessary action must be taken to avoid or effectively manage clinical deterioration. The expert nurse is also able to apply this knowledge to other client care settings when needed.

Knowledge of potential nursing actions assists both the novice and the expert nurse when preparing to take actions. Through basic nursing education experiences, nursing students learn the foundational knowledge of potential nursing actions. When practicing as a nurse, the nurse has the opportunity to generate a wide scope of knowledge of potential nursing actions through experience with different client care situations. This knowledge base helps the nurse to create a mental "database" of potential solutions for taking action. The nurse then draws from these proven potential nursing actions to rapidly and effectively take actions without delay or need to seek out resources.

As with any health care profession, the *physical and mental health* of the nurse greatly impact the ability to take actions. Nursing practice is physical and mental work that is at times stressful and challenging. Taking actions in a timely manner can take physical strength and dexterity. Lacking strength or dexterity puts both the nurse and the client at risk for potential harm or injury. For example, physical strength is required when taking actions to reposition or transfer a client. The Centers for Disease Control: National Institute for Occupational Safety and Health (2023) report that the single greatest risk factor for overexertion injuries in nursing is manual client handling. Strength is also required when working with heavy technology or equipment that may need to be lifted, pushed, or pulled. Dexterity is required when manipulating equipment such as establishing peripheral venous access or removing sutures. Without strength and/or dexterity to safely perform needed physical actions, the nurse is at high risk for personal injury and the client is at risk for negative outcomes. Don't forget, though, to follow agency policies to prevent back and other types of personal injury.

It is widely known that persons who are physically and mentally healthy are much more resistant to potential injury or development of disease. Therefore, make physical and mental health a priority and take time for personal care. This practice will ensure that you have the physical and mental capabilities needed for taking actions, and will have decreased risk for suffering harm, acquiring infectious disease, or sustaining an injury.

System Factors

System or organizational factors that impact other clinical judgment cognitive skills discussed throughout this book also impact the ability of the nurse to take actions. Alaseeri et al. (2021) found that nurses report workload, availability of resources, and consistency of policies as major system factors that influence their ability to make safe clinical judgments. An impaired decision-making ability includes an inability to take actions that are timely and safe. As a result, needed actions could be delayed and client conditions may deteriorate.

The *workplace environment* is a factor that greatly impacts the ability of the nurse to take actions. Unfortunately, bullying and violence in the health care environment are widely prevalent for nurses. TJC (2021) reports that 44% of nurses have experienced bullying, and that nurses tend to accept nurse-on-nurse bullying as part of the job, especially for new nurses. The ANA (American Nurses Association, n.d., b) defines **bullying** as "repeated, unwanted, harmful actions intended to humiliate, offend and cause distress." Additionally, nurses often experience violence in the workplace setting. **Workplace violence** is defined as an actual act or threat of physical violence, harassment, or intimidation. Violence can be perpetrated by clients, family members, and hospital personnel. Nurses have experienced not only physical violence but sexual and

psychological assault as well. The ANA (n.d., b) reports that one in four nurses have suffered assault. TJC (2021) reports the most common settings for bullying include:
- Behavioral Health units
- Emergency Departments
- Intensive Care Units
- Long-Term Care on evening and night shifts

Additionally, bullying can result in:
- Low morale
- Lower productivity
- Increased absenteeism
- Increases in client harm, errors, infections, and costs of health care
- Burnout resulting in nurses leaving the profession

Workload is perhaps the most overwhelming factor when trying to take actions. Chapter 4 discusses how work can even be left undone, resulting in important actions not being implemented due to lack of time or competing priorities. Degroot et al. (2022) report that nurses in the United States spend 25%–41% of their time in documentation and feel that this task contributes to the perception of an overwhelming workload.

Additionally, *lack of available resources and staff* impacts the ability of a nurse to take actions. Care is delayed when there are not enough nurses to care for the number of clients or when clients require high acuity, complex care. Care is also delayed when needed equipment or resources are unavailable. In this case, the nurse must take valuable time to find needed equipment or find an alternative solution for implementation that may not be as desirable.

To support efforts to improve the environment for nursing, the ANA (n.d., a) has developed The Nurses Bill of Rights for a Healthy Work Environment. This document states that nurses have the right to an environment of safety for themselves and the clients for whom they care. Additionally, it states that nurses have the right to freely and openly advocate for themselves and their clients (ANA, n.d., a). Nurses need to advocate for environments that have adequate resources, maintain evidence-based practices, and are free from bullying and abuse. Advocating for a safe workplace environment will ultimately result in nurses who are better able to take appropriate action to improve client outcomes.

Role of Nursing Knowledge Base

Chapter 3 discusses the fundamental knowledge needed for making clinical judgments. Gillespie (2010) describes key areas of foundational knowledge (summarized in Table 3.3) that include knowledge of:
- The nursing profession
- Yourself
- The clinical situation
- The client's clinical condition and assessment data
- The person's (client's) past experiences with health care and responses to condition and treatment

This basic foundational knowledge is essential for taking actions to make safe clinical judgments. The nurse must be aware of nursing knowledge to be familiar with actions that are reflective of current, evidence-based practices and protocols. The nurse must recognize personal strengths, experiences, biases, and lack of experience when taking actions and not take actions that are unfamiliar. Foundational knowledge of clinical conditions requires that you know the appropriate pathophysiology, common clinical cues, patterns of typical cases, predicted outcomes, and potential client responses to determine safe actions for improving outcomes. The nurse must know the client's assessment data, and personal preferences and experiences with health care to take safe nursing actions that are client-centered.

Chapter 4 reminds us that in addition to foundational knowledge, nurses need knowledge of priority-setting approaches and models. These approaches and models are also relevant when taking action. Nurses must be able to use evidence-based methods of prioritization such as the ABCVL or CURE models when determining in which order to take needed actions. Emergent needs must be addressed first. Knowledge of priority setting methods will enable you to take actions in the most efficient and effective order to achieve optimal client outcomes.

CLINICAL JUDGMENT TIP

Remember: Knowledge of client conditions and priority setting methods will help you take actions in the most efficient and effective order to achieve optimal client outcomes.

Role of Client Condition and Context

Nurses need to consider not only the role of the client condition but also the context in which the condition is occurring when determining how to take actions. Clients may have mental health needs or physical health needs. In most cases, clients are complex and have both mental health and physical needs. Chapter 4 reminds us that it is important to utilize prioritization tools to determine the most urgent need, whether it be mental or physical. The nurse should take actions on first-level priorities immediately whether it be a mental health priority such as risk for suicide or a physical priority such as labored breathing and retractions. Remember, the nurse needs to be familiar with and be prepared for taking actions quickly on first-level priorities as the client is at risk for immediate harm or even death.

Physical Health Needs

Physical health needs of clients resulting in client conditions have been discussed extensively throughout this book. Client conditions cause impairment or dysfunction of a wide range of body systems impacting the overall functioning and health of the client. Examples of physical client conditions include:

- Dysrhythmias
- Dyspnea
- Pain
- Infection
- Fracture
- Stroke
- Hemorrhage
- Fluid and electrolyte imbalances

Nurses must be familiar with these various client conditions and a wide range of solutions for addressing them. Then the nurse is better able to utilize clinical judgment cognitive skills to prioritize needs and take appropriate actions in a timely manner to prevent potentially life-threatening clinical deterioration.

Mental Health Needs

The mental or behavioral health needs of the client also help the nurse determine which actions to take. As stated previously, clients usually present with both mental and physical health needs. Physical client conditions often cause a high level of stress and anxiety for clients which results in mental health needs. Conversely, mental health needs can result in failing to care for self, which can result in physical health conditions. A large number of clients are impacted by serious mental health needs, which can be debilitating or life-threatening. The National Alliance on Mental Illness (Brister, 2018) reports that one in five adults will experience mental illness in a given year and that depression, dysthymic disorder, and bipolar disorder are the third most common causes of hospitalization in the US. Brister (2018) also reports that clients with mental illness have an increased risk of having chronic medical conditions and have a shorter life span often due to treatable medical conditions. Therefore, when taking actions, be sure to consider both the client's physical and mental health, prioritize all client conditions, and take appropriate actions as needed.

CLINICAL JUDGMENT TIP

Remember: When prioritizing health conditions for determining actions, do not overlook the serious potential complications that mental health conditions have the potential to cause.

Contextual Considerations

Nurses should be very familiar with the environment in which they are providing care so that they can be prepared to know which resources are available for taking actions. For example, a nurse in the Emergency Department (ED) is well equipped with resources to manage a wide range of life-threatening emergencies. The ED nurse coordinates the care of the client through use of these easily available resources to manage physical crises. But the nurse is not as well equipped to manage an older client with delirium or a client experiencing psychoses because the environment is usually not set up to provide for these types of health needs. Oftentimes, it becomes necessary for a client with these types of conditions to be managed for extended periods in the ED as the client waits for an acute care bed to become available. The emergency nurse must take actions to create a safe environment for this client by removing potentially dangerous medical equipment, decreasing stimuli in the environment, providing a staff member to sit with the client, and frequently monitoring the client until the bed becomes available.

Actions that a nurse is able to take can also be limited by what is available to the nurse. For example, a school nurse does not have the same supplies, staff, or providers available as in an acute care setting. Yet, school nurses must deal with daily urgent health needs which may include:

- Allergic reactions
- Hyper-/hypoglycemia
- Seizures
- Injuries such as fractures or lacerations

The nurse in the school setting may have some emergency supplies such as an epinephrine pen or dressings for bleeding, but the nurse is limited in taking actions by the equipment available. For example, the nurse may not have a provider available to suture lacerations, but will need to use available resources to stabilize the wound while waiting for the child to be taken to the ED or urgent care.

The nurse should prepare in advance for what actions would most likely be needed in the particular context of care by reviewing:

- Types of conditions commonly occurring in the population
- Types of injuries commonly seen in the population (different types of injuries/emergencies; must be familiar with developmental needs for safety)
- Types of evidence-based actions generally needed for these types of conditions and injuries
- Equipment on hand to be prepared to stabilize these conditions and injuries

It is especially important to remember that taking actions is not a "one size fits all." What works in one situation may not work in another. For example, caring for children and adults with the same condition results in taking some actions that are similar and some that are different. Additionally, a medication that may have worked well for one client may not work for another. Actions depend not only on the context of the setting but also the context of the individual client and family.

CLINICAL JUDGMENT TIP

Remember. There is no "one size fits all" when taking actions to improve client outcomes or prevent deterioration. Be sure to consider the context of the client and setting when determining which actions to take.

Strategies for How to Take Actions

This chapter has explored the process for taking actions and the factors that affect your ability as a nurse to use this clinical judgment cognitive skill. This discussion highlights the strategies you should use to accurately take actions as a client's condition changes or deteriorates (Box 6.2).

BOX 6.2 Strategies for Taking Action

- Generate solutions for client condition priorities and expected outcomes through recognition of relevant cues, analysis of cues, and prioritization of hypotheses
- Use an appropriate model for selecting and prioritizing which actions should be implemented and in what order
- Take immediate actions on any emergent Level 1 conditions
- Take actions using solutions that will impact the most urgent client condition

---

Generate Solutions for Client Condition Priorities

Chapter 2 discusses recognizing relevant cues as the initial step in determining whether the client is currently or is at risk for experiencing clinical deterioration. Chapter 3 describes the process for analyzing relevant cues through clustering and recognizing relationships between the cues to create hypotheses about potential client conditions. Chapter 4 provides strategies for determining how to prioritize which client conditions are highest priority through the use of evidence-based prioritization models. Using these three cognitive skills and appropriate evidence-based tools (e.g., ABCDE Prioritization Model), the nurse is able to determine which client condition should be a priority for generating solutions to take action.

After priority conditions have been determined, the nurse can then generate potential solutions for implementation aimed at addressing the client's highest priority needs to prevent or manage clinical deterioration. Chapter 5 discusses the importance of generating solutions that are evidence-based, inclusive of client and family priorities, and aimed at achieving desired clinical outcomes.

Use a Model to Select and Prioritize Nursing Actions

Once solutions have been generated, the nurse selects the most appropriate, evidence-based action to prevent clinical deterioration or address the client's immediate needs. The nurse can use the same models for prioritizing client conditions to prioritize the order for taking this action. For example, the ABCDE model for prioritization of client conditions also provides direction for prioritizing taking actions (see Chapter 4) and is a mnemonic for:

- **A**irway
- **B**reathing

- Circulation
- Disability
- Exposure

This model indicates that the airway is the highest priority for the client; without a patent airway, the client is in a life-threatening situation. Through use of this mnemonic, the nurse can prioritize actions that establish a client's airway.

The CURE model discussed in Chapter 4 also provides direction for the order that actions should be taken. This model categorizes priorities in client conditions as:

- **C**ritical acute, life-threatening conditions that require immediate intervention; emergent, Level 1 priorities
- **U**rgent conditions that place the client at significant safety risk and require prompt action (similar to Level 2 priorities)
- **R**outine maintenance care needed for chronic stable client conditions
- **E**xtra action or care that is not essential for client safety but important for nurses to provide (similar to Level 3 priorities)

Using the CURE model, the nurse would direct actions first toward any client conditions in the critical, emergent category because they are highly likely to result in immediate client harm. Then the nurse would examine all other priority client conditions, and take actions by addressing urgent issues. Once the client's condition stabilizes, the nurse would be able to take actions on routine maintenance stable chronic conditions and conditions that require extra action.

When caring for any client, the nurse should not overlook mental health conditions when setting priorities for taking actions. Use of an evidence-based prioritization method can assist in determining if there is a Level 1 mental health condition that requires immediate action(s). Table 4.3 in Chapter 4 provides a summary of four crisis phases (client conditions) with a description of each phase and clinical cues to assist with categorizing the urgency of each condition. For example, clients in Phase 4 exhibit characteristics for extremely urgent, Level 1 intervention such as:

- Clients may pace; clench their fists; perspire heavily; and/or demonstrate rapid, shallow, panting breathing.
- Clients demonstrate emotional lability and possible psychotic thinking.
- *Clients may be a danger to themselves or others.*

This model is a useful tool for determining in which order actions should be taken to address mental health clinical conditions.

Take Actions on Emergent Level 1 Priorities

As discussed previously in this chapter, remember that you must take actions on Level 1 priorities first. Examples of Level 1 emergent priorities include:

- Absence of pulse or respirations
- Obstructed airway
- Potential harm to self or others
- Crushing chest pain with bradycardia
- Retractions with nasal flaring

As previously discussed, Padilla and Mayo (2018) remind nurses to be highly vigilant and prepared to take immediate action on clients who:

- Are emergency admissions
- Have acute or preexisting health conditions
- Have had recent surgeries
- Are recovering from critical illnesses

The nurse must take actions to immediately address all Level 1 life-threatening priorities before moving to take actions on Level 2 urgent priorities.

Take Actions to Impact the Most Urgent Client Need

Once all Level 1 priorities have been addressed and the client's conditions are no longer life-threatening, the nurse then uses a prioritization model to take actions on other client conditions in order of urgency. Chapter 4 describes urgent Level 2 conditions as those that pose a significant safety risk and have the potential to cause client deterioration. These Level 2 conditions should be targeted for action once emergent, critical needs have been stabilized. After all Level 2 priorities have been addressed or stabilized, the nurse can then take actions on all remaining priority client conditions that do not pose a risk to client safety. Table 6.5 provides examples of actions for urgent and nonurgent conditions for contrast and comparison.

TABLE 6.5 Examples of Taking Actions for Urgent and Nonurgent Conditions by Body System/Type

Body System/Type	Urgent Actions	Nonurgent Actions
Respiratory	• Monitoring chest X-ray results for client with COPD • Assisting with procedure for insertion of chest tubes • Administering nebulizer treatment for acute respiratory wheezing	• Providing education on smoking cessation • Administering pneumonia and influenza vaccines • Administering maintenance inhaler medications
Cardiac/perfusion	• Notifying provider for neurovascular impairment in a casted limb • Monitoring cardiac enzyme values in client with chest pain • Administering intravenous anticoagulants for VTE	• Elevating edematous limbs to promote circulation • Applying compression stockings • Administering maintenance antihypertensive medications
Immunity	• Assisting with lumbar puncture for suspected meningitis • Implementing appropriate infection control measures for client with infectious disease • Monitoring vital signs, especially temperature for clients who are immunocompromised	• Providing education on use of epipen for allergic reactions • Administering vaccines (e.g., Tdap) • Administering biologic medications for those with chronic immune disorders
Neurological	• Assessing head injury client for signs and symptoms of increased intracranial pressure (ICP) • Preventing falls in client with vertigo • Providing for safety and maintaining airway during seizures	• Administering long-term medication management for seizure disorder • Assisting client with physical and occupational therapy exercises for impairments from stroke • Providing education on use of assistive devices for clients with impairments

Continued

TABLE 6.5   Examples of Taking Actions for Urgent and Nonurgent Conditions by Body System/Type—cont'd

Body System/Type	Urgent Actions	Nonurgent Actions
Mental/behavioral health	• Deescalating severe agitation and/or aggression • Administering depression screenings for clients with complaints of acute symptoms • Assessing risk for self-harm • Providing for safety in client experiencing psychoses	• Providing education on self-care to promote mental health • Administering long-term depression medication • Monitoring relevant lab results such as lithium levels

Adapted from Ignatavicius, D.D., Rebar, C.R., & Heimgartner, N.M. (2024). *Medical-surgical nursing: Concepts for interprofessional collaborative care* (11th ed.). Elsevier; Brister, T. (2018). *Navigating a mental health crisis: A NAMI resource guide for those experiencing a mental health emergency*. National Alliance on Mental Illness. Retrieved from https://www.nami.org/Support-Education/Publications-Reports/Guides/Navigating-a-Mental-Health-Crisis/Navigating-A--Mental-Health-Crisis?utm_source=website&utm_medium=cta&utm_campaign=crisisguide

Thinking Exercise 6.4 will help you practice what you've learned in this chapter about taking action(s). The answer and rationale for the exercise are located at the end of this book.

THINKING EXERCISE 6.4

The nurse is caring for an 18-year-old client in an acute care mental health setting.

History and Physical	Nurses Notes	Orders	Laboratory Results

2000:   Client with history of bipolar disorder admitted yesterday with report of ongoing depression despite medication therapy. Client states depression has worsened over the last 6 weeks resulting in loss of employment due to overwhelming fatigue and inability to arrive for early morning shifts. Client has been on aripiprazole daily for 9 months, although client reports nonadherence at times with medication due to "forgetting." Reports increased incidence of alcohol abuse at 3–4 beers/alcoholic drinks/day. Client states risk for losing housing as mother has become frustrated with his increased alcohol intake, lack of ability to sustain employment, and extremes in mood swings. Client's mother reports feeling "afraid at times" due to the extreme agitation client occasionally exhibits. Describes having a serious relationship that recently ended as partner "was tired of unstable mood and depression." At this time, client is extremely agitated and talking in a loud volume of voice to another client on the unit. Client states "If this guy doesn't quit talking, I am going to lose it and hurt somebody." Client's hands are shaking, face is red; standing in hallway near other clients.

Which of the following actions would the nurse take? **Select all that apply.**
○ Maintain continuous eye contact
○ Move quickly
○ Keep voice calm
○ Raise voice to gain client's immediate attention
○ Offer options for what the client might want
○ Take control
○ Give the client space
○ Gently announce actions before initiating them
○ Initiate a concealed "Code White" to alert security

END-OF-CHAPTER EXERCISES

Additional End-of-Chapter Exercises will help you apply what you've learned in this chapter. The answers and rationales for these exercises are located at the end of this book.

↯ END-OF-CHAPTER THINKING EXERCISE 6.1

The nurse is caring for an 83-year-old client in an acute care setting.

History and Physical	Nurses Notes	Orders	Laboratory Results

1700:   Client admitted yesterday for surgical reduction and stabilization of fractured right femur. States pain is 2/10; denies need for pain medication at this time. S_1 and S_2 present; rate regular. Breath sounds clear throughout lung fields; respirations nonlabored. Abdomen soft; bowel sounds present × 4 quadrants. Alert and oriented × 4, PERRLA. Right leg splint dry and intact; toes warm, pink, and mobile with cap refill <3 seconds. Client instructed on use of incentive spirometer. VS: T 99.0°F (37.2°C); HR 80 beats per minute; RR 16 breaths per minute; B/P 130/80 mmHg; SpO_2 98% on RA.

1830:   Client reports "My chest hurts. I just don't feel right." Very anxious and asking for doctor. Client is dyspneic with dry cough. Skin warm and diaphoretic with usual pigmentation. S_1, S_2, and S_3 sounds present with tachycardia. Breath sounds clear in right lung, crackles in left lower lobe anterior and posterior. Slight circumoral cyanosis present. Capillary refill sluggish. VS: T 99.0°F (37.2°C); HR 110 beats per minute; RR 36 breaths per minute; B/P 90/68 mmHg; SpO_2 88% on RA.

For each body system/need below, specify the potential nursing actions that would be appropriate for the care of the client. Each body system/need may support more than one nursing action.

Body Systems/Needs	Potential Nursing Actions
Respiratory	☐ Place client in high-Fowler's (sitting) position
	☐ Administer oxygen
	☐ Administer albuterol via nebulizer
Cardiovascular	☐ Initiate continuous telemetry monitoring
	☐ Administer anticoagulants
	☐ Administer nitroglycerin sublingual prn chest pain; repeat as needed every 5 minutes for up to 15 minutes
Mental health	☐ Reassure client everything will be fine
	☐ Speak in a calm voice
	☐ Keep room stimulation level low

END-OF-CHAPTER THINKING EXERCISE 6.2

The nurse is caring for an 18-month-old client in an acute care setting.

History and Physical	Nurses Notes	Orders	Laboratory Results

0500:   18-month-old client admitted last evening for gastroenteritis and dehydration. Child has had history of nausea, vomiting (2–3 times/day) and diarrhea (6–8 watery stools/day) × 4 days with elevated temperatures. Client sleeping. Has IV of D_5/0.45% normal saline at 50 mL per hour in the right hand. IV site has good blood return, no redness or swelling noted. S_1 and S_2 present. Breath sounds clear throughout lung fields. Abdomen soft with hyperactive bowel sounds present × 4 quadrants. Last bowel movement was at 2200. Skin warm and dry with usual pigmentation, turgor elastic. Last void was at 1600. VS: T 101.0°F (38.3°C); HR 100 beats per minute; RR 20 breaths per minute; B/P 90/65 mmHg; SpO_2 99% on RA. Wt. 26 lbs. (68.2 kg).

0730:   Child's parent states "I'm not sure what's wrong, but the bed feels really wet. He just woke up crying. I think he's hungry, can he eat?" Child crying; has had large, watery diarrhea stool, diaper saturated. IV site leaking clear fluid, dressing saturated. Right hand cool to touch and edematous. VS: T 100.8°F (38.2°C); HR 120 beats per minute; RR 24 breaths per minute; B/P 100/75 mmHg; SpO_2 99% on RA. Wt. 26 lbs. (11.8 kg).

Select whether the following potential nursing actions are indicated or not indicated for the client at this time.

Potential Nursing Actions	Indicated	Not Indicated
Remove dressings; resecure IV catheter and reapply dressing		
Decrease IV rate to 10 mL per hour and monitor		
Check for blood return from IV site		
Remove intravenous catheter and dressings; apply pressure to site		
Elevate affected limb		
Apply warm pack to IV site		
Notify provider		
Administer acetaminophen		
Administer clear liquids		

END-OF-CHAPTER THINKING EXERCISE 6.3

The nurse is caring for a 19-year-old client in the Urgent Care Center.

History and Physical	Nurses Notes	Orders	Laboratory Results

1900:   Client lethargic. Reports having an "excruciating headache and stiff neck." Client holding sides of head. Client reports photophobia. States has been having nausea and vomited five times today. Reports has been unable to retain sips of fluids. Reports generalized muscle aches, joint aches, and overall weakness. Parent states client has had a fever of 101°–103° F (38.3°–39.4°C) which started yesterday and has a rash on his hands and feet. Petechiae noted on palms of hands and soles of feet. Parent reports client recently returned from traveling to Ethiopia to see family. VS: T 103.8°F (39.9°C); HR 110 beats per minute; RR 28 breaths per minute; B/P 138/88 mmHg; SpO_2 95% on RA.

END-OF-CHAPTER THINKING EXERCISE 6.3—cont'd

Which of the following **priority** actions would the nurse take? **Select all that apply.**
- ○ Place client on droplet precautions
- ○ Place client on contact precautions
- ○ Notify physician of client's condition
- ○ Obtain neurological assessment
- ○ Prepare parent to transport client to acute care emergency department
- ○ Prepare client for transfer to acute care emergency department
- ○ Administer acetaminophen orally
- ○ Initiate intravenous access and fluids

END-OF-CHAPTER THINKING EXERCISE 6.4

The nurse is caring for a 22-year-old female client in an acute care setting.

History and Physical	Nurses Notes	Orders	Laboratory Results

0700: Client has history of acute lymphocytic leukemia (ALL) ×3 months being treated with chemotherapy regimen. States "I don't feel as good as yesterday." Client alert, oriented ×4. PERRLA. Grips equal; strong, gait steady. Central line dressing dry and intact. No redness or swelling at site. CBC drawn from central line; sent to lab. S_1 and S_2 present; rate regular. Breath sounds clear throughout lung fields. Abdomen soft, flat, bowel sounds present ×4. Client denies pain. Voided 200 cc clear, straw-colored urine. Reports feeling slightly nauseated, drank 120 mL apple juice without emesis. VS: T 99.0°F (37.2°C); HR 100 beats per minute; RR 24 breaths per minute; B/P 100/75 mmHg; SpO_2 99% on RA. Wt. 100 lbs. (45.5 kg).

History and Physical	Laboratory Results	Orders	Nurses Notes

Serum Laboratory Test and Reference Range	Results Today at 0700
RBC	$3.7 \times 10^6/\mu L$ (3.7×10^{12} cells/L)
Female: $4.2–5.4 \times 10^6/\mu L$ ($4.2–5.4 \times 10^{12}$ cells/L)	
Male: $4.7–6.1 \times 10^6/\mu L$ ($4.7–6.1 \times 10^{12}$ cells/L)	
WBC (5000–10,000/mm³ [$5.0–10.0 \times 10^9$ cells/L])	3000/mm³ (3.0×10^9 cells/L)
Platelet count (150,000–440,000/mm³ [$150–400 \times 10^9$/L])	15,000/mm³ (15×10^9/L)
Hemoglobin	10.0 g/dL (6.21 mmol/L)
Female: 12.0–15.0 g/dL (7.4–9.9 mmol/L)	
Male: 14.0–18.0 g/dL (8.7–11.2 mmol/L)	
Hematocrit	26% (0.26 volume fraction)
Female: 37%–47% (0.37–0.47 volume fraction)	
Male: 42%–52% (0.42–0.52 volume fraction)	
Absolute neutrophil count	600 cells/mm³ (600 cells/μL)
Mild neutropenia: 1000–1500 cells/mm³ (1000–1500 cells/μL)	
Moderate neutropenia: 500–1000 cells/mm³ (500–1000 cells/μL)	
Severe neutropenia: less than 500 cells/mm³ (500 and below cells/μL)	

Continued

END-OF-CHAPTER THINKING EXERCISE 6.4—cont'd

Select **2 priority** nursing actions the nurse should take.
- Place the client in a negative-pressure room
- Place the client in a positive-pressure room
- Place client on contact precautions
- Start a peripheral IV
- Administer an iron supplement
- Manage the client's pain
- Place client on bleeding precautions
- Provide education on prevention of mouth sores

END-OF-CHAPTER THINKING EXERCISE 6.5

The nurse is caring for an 84-year-old client in an acute care setting.

History and Physical	Nurses Notes	Orders	Laboratory Results

1200: Client with history of stroke resulting in cognitive impairment and limited mobility. Has gastrostomy tube to abdomen, site dry, intact, tube patent. Receiving continuous enteral feedings at 75 mL per hour per Kangaroo pump. Client vomited 100 mL of milky formula-type emesis. Abdomen is distended; bowel sounds present and hypoactive × 4. Last bowel movement this am at 0800, soft, brown. Lung sounds have scattered crackles in lower lobes. Client is coughing, nonproductive. Alert and oriented to person only. Skin warm, slightly diaphoretic, with usual pigmentation. VS: T 98.0°F (37.2°C); HR 100 beats per minute; RR 28 breaths per minute; B/P 140/88 mmHg; SpO$_2$ 94% on RA.

Select **3 priority** nursing actions the nurse should take.
- Slow feeding to 50 mL per hour
- Stop the tube feeding
- Change the tube feeding to water only
- Notify physician or advanced practice provider
- Check the gastrostomy for residual feeding
- Flush the gastrostomy tube to determine patency

END-OF-CHAPTER THINKING EXERCISE 6.6

The nurse is caring for a 3-year-old client in the Emergency Department (ED).

History and Physical	Nurses Notes	Orders	Laboratory Results

0215: Client presents to ED accompanied by parents. Mother states child was "a little fussy all day, but otherwise ok." Mother reports client woke up at 0100 crying and complaining of severe throat pain; child inconsolable, talking with "thick voice" and making a "weird noise" when breathing. Client alert, crying, moves all extremities equal. Child unwilling to lie on stretcher, sitting in tripod position, mouth open, tongue protruding, and drooling. Has an anxious frightened expression. Suprasternal and substernal retractions are present. S$_1$ and S$_2$ present. Breath sounds clear throughout lung fields with occasional scattered crackles; audible "croaking" sound on inspiration; no cough. Abdomen soft; bowel sounds present × 4. Mother states child has not been vaccinated with routine childhood vaccines due to personal beliefs. VS: T 102.8°F (39.3°C); HR 120 beats per minute; RR 28 breaths per minute; B/P 100/75 mmHg; SpO$_2$ 97% on RA.

END-OF-CHAPTER THINKING EXERCISE 6.6—cont'd

For each body system below, specify the **priority** nursing actions that the nurse would take for the care of the client. Each body system may support more than one nursing action.

Body Systems	Potential Nursing Actions
Respiratory	☐ Initiate rapid response
	☐ Administer humidified oxygen
	☐ Administer albuterol via nebulizer
Ears/nose/throat	☐ Assess tonsils using tongue blade and flashlight
	☐ Prepare intubation equipment at the bedside
	☐ Assess ears using otoscope
Immune	☐ Administer haemophilus influenza and pneumococcal vaccines
	☐ Administer ceftriaxone sodium
	☐ Take temperature using oral method due to developmental stage

Answers and Rationales for Thinking Exercises

CHAPTER THINKING EXERCISES

THINKING EXERCISE 6.1

Answer:

Anticipated Orders	Indicated	Not Indicated
Obtain serum creatinine, BUN, and potassium	X	
Insert indwelling urinary catheter		X
Obtain abdominal/renal CT scan	X	
Prepare client for renal biopsy	X	
Administer increased doses of immunosuppressive drugs	X	
Initiate intravenous steroids	X	
Prepare client for emergency surgery to remove kidney		X
Prepare client for dialysis		X

Continued

⚡ **THINKING EXERCISE 6.1—cont'd**

Rationale: The client has evidence of an acute rejection of the transplanted kidney which usually occurs 1 week to any time after surgery. Symptoms of rejection include oliguria, increased temperature, increased blood pressure, and an enlarged and/or tender kidney. Clients also experience lethargy and fluid retention. It would be anticipated that a serum creatinine, BUN, and potassium level would be obtained to determine if this was an acute rejection or an acute kidney injury. Additionally, a CT scan of the kidneys and abdomen, and kidney biopsy will likely be ordered to diagnose the rejection. Increased immunosuppressive drugs with intravenous steroids would be prescribed to inhibit the rejection. At this time, an indwelling urinary catheter, surgical removal of the kidney, or dialysis are not indicated. However, if initial actions are not effective, more invasive actions may be required.

⚡ **THINKING EXERCISE 6.2**

Answer:

Potential Nursing Actions	Indicated	Not Indicated
Initiate intravenous fluids	X	
Administer oral glucose		X
Initiate intravenous regular insulin	X	
Initiate intravenous long-acting insulin		X
Initiate cardiac monitoring	X	
Obtain bedside glucose and ketone samples	X	
Obtain glucose, electrolytes, and blood gases	X	
Obtain BUN, creatinine, and liver enzymes		X
Administer oral carbohydrates (e.g., orange juice)		X

Rationale: This client is exhibiting symptoms of diabetic ketoacidosis (DKA) due to hyperglycemia which likely developed as a result of limited access to insulin. The client has diabetes mellitus type 1 and is unable to produce insulin. The nurse should be aware that transgender clients are at increased risk for being unhoused, which results in difficulty in accessing needed health care. This limited access to insulin and needed supplies has likely resulted in the client developing DKA. The nurse would anticipate needing rapid assessment of the client's blood glucose and ketone levels so a blood draw would be obtained at the bedside. Additionally, serum glucose, electrolytes, BUN, and blood gases would be obtained to determine if the client is experiencing metabolic acidosis, dehydration, or electrolyte imbalances. Intravenous fluids would be administered to correct dehydration (intravenous electrolytes may also be needed). Intravenous regular insulin would be anticipated to reduce the client's glucose level. Cardiac monitoring would be indicated as this client may be experiencing serious electrolyte imbalance which could result in dysrhythmias. Oral glucose or oral carbohydrates would not be indicated as this would increase the severity of the hyperglycemia. CBC and liver enzymes are not necessary at this time. Only short-acting (regular) insulin is given intravenously; therefore, long-acting intravenous insulin is not indicated.

THINKING EXERCISE 6.3

Answer:
Select **3** actions the nurse should take **immediately**.
X Ask another nurse team member to initiate rapid response and notify provider
X Insert gloved fingers into vaginal canal to manually relieve compression of the cord
○ Place client into side-lying position
○ Ask a nurse team member to administer oxygen 2 L by nasal cannula
X Ask a nurse team member to start or increase intravenous fluids
○ Ask a nurse team member to prepare for forceps delivery

Rationale: The fetus is experiencing distress as a result of a compressed, prolapsed umbilical cord. The distress can be seen in the varying heart rate and variable decelerations. This client situation is considered an emergency situation for the fetus because oxygenation and perfusion are being compromised and can result in fetal harm. It would be most important for the nurse to remain with the client and ask a nurse team member to initiate a rapid response and notify the provider. The nurse should immediately use a gloved hand to manually relieve compression of the cord and promote fetal circulation. The nurse should also ask a nurse a team member to start or increase intravenous fluids or have a team member do this as soon as possible. It is not appropriate to have the client in a side-lying position as this will not relieve the cord compression. The client should be placed in an extreme Trendelenburg or a modified Sims' position or a knee-chest position. While it would be important to delegate application of oxygen therapy, oxygen is indicated but at a much higher flow-rate, 8–10 L/minute using a nonrebreather mask until birth is accomplished. The nurse should ask a nurse team member to prepare for an immediate cesarean delivery since the cervix is not fully dilated. Therefore, a forceps delivery is not indicated in this situation.

THINKING EXERCISE 6.4

Answer:
Which of the following actions would the nurse take? **Select all that apply.**
○ Maintain continuous eye contact
○ Move quickly
X Keep voice calm
○ Raise voice to gain client's immediate attention
X Offer options for what the client might want
○ Take control
X Give the client space
X Gently announce actions before initiating them
X Initiate a concealed "Code White" to alert security

Rationale: The client is experiencing depression and anxiety related to bipolar disorder that is not being controlled by medication. This is likely due to the client's nonadherence with the medication regimen. Additionally, this drug may be ineffective for this particular client. The client is experiencing life-stressors that are worsening the condition such as loss of employment, lack of family support, risk for being unhoused, and loss of partner. These factors are impacting the mental well-being of the client resulting in periods of increased depression and agitation. Currently, the client is agitated and is a potential risk to the safety of other clients on the unit. The situation is in need of deescalation techniques for calming the client and preventing harm to others. The nurse should maintain a calm voice, move slowly, and give the client space. It is important not to maintain continuous eye contact as that can increase fear and aggressive behaviors in the client. The nurse should announce any actions before initiating them to prevent surprising or startling the client. Avoid making rapid movements as this can increase agitation. The nurse should offer the client options to increase the client's sense of autonomy and potentially decrease agitation rather than trying to take control of the client. The nurse should also initiate a concealed "Code White" rather than an overhead page so that security team members can be alerted to assist with a potentially dangerous situation without escalating the agitation of the client by making an overhead announcement.

END-OF-CHAPTER THINKING EXERCISES

END-OF-CHAPTER THINKING EXERCISE 6.1

Answer:

Body Systems/Needs	Potential Nursing Actions
Respiratory	☒ Place client in high-Fowler's (sitting) position
	☒ Administer oxygen
	☐ Administer albuterol via nebulizer
Cardiovascular	☒ Initiate continuous telemetry monitoring
	☒ Administer anticoagulants
	☐ Administer nitroglycerin sublingual prn chest pain; repeat as needed every 5 minutes for up to 15 minutes
Mental health	☐ Reassure client everything will be fine
	☒ Explain rationale when providing care
	☒ Keep room stimulation level low

Rationale: This client is experiencing signs and symptoms of pulmonary embolism, which is a potentially life-threatening complication following orthopedic surgery. The classic signs and symptoms which the client is demonstrating include: hypotension, tachycardia, extra heart sounds, dyspnea, decreased SpO_2, anxiety and feeling of impending doom, crackles, dry cough, chest pain, and diaphoresis. The nurse should place the client high-Fowler's (sitting) position and administer oxygen to help relieve dyspnea. Bronchodilators will not be useful as symptoms are a result of impaired perfusion rather than constricted bronchioles. The client should be on continuous telemetry monitoring and anticoagulants should be started as soon as prescribed. Nitroglycerin is not indicated at this time as pain is not due to angina but is related to a clot in the circulatory system in the lungs. The nurse should try to alleviate the client's anxiety related to feelings of impending doom by maintaining a calm environment and explaining rationale of treatments and interventions. The nurse should not give false hope by saying "everything will be fine" but should acknowledge the client's fear and reassure the client effective measures are being quickly taken.

END-OF-CHAPTER THINKING EXERCISE 6.2

Answer:

Potential Nursing Actions	Indicated	Not Indicated
Remove dressings; resecure IV catheter and reapply dressing		X
Slow IV rate to 10 mL per hour and monitor		X
Check for blood return from IV site		X
Remove intravenous catheter and dressings; apply pressure to site	X	
Elevate affected limb	X	
Apply warm pack to IV site	X	
Notify provider	X	
Administer acetaminophen	X	
Administer clear liquids by mouth		X

Rationale: This child has symptoms of an intravenous infiltration: edema and leaking at site, cool skin, and pain. The nurse should intervene quickly by immediately discontinuing IV site and applying pressure to wound. The affected limb should be elevated to decrease edema. A warm pack should be applied along with acetaminophen for helping with discomfort. The physician or other provider needs to be notified. This IV should be restarted in an alternate site. It would be inappropriate to attempt to resecure/redress the IV site, to check the site for blood return, or to continue to allow any further fluids to go through this site by decreasing the flow rate. When IV sites infiltrate, the intravenous fluids are not going into the vein but are going directly into surrounding tissues causing pain and edema. Infiltrated IV sites need to be immediately discontinued to prevent further harm to the client. It would be inappropriate to provide clear liquids as the child is NPO.

END-OF-CHAPTER THINKING EXERCISE 6.3

Answer:
Which of the following **priority** actions would the nurse take? **Select all that apply.**

X Place client on droplet precautions

○ Place client on contact precautions

X Notify physician or advanced practice provider of client's condition

X Obtain neurological assessment

○ Prepare parent to transport client to acute care emergency department

X Prepare client for transfer to acute care emergency department

○ Administer acetaminophen orally

X Initiate intravenous access and fluids

Rationale: This client is showing signs and symptoms of meningococcal meningitis caused by *Neisseria meningitidis* which commonly occurs in sub-Saharan Africa where Ethiopia is located. Clients aged 16–23 are at high risk for this condition. The most relevant signs and symptoms the client is exhibiting indicating meningococcal meningitis are:

○ Photophobia

○ Severe headache with stiff neck

○ Nausea and vomiting

○ Weakness; muscle and joint pain

○ Fever, tachycardia, tachypnea

○ Petechiae rash (this is possibly the most ominous symptom and indicates damage to blood vessels resulting from the rapidly advancing infection)

Meningococcal meningitis is an emergency condition with a high risk for morbidity and mortality. It is also highly contagious and is spread through respiratory secretions. The nurse should immediately protect everyone in the clinic by placing the client on droplet precautions. The nurse should immediately notify the physician or advanced practice provider of the urgent condition of the client, and begin to prepare the client to be transferred to an acute care emergency department. Due to the client's acute illness, the nurse should limit unnecessary assessments at this time. Neurological assessments need to be completed to monitor the client's condition and assess for potential deterioration while awaiting the transport team. The nurse should anticipate initiating intravenous access and fluids in preparation for transferring the client as the client will require urgent administration of intravenous antibiotics. It would be ineffective to place the client on contact precautions because the disease is spread via the respiratory tract. It would not be safe for the parent to transport the client to the emergency department because the condition of the client is too critical and the client requires constant medical supervision. Oral acetaminophen would not be helpful at this time due to the client's inability to retain sips of fluids; intravenous acetaminophen would more likely be used.

END-OF-CHAPTER THINKING EXERCISE 6.4

Answer:
Select **2 priority** nursing actions the nurse should take.
○ Place the client in a negative-pressure room
X Place the client in a positive-pressure room
○ Place the client on contact precautions
○ Start a peripheral IV
○ Administer an iron supplement
○ Manage the client's pain
X Place the client on bleeding precautions
○ Provide education on prevention of mouth sores

Rationale: This client is experiencing neutropenia, anemia, and thrombocytopenia, likely a result of the disease process and chemo-therapy treatment. The absolute neutrophil count and platelet counts are critically low. Neutropenia places the client at critical risk for infection, which is potentially life-threatening. The client should be placed on protective isolation precautions to prevent acquiring any potential infections which would be life-threatening. This situation would require the nurse to place the client in a positive air-pressure room. When the door is opened to the room, potentially contaminated air from the hallway will not enter the room and infect the client. Additionally, with the low platelet count, the client is at great risk for bleeding, and bleeding precautions would be a priority. The client should not be placed in a negative air-pressure room as this environment is designed to protect people outside the room from any organ-isms in the room. Every time the door opens, outside air from the hall would enter the room and potentially bring in pathogens. Contact precautions are not indicated as the client does not have evidence of infectious disease or symptoms. It would not be indicated to start a peripheral IV due to the risk for bleeding. Iron supplements or providing education at this time are not priority measures. The client is not reporting pain at this time so this is not a priority action.

END-OF-CHAPTER THINKING EXERCISE 6.5

Answer:
Select **3 priority** nursing actions the nurse would anticipate implementing.
○ Slow feeding to 50 mL per hour
X Stop the feeding
○ Change the feeding to water only
X Notify physician or advanced practice provider
X Check the gastrostomy for residual feeding
○ Flush the gastrostomy tube to determine patency

Rationale: The client is exhibiting signs of overfeeding including vomiting and abdominal distention. The client may also be exhibiting signs of potential aspiration due to the overfeeding, cough, and crackles. The nurse should take action to stop the feeding and check for residual to determine the amount the client has been overfed. It would be important to notify the provider so that they provide guidance as to how to proceed with feedings. Continuing the feeding or providing water would worsen the condition and should be avoided. There is no evidence that the gastrostomy tube is not patent, so checking for patency is not needed at this time.

⚡ **END-OF-CHAPTER THINKING EXERCISE 6.6**

Answer:

Body Systems	Potential Nursing Actions
Respiratory	☒ Initiate rapid response
	☒ Administer humidified oxygen
	☐ Administer albuterol via nebulizer
Ears/nose/throat	☐ Assess tonsils using tongue blade and flashlight
	☒ Prepare intubation equipment at the bedside
	☐ Assess ears using otoscope
Immunity	☐ Administer haemophilus influenza and pneumococcal vaccines
	☒ Administer ceftriaxone sodium
	☐ Take temperature using oral method due to developmental stage

Rationale: This client is showing classic signs and symptoms of epiglottitis which occurs in children ages 2–5 and is a life-threatening emergency. The epiglottis becomes red and edematous and potentially can totally occlude the client's airway. The nurse should initiate a rapid response, place the child on humidified oxygen via mask or blow by if the mask agitates the child. The nurse should have intubation equipment at the bedside and be prepared to initiate IV antibiotics such as ceftriaxone sodium to treat the infection. With this condition, the epiglottis is very large and unstable. It is important to keep the client calm and comfortable. It is very important not to examine the throat or place anything in the mouth (e.g., thermometer) until the advanced practice provider can stabilize the airway. Examining the ears at this time is contraindicated and will cause unnecessary distress for the client. Albuterol is not useful in this situation because the situation is not a bronchiole constriction issue. While epiglottitis is usually caused by *H. influenzae*, vaccines are preventive but not curative for active infections and would not be useful at this critical time.

REFERENCES

Agency for Healthcare and Research Quality (AHRQ). (2020). Toolkit for reducing catheter-associated urinary tract infections in hospital units: Implementation Guide, Appendix M. Example of a nurse-driven protocol for catheter removal. https://www.ahrq.gov/hai/cauti-tools/impl-guide/implementation-guide-appendix-m.html.

Alaseeri, R., Rajab, A., & Banakhar, M. (2021). Do personal differences and organizational factors influence nurses' decision making? A qualitative study. *Nursing Reports, 11*(3), 714–727.

American Nurses Association (ANA). (n.d., a). Healthy work environment: The Nurses bill of rights. https://www.nursingworld.org/practice-policy/work-environment/.

American Nurses Association (ANA). (n.d., b). Protect yourselves, protect your clients. https://www.nursingworld.org/practice-policy/work-environment/end-nurse-abuse/.

Barto, D. (2019). Nurse-driven protocols. *Nursing in Critical Care, 14*(4), 18–24.

Brister, T. (2018). *Navigating a mental health crisis: A NAMI resource guide for those experiencing a mental health emergency*. National Alliance on Mental Illness. https://www.nami.org/Support-Education-Publications-Reports/Guides/Navigating-a-Mental-Health-Crisis/Navigating-A-Mental-Health-Crisis?utm_source=website&utm_medium=cta&utm_campaign=crisisguide.

Centers for Disease Control: National Institute for Occupational Safety and Health (CDC: NIOSH). (2023). *Safe client handling and mobility.* https://www.cdc.gov/niosh/topics/safeclient/default.html.

Center for Medicaid and Medicare Services (CMS). (2022). *Hospital-acquired condition reduction program.* https://www.cms.gov/medicare/payment/prospective-payment-systems/acute-inpatient-pps/hospital-acquired-condition-reduction-program-hacrp.

De Groot, K., De Veer, A. J. E., Munster, A. M., Francke, A. L., & Paans, W. (2022). Nursing documentation and its relationship with perceived nursing workload: A mixed-methods study among community nurses. *BMC Nursing, 21*(1), 34.

*Gillespie, M. (2010). Using the situated clinical decision-making framework to guide analysis of nurses' clinical decision-making. *Nurse Education in Practice, 10,* 333–340.

I-PASS Client Safety Institute. (2022). *A Closer look at SBAR vs. the I-PASS handoff method. I-PASS Blog.* https://news.ipassinstitute.com/news/a-closer-look-at-sbar-vs.-the-i-pass-handoff-method.

Ignatavicius, D. D., Rebar, C. R., & Heimgartner, N. M. (2024). *Medical-surgical nursing: Concepts for interprofessional collaborative care* (11th ed.). Elsevier.

Kelly, D., Campbell, P., Torrens, C., Caralambous, A., Ostlund, U., Eicher, M., Larsson, M., Nohavova, I., Olsson, C., Simpson, M., Patiraki, E., Sarp, L., Wiseman, T., Oldenmenger, W., & Wells, M. (2022). The effectiveness of nurse-led interventions for cancer symptom management 2000-2018 A Systematic review and meta-analysis. *Health Sciences Review, 4,* 1–11.

*Levett-Jones, T., Hoffman, K., Dempsey, J., Yeun-Sim Jeong, S., Noble, C. A. N., et al. (2010). The 'five rights' of clinical reasoning: An educational model to enhance nursing students' ability to identify and manage clinically 'at risk' clients. *Nurse Education Today, 30*(6), 515–520.

*Padilla, R. M., & Mayo, A. M. (2018). Clinical deterioration: A concept analysis. *Journal of Clinical Nursing, 27,* 1360–1368.

Potter, P., Griffin Perry, A., Stockert, P., & Ostendorf, W. (2021). *Fundamentals of nursing* (10th ed.). Elsevier Health Sciences (US).

TJC (The Joint Commission). (2021). *Quick safety Issue 24: Bullying has no place in health care.* https://www.jointcommission.org/resources/news-and-multimedia/newsletters/newsletters/quick-safety/quick-safety-issue-24-bullying-has-no-place-in-health-care/bullying-has-no-place-in-health-care/.

*TJC (The Joint Commission). (2017). *Sentinel event alert: Inadequate hand-off communication, Issue 58.* https://e-handoff.com/wp-content/uploads/2017/09/Joint-Commision-Handoff-Communication-Alert.pdf.

*Denotes classic reference.

7

How to Evaluate Outcomes

LEARNING OUTCOMES

1. List nursing competencies needed for evaluating outcomes.
2. Briefly describe the role of observation, physical assessment, and communication in evaluating outcomes.
3. Describe four steps of the client evaluation process.
4. Differentiate nurse, client, and system factors that can affect the ability to evaluate outcomes.
5. Identify strategies for evaluating outcomes to make safe, appropriate clinical judgments.

KEY TERMS

Client experience: Client-centered care and client–staff interactions during all episodes of care.

Clinical outcomes: Measurable changes in signs and symptoms, health, ability to function, quality of life, or survival.

Evaluation: The process of determining the progress toward attainment of expected outcomes, including the effectiveness of care.

Expected clinical outcomes: Client changes or results that are desirable and observable in response to evidence-based nursing actions.

Focused assessment: Provides specific information related to a client's results or change in condition when evaluating outcomes.

Functional ability: Client ability to perform activities of daily living (ADLs) and independent living skills.

Inference: The process of drawing conclusions based on interpretation of client findings using clinical reasoning.

Objective clinical cues: Client observations made by the nurse or other member of the interprofessional health care team; also called signs.

Observation: The purposeful gathering of clinical cues from clients and/or family members to inform the effectiveness of clinical judgments.

Reflective practice: A thinking skill in which nurses examine a situation with an awareness of their own values and practices, enabling them to learn from each experience.

Subjective clinical cues: Self-reports of the client's condition or family's reports of client changes; also called symptoms.

Evaluating clinical outcomes involves determining if the nursing actions implemented for the client effectively managed the client's condition. In other words, *did the action(s) help?*

EVALUATING CLINICAL OUTCOMES

Introduction to Evaluation

Making sound clinical judgments is the foundation of professional nursing practice, positively influencing clinical outcomes and ensuring client safety (Manetti, 2019). According to the most recent American Nurses Association's (ANA) *Nursing Scope and Standards of Practice*, evaluation is defined as "the process of determining the progress toward attainment of expected outcomes, including the effectiveness of care" (ANA, 2021, p. 111).

As defined in Chapter 5, clinical outcomes are measurable changes in signs and symptoms, health, ability to function, quality of life, or survival. Expected clinical outcomes are *positive* client changes or results that are desirable and observable in response to evidence-based nursing actions. Expected outcomes are, therefore, sometimes referred to as desired outcomes.

According to the ANA, expected outcomes should be developed in partnership with the client and family. Additional examples of ANA evaluation competencies are listed in Box 7.1.

BOX 7.1   Examples of ANA Competencies for Standard 6: Evaluation

- Conducts a systematic, ongoing, and criterion-based evaluation of the goals and outcomes in relation to the structure, processes, and time line prescribed in the plan [of care].
- Collaborates with the health care consumer, stakeholders, interprofessional team, and others involved in the care or situation in the evaluation process.
- Documents the results of the evaluation.
- Reports evaluation data in a timely fashion.
- Shares evaluation data and conclusions with the health care consumer and other stakeholders to promote clarity and transparency in accordance with state, federal, organizational, and professional requirements.

Adapted from American Nurses Association (ANA). (2021). *Nursing scope and standards of practice* (4th ed.). ANA.

The primary objectives of evaluating client outcomes are to:
- Analyze current client findings.
- Determine if nursing actions are helping clients achieve expected clinical outcomes.
- Verify the quality of the nursing care provided.
- Promote nursing accountability.

Nurses are accountable for the quality of their practice (ANA, 2021). Koy et al. (2015) found that good nursing care quality is a process that consists of six core elements needed to achieve positive clinical outcomes:
- Holistic approach that is client-centered and continuous
- Nursing efficiency and effectiveness combined with humanity and compassion
- Professional, high-quality evidence-based practice
- Safe, effective, and prompt nursing actions
- Client empowerment, support, and advocacy
- Seamless care through effective teamwork with other professionals

Role of Observation, Physical Assessment, and Communication

Nurses use observation, physical assessment skills, and communication to determine the client's progress toward achieving expected outcomes (Potter et al., 2023). As discussed in Chapter 2, observation is the purposeful gathering of clinical cues from clients and/or significant others/family members to inform the effectiveness of clinical judgments. As part of evaluating outcomes, observation helps to determine if the client improved as a result of implementing the plan of care.

As a brief review, the core principles of observation as delineated in Table 2.4 in Chapter 2 include that observation:

- Is comprehensive, meaning that all senses should be used.
- Is a critical part of client assessment and evaluation.
- Requires interactive communication with the client.
- Is affected by the health care environment.
- Needs to be communicated and documented.

CLINICAL JUDGMENT TIP

Remember: Nurses use observation, physical assessment, and communication skills to determine the client's progress toward achieving expected outcomes.

Recognizing changes in the client's condition or clinical state depends on your ability to identify relevant objective and subjective clinical cues as part of physical assessment. Distinguishing relevant from irrelevant (not relevant) cues can be described as deciding what client information is important to understanding specific health concerns and what information is not important. Objective clinical cues, also called signs, are client observations made by the nurse or other member of the interprofessional health care team. In addition to physical assessment data, these findings include diagnostic test results. Subjective clinical cues, also called symptoms, are self-reports of the client's condition or family's reports of client behaviors.

Nursing competence in *physical assessment* is essential for determining the client's progress toward achieving expected clinical outcomes in any health care setting (Liyew et al., 2021). When a client's condition or clinical state changes, you must be able to perform relevant focused assessments consistent with the parameters you planned to monitor when implementing actions. A focused assessment provides specific information related to a client's results or change in condition when evaluating outcomes. Examples of focused assessments are listed in Table 7.1.

TABLE 7.1   Examples of Focused Physical Assessments to Evaluate Outcomes

Body System	Parameters to Monitor
Neurologic	• Level of consciousness • Orientation • Pupil size, symmetry, shape, and reaction • Muscle strength and ability to move extremities • Communication ability • Swallowing ability • Pain intensity and quality

Continued

TABLE 7.1   **Examples of Focused Physical Assessments to Evaluate Outcomes—cont'd**

Body System	Parameters to Monitor
Respiratory	• Breath sounds • Respiratory effort • Presence and quality of sputum • Peripheral oxygen saturation (SpO_2)
Cardiovascular	• Heart rate quantity and quality • Heart sounds • Peripheral pulse strength and quality • Capillary refill • Blood pressure • Edema
Renal/urinary	• Voiding amount and pattern • Urine color and clarity
Gastrointestinal	• Abdomen contour • Distention • Bowel sounds
Immunologic	• Body temperature • Wound characteristics
Integumentary	• Color • Integrity • Turgor • Lesions

Because nurses often rely on self-reports of clients and their families regarding the client's condition, the nurse's skill in therapeutic *communication* is very important. Interviewing the client and/or family helps to determine the effectiveness of nursing care and the client's satisfaction with the outcome of that care. Client satisfaction is discussed later in this chapter.

Thinking Exercise 7.1 will help you practice what you've learned in this chapter about evaluating outcomes. The answer and rationale for the exercise are located at the end of this book.

THINKING EXERCISE 7.1

The nurse is caring for a 50-year-old client in the Emergency Department (ED).
  Highlight the findings in the 2220 note that demonstrate the client's condition is **improving**.

History and Physical	Nurses Notes	Orders	Laboratory Results

2110:   Family brought client to ED due to client's severe right back pain, fever, chills, and vomiting which started early this morning. No significant medical history. Client alert and oriented ×4, but wincing in severe pain rated at 10/10 on a 0–10 pain intensity scale. Breath sounds clear throughout lung fields; no dyspnea. S_1 and S_2 present. Bowel sounds present ×4; abdomen soft. VS: T 101.8°F (38.8°C); HR 112 beats per minute and regular; RR 28 breaths per minute and shallow; BP 148/92 mmHg; SpO_2 95% on RA.

2135:   Voided urine with gross hematuria. Sample sent to lab. IV morphine administered.

2220:   States feeling "a little better"; pain level now 6/10. VS: T 102°F (38.9°C); HR 94 beats per minute and regular; RR 20 breaths per minute and regular; BP 130/86 mmHg; SpO_2 96% on RA. Transferred for kidney ultrasound.

PROCESS FOR EVALUATING OUTCOMES

Evaluating outcomes focuses on the effectiveness of implemented nursing actions by determining if expected outcome(s) that address the priority client condition were met. Each step of the evaluation process requires higher order thinking to analyze and interpret relevant clinical cues (Fig. 7.1).

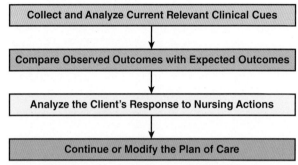

FIG. 7.1 Process for evaluating outcomes.

Collect and Analyze Relevant Clinical Cues

Evaluating nursing care begins with identifying which current clinical cues (parameters), should be collected and analyzed based on the priority client condition. As discussed in Chapter 1, cues to indicate improved clinical condition have been underreported in the literature. Decreasing pain is the most common cue used to identify client improvement, but other data, such as vital signs, are more useful in determining whether a client's condition has improved or worsened (Burdeu et al., 2021).

Recall that priority client conditions are emergent (life-threatening) or urgent (serious), as discussed in Chapter 4. Organize and cluster those client findings that provide information about the status of the priority condition—either improved or not, or possibly worsened. Recall that clustering cues is the process of classifying data to enhance the ability of determining relationships between and among those findings. For example, if a client experiences severe dehydration as evidenced by hypotension and tachycardia, you would want to monitor vital signs for changes after actions are implemented. Analysis of these clustered relevant clinical cues, or client findings, helps you decide whether the client's condition has improved.

Determining *when* to monitor physical/biological or behavioral changes in a client depends on several factors, including the severity of the client condition, established best practices or protocols, and the ability of the nurse to collect these data. In an emergent clinical situation, clients need to be monitored at frequent intervals per protocol or policy, perhaps as often as every 5 minutes or continuously. The nurse needs to be available to perform this monitoring, and would *not delegate* these assessments to assistive personnel or unregulated health care workers because emergent clients are unstable and need nurses to interpret clinical findings.

Compare Observed Outcomes with Expected Outcomes

As defined by ANA (2021), evaluating outcomes involves determining the progress toward attainment of expected (desired) outcomes, including the effectiveness of care. To evaluate the client's progress, collected client findings must be analyzed to determine any differences from initial or earlier assessments.

Many physical assessment findings are *objective* clinical cues collected using evidence-based tools that can identify trends in client data. Examples of these commonly used tools include:

- Vital signs (VS)
- Modified early warning system (MEWS) (see Chapter 2)
- Glasgow Coma Scale (GCS)
- Pain intensity scale (0–10)

Determining the amount or degree of change in a client's condition can be interpreted using any of these tools by comparing the client's score or numerical value before and after nursing action(s). This interpretation then leads to an inference, which can be defined as drawing conclusions based on interpretation of client findings using clinical reasoning. For example, if the client's blood pressure was initially 230/120 mmHg and then decreased to 142/88 mmHg after nursing actions were implemented, the nurse would infer the client's condition *improved* and the care was effective. If a client's GCS was initially 13 and then 10 after actions were implemented, the nurse would infer that the client's condition *worsened*. In this case, though, the nurse should not conclude that care was ineffective. Instead, a declining GCS score indicates the client is experiencing a decreasing level of consciousness, a sign of clinical deterioration.

CLINICAL JUDGMENT TIP

Remember. Making inferences can be defined as drawing conclusions based on interpretation of client findings using clinical reasoning.

Subjective clinical cues, such as dyspnea, nausea, and anxiety, are more challenging to measure and quantify. Therefore, it is more difficult to make comparisons between initial assessment findings and those data collected after actions are implemented.

Objective and subjective clinical cues provide supporting evidence for whether expected outcomes are met or not met. For example, if a young adult initially experiences acute respiratory distress as evidenced by a low SpO_2, tachypnea, and shortness of breath, the expected or desired outcome is that the client will have a normal SpO_2 (95% or higher), a respiratory rate between 14–20 breaths per minute, and no shortness of breath after interventions are implemented. If this outcome is met, the client's condition improved and the vital signs, in this case, returned to a normal range. In other cases, the expected outcomes might include that the vital signs return to the client's baseline. Remember that the client's baseline findings may not be within the normal range due to the presence of chronic health conditions. If the client's condition did not improve to either normal or baseline range, you would want to determine the reason(s) why.

CLINICAL JUDGMENT TIP

Remember. To evaluate the client's progress, collected client findings must be analyzed to determine any differences from initial or earlier assessments.

As part of evaluating outcomes, you would want to infer from relevant clinical cues whether the client's condition improved, has not changed, or worsened. If the client's condition has not changed or worsens, identify relevant client findings and take action immediately.

CLINICAL JUDGMENT TIP

Remember. If the client's condition has not changed or worsens, identify relevant client findings and take action *immediately.*

Common reasons why expected clinical outcomes may not be met or partially met include:
- Initial assessment to recognize relevant cues was incomplete or inaccurate.
- All of the most relevant clinical cues were not initially recognized.
- The priority client condition was not identified or correctly identified.
- Expected (desired) outcomes were not realistic or achievable.
- Not enough time elapsed for the expected outcomes to be evaluated.
- Nursing actions were not appropriate or adequate for the client condition or the severity of the condition.

In some cases, the client's condition worsens or does not improve despite implementation of an evidence-based plan of care.

Analyze the Client's Response to Nursing Actions

When evaluating outcomes, include an assessment of the client experience. **Client experience** includes client-centered care and client–staff interactions during all episodes of care (Avlijas et al., 2023). When analyzing the client experience, ask yourself these questions:
- Is the client safe?
- Is the client functional?
- Is the client (and family) satisfied with the outcome?

Client *safety* is always the desired priority result of nursing care. When evaluating outcomes and the effectiveness of care for a client experiencing clinical deterioration or medical complication, monitor the client carefully and frequently to ensure client safety.

CLINICAL JUDGMENT TIP

Remember. Client safety is always the desired priority result of nursing care!

If the client loses *function* as a result of clinical deterioration or complication, perform a functional assessment as part of the evaluation process. **Functional ability** refers to the client's ability to perform activities of daily living (ADLs) and independent living skills, sometimes referred to as instrumental activities of daily living (IADLs). Box 7.2 lists examples of these skills and abilities.

BOX 7.2   Examples of ADLs and Independent Living Skills

ADLs (needed for self-care)
- Eating/feeding
- Bathing/grooming
- Dressing
- Toileting
- Ambulating
- Using stairs
- Transferring

IADLs (needed for independent community living)
- Shopping
- Meal preparation
- Housekeeping/home maintenance
- Laundry
- Managing finances
- Taking medications
- Using transportation

Both clinical safety and function help to promote client (and family) *satisfaction*. Client satisfaction is determined by expectations and if those expectations were met. The client experience is consistently positively associated with expectations of safety and clinical effectiveness (Doyle et al., 2012).

Continue or Modify the Plan of Care

If expected outcomes are met and/or the client and family are satisfied, the client likely demonstrated improvement. As a result, you would either continue with the plan of care and monitor the client for additional changes, or discontinue the plan because the client condition was resolved. If expected outcomes are *not* met and/or the client and family are *not* satisfied, you would likely want to modify the plan of care. If any of the nursing actions were inadequate or inappropriate, more appropriate evidence-based actions would need to be planned and implemented.

Thinking Exercise 7.2 will help you practice what you've learned in this chapter about evaluating outcomes. The answer and rationale for the exercise are located at the end of this book.

THINKING EXERCISE 7.2

The nurse is caring for a 62-year-old client who had a left below-the-knee amputation (BKA).

History and Physical	Nurses Notes	Orders	Laboratory Results

0815: Had left BKA yesterday due to complications of diabetes mellitus type 2. Alert and oriented ×4. Left leg and foot pain described as sharp with a "pins and needles" feeling; reports 9/10 pain now. PCA shows inadequate dosing by the client. Breath sounds clear throughout lung fields; no dyspnea. Abdomen soft, round, and nontender. Skin dry with usual pigmentation. Saline lock in place. Bowel sounds present in all quadrants. Cap refill >3 seconds right foot. Bulky dressing on left residual limb dry and intact. Small amount of serosanguinous drainage in Jackson–Pratt (JP) drain. VS: T 98.8°F (37.1°C), HR 98 beats per minute and regular, RR 22 breaths per minute, BP 128/74 mmHg, SpO$_2$ 97% on RA. FSBG 108 mg/dL (5.99 mmol/L) at 0700. (Normal range 70–110 mg/dL [3.89–6.11 mmol/L].)

1210: Used PCA more often this morning; pain reported at 6/10 now. Moderate amount of new bright red blood on surgical dressing. VS: 98.8°F (37.1°C), HR 108 beats per minute and regular, RR 26 breaths per minute, BP 106/54 mmHg, SpO$_2$ 96% on RA. FSBG 100 mg/dL (5.55 mmol/L). (Normal range 70–110 mg/dL [3.89–6.11 mmol/L].)

1245: Surgeon notified about changes in vital signs and new bright red blood on dressing.

1255: Left residual limb elevated on two pillows with elastic wrap to provide pressure on the surgical site. No blood or dampness under residual limb. Peripheral IV fluids started via saline lock. Client to stay in bed today. PCA discontinued.

1440: VS: T 98.6°F (37°C), HR 86 beats per minute and regular, RR 18 breaths per minute, BP 122/76 mmHg, SpO$_2$ 97% on RA. States left foot pain is becoming more painful again at 10/10, even after taking analgesic. No new bleeding noted on surgical dressing.

For each current client finding, select whether the finding indicates that the client's condition has improved or worsened by 1440.

Client Findings	Improved	Worsened
Heart rate		
Pain intensity		
Respiratory rate		
Blood pressure		
Bleeding from surgical site		

EVALUATING OUTCOMES TO MAKE SAFE CLINICAL JUDGMENTS

Evaluating outcomes requires higher order thinking to determine the client's progress in a given clinical situation. A number of factors can affect the ability of nurses to evaluate outcomes when caring for clients who are experiencing medical complications or clinical deterioration.

Factors that Influence the Ability of Nurses to Evaluate Outcomes

Nurses make clinical judgments that are affected by many factors in today's complex multilayered health care settings. Being aware of these factors can help you understand their impact on how you evaluate outcomes and make inferences. These factors can be categorized into nurse factors, client factors, and system factors.

Nurse Factors

The *work experience* of nurses and how it influences decision-making has been one of the most explored factors. Orique et al. (2019) found that new nursing graduates were technically competent but missed clinical cues that could have prevented client harm due to lack of work experience. Experienced nurses learn from each client interaction and can transfer that learning from one clinical situation to another.

Experienced nurses understand their clients' clinical status by developing relationships with clients and spending time with them. Physical nurse presence is vital to evaluating outcomes and analyzing the client's response as part of situational awareness. Knowing the client includes (1) performing and documenting frequent assessments, especially client observations and vital signs (Nibbelink & Brewer, 2018), and (2) recognizing the client's pattern of responses or trends in data to support the achievement of expected outcomes.

Experienced nurses are also able to reflect on their clinical decision-making as part of evaluating outcomes. Reflective practice is a thinking skill in which nurses examine a situation with an awareness of their own values and practices, enabling them to learn from each experience. This learning is then used to improve client outcomes which leads to new knowledge development (Patel & Metersky, 2022). As described in Chapter 1, reflective thinking is also known as abductive reasoning, which is the ability to reflect on the explanation for a conclusion or observation about a client. *Reflection on practice* is critical for the development of clinical knowledge and improvement in clinical reasoning.

The nurse's ability to effectively *communicate* can markedly affect outcome achievement. As discussed in Chapter 2, identifying relevant cues during client re-assessment requires effective and respectful communication with the client and/or family members. Remember that observation requires interactive communication with the client.

CLINICAL JUDGMENT TIP

Remember: The nurse's ability to effectively *communicate* can markedly affect outcome achievement. Remember that observation requires interactive communication with the client.

Client Factors

In their classic research, Liu et al. (2014) identified factors about clients that influence the ability to meet expected outcomes, including the client's:

- Age
- Degree of illness, injury, or condition
- Ability to communicate

A good example of the influence of *age* is the older client. Normal physiologic changes associated with aging can impact the ability of clinically deteriorating clients to achieve expected outcomes. Table 7.2 includes examples of common changes of aging that can affect outcomes achievement (Touhy & Jett, 2022).

In addition to age, the *severity or degree of illness, injury, or condition* can affect the achievement of expected outcomes. Some conditions rapidly become severe and may not be reversible, even after implementing prompt, evidence-based actions. Examples of these conditions include shock, sepsis, and disseminated intravascular coagulation (DIC). Therefore, noticing early or subtle clinical cues is essential to promote positive or optimal client outcomes. Recall in Chapter 2 that failure to rescue (FTR) can result when early or subtle signs and symptoms are not noticed (*failure to recognize cues*) or accurately interpreted, and therefore action to improve the client's condition is not implemented (*failure to escalate*).

TABLE 7.2 Examples of Common Major Physiologic Changes of Aging that Can Impact Expected Outcome Achievement

Body System or Function	Major Physiologic Changes of Aging Examples
Immune system	Decline in immune function, decreasing protection against infections and cancers
Neurological system	Decreased balance and proprioception, increasing risk of falls
Cardiovascular system	Decreased elasticity of arterial walls and narrowing of arteries, decreasing blood flow to major organs
Respiratory system	Less efficient alveolar gas exchange and elasticity, decreased cough reflex, and decreased cilia function, increasing risk of infection
Renal system/fluid balance	Decreased glomerular filtration rate and the ability to regulate body fluid; decreased fluid volume, leading to high risk for dehydration
Gastrointestinal system	Decreased function of intestinal villa causing decrease in absorption of nutrients; decreased GI motility, causing high risk of gastroesophageal reflux disease (GERD) and intestinal obstruction

The ability to effectively *communicate* is crucial for the client and/or family to adequately and accurately evaluate outcomes. If the client's primary language differs from yours, be sure to seek a translator who can facilitate prompt and accurate communication. If the client wears glasses, contact lenses, and/or hearing aids, be sure they are in place. Be aware of any potential communication barriers that may be present. For example, many hearing-impaired clients have increased difficulty communicating with staff who are wearing masks.

System Factors

Similar to the discussion about system factors in other chapters, system factors such as nursing workload can also impact your ability to evaluate outcomes. As a result of heavy *workload*, nurses are often overworked, have insufficient time to determine if client conditions have improved or worsened, experience cognitive overload, and have minimal opportunity for self-care. Chapter 2 discusses these factors in detail. Additional system factors reported by nurses include lack of organizational support, lack of available technological resources to measure client outcomes, and inadequate policies and procedures (Alaseeri et al., 2021).

Role of Nursing Knowledge Base

Similar to the knowledge needed for the other clinical judgment cognitive skills, to evaluate outcomes, nurses need to know how to:
- Make timely and accurate observations
- Perform appropriate physical assessment skills

- Communicate effectively
- Use appropriate higher order critical thinking and clinical reasoning skills to make accurate inferences from observations and physical assessments

Making correct inferences requires knowledge of:

- Signs and symptoms of common complications and health conditions
- The common needs of vulnerable populations (e.g., older adults, members of the LGBTQI+ community)
- Cultural and spiritual influences on communication and other interactions
- Knowledge of the client as a person
- Anatomy, pathophysiology, pharmacology, medical-surgical nursing, and specialty nursing practice (e.g., pediatrics)

Strategies for How to Evaluate Outcomes

This chapter has explored the process for evaluating outcomes and the factors that affect your ability as a nurse to use this clinical judgment cognitive skill. This discussion highlights the strategies you should use to accurately evaluate outcomes to determine if expected or desired outcomes were met (Box 7.3).

BOX 7.3   Strategies for Evaluating Outcomes

- Determine the parameters to monitor based on the expected outcome and implemented action.
- Collect and analyze client findings consistent with the priority client condition.
- Compare observed outcomes (based on collected relevant findings) with expected outcomes for managing the client condition.
- Make an inference about the current status of the client condition to determine outcome achievement.
- Continue, modify, or discontinue the plan of care.
- Reflect on your own practice related to the client situation.

Determine the Parameters to Monitor

Nurses need to make safe, appropriate clinical judgments when clients experience either clinical deterioration or a medical complication. When planning to take action, determine which parameters or client findings need to be monitored as a result of intervention. For example, if the client is experiencing bleeding and losing significant fluid volume, the client would likely be hypotensive. After taking action, such as fluid replacement, you would continue to monitor the client's vital signs to determine if the expected outcome of increasing the blood pressure to a normal or baseline range was achieved. In this case, the client's blood pressure is the most important parameter to monitor. Likewise, the client experiencing respiratory distress with an SpO_2 of 88% would be expected to have an increase in SpO_2 after administering supplemental oxygen unless the client has chronic obstructive pulmonary disease (COPD).

Collect and Analyze Client Findings

After action is taken to manage the client's priority condition, the predetermined relevant client findings (parameters) are collected using your observation, physical assessment, and communication skills. These findings include subjective and objective data, including the results of laboratory and other diagnostic testing. To evaluate the client's progress, collected client findings must be analyzed to determine any differences from initial or earlier assessments. Use higher order thinking based on your knowledge, experience, and expertise to interpret client findings. If needed, collaborate with other health care team members to help with the analysis of client findings.

Compare Observed Outcomes with Expected Outcomes

The relevant findings collected and analyzed as the result of taking action for clients who are clinically deteriorating or experiencing a medical complication are supporting evidence for whether expected outcomes are met or not. Compare the observed clinical outcome(s) with expected or desired outcome(s). Using the earlier example, if a client's blood pressure is low due to decreased fluid volume, the expected outcome would be to achieve a blood pressure within the normal range. Following action by implementing fluid replacement, the nurse would expect the client's blood pressure to increase to the normal range or client's baseline.

CLINICAL JUDGMENT TIP

Remember: The relevant findings you collect and analyze as the result of taking action for clients who are clinically deteriorating or experiencing a medical complication are supporting evidence for whether expected outcomes are met or not.

Make an Inference to Determine Outcome Achievement

As defined earlier, an inference is a conclusion based on interpretation of client findings using clinical reasoning, or higher order thinking. For example, following fluid replacement, the nurse would expect the blood pressure of a client experiencing fluid deficit to increase to the normal range or client's baseline. If the initial blood pressure was 82/50 mmHg *before* fluid replacement and 110/74 mmHg *after* fluids were administered, the nurse would infer that the client's expected outcome was met or achieved. If the blood pressure only increased to 88/56 mmHg, the expected outcome would be considered partially met because the BP increased but not to the desired level.

Continue, Modify, or Discontinue the Plan of Care

Making inferences helps determine whether to continue, modify, or discontinue the plan of care. If expected outcomes are met, you may want to either maintain or discontinue the plan of care. If expected outcomes are not met or partially met, the plan of care may need to be continued until the client improves, or modified to add or change the planned interventions to be implemented. For example, if the blood pressure of a client who has a fluid volume deficit only increased to 88/56 mmHg, the expected outcome would be considered partially met because the BP increased but not to the desired level. Unless contraindicated due to heart or end-stage chronic kidney disease, the rate of fluid replacement then may be increased to more rapidly increase the client's fluid volume and bring up the blood pressure to a normal level.

Regardless of how the plan of care may or may not be altered, be sure to inform the client and family, and ask them about their perception of the situation. If needed, also collaborate with appropriate health care team members.

Reflect on Your Own Practice Related to the Client Situation

As discussed earlier in this chapter, nurses are also able to reflect on their clinical decision-making as part of evaluating outcomes, especially as they become more experienced. Reflective practice is a thinking skill in which nurses examine a situation with an awareness of their own values and practices, enabling them to learn from each experience. This learning is then used to improve client outcomes, which leads to new knowledge development

(Patel & Metersky, 2022). As you encounter each clinical situation in which a client clinically deteriorates or has a medical complication, you will likely strengthen your knowledge base and expertise.

> **CLINICAL JUDGMENT TIP**
>
> *Remember.* Reflective practice is a thinking skill in which nurses examine a situation with an awareness of their own values and practices, enabling them to learn from each experience. This learning is then used to improve client outcomes, which leads to new knowledge development.

Thinking Exercise 7.3 will help you practice what you've learned in this chapter about evaluating outcomes. The answer and rationale for the exercise are located at the end of this book.

THINKING EXERCISE 7.3

The nurse is caring for a 38-year-old client in the trauma center.

History and Physical	Nurses Notes	Orders	Laboratory Results

0430:   Admitted to trauma unit yesterday afternoon with bilateral lower extremity trauma and fractured left wrist as a result of a motor vehicle crash. Being frequently monitored for chest or pelvic injuries. No chest or abdominal pain; no report of headache. Alert and oriented ×4, PERRLA. Moves both upper extremities without problem. Breath sounds clear throughout lung fields. S_1 and S_2 present. Client crying and asking for family who left briefly to obtain food. Left leg with multiple bruising and superficial cuts; left ankle fracture treated with splint until swelling decreases; surgical repair not yet scheduled. Extensive right leg muscle and soft tissue damage with fractured tibia; long leg splint in place. Cap refill >3 seconds in right foot; <3 seconds in left foot. Client states feelings of numbness and tingling in right foot and lower leg. Unable to move toes in right foot; movement normal in left foot. Right foot very cool and pale when compared to right with no palpable pedal pulse. 1+ pedal pulses palpated at 0230. VS: T 98.8°F (37.1°C), HR 88 beats per minute and regular, RR 20 breaths minute, BP 118/70 mmHg, SpO_2 95% on RA. Reports pain in right leg getting worse; is now 10/10. Surgeon notified.

0705:   Transferred to OR for right leg fasciotomy.

1035:   Returned from OR with open fasciotomy on anterior right calf. Pedal pulses bilaterally 1+. Both feet cool but right foot cooler than left. Color same in both feet; cap refill <3 seconds bilaterally. Right leg pain reported at 5/10. VS: T 98.6°F (37°C), HR 76 beats per minute and regular, RR 16 breaths per minute, BP 106/64 mmHg, SpO_2 96% on RA. Analgesic administered.

Select **4** client findings that indicate the client's condition has **improved** following surgery.
- Pulses
- SpO_2
- Foot color
- Foot temperature
- Right leg pain
- Capillary refill
- Blood pressure

END-OF-CHAPTER THINKING EXERCISES

These additional End-of-Chapter Thinking Exercises will help you apply what you've learned in this chapter about evaluating outcomes. The answers and rationales for these exercises are located at the end of this chapter.

⟩ END-OF-CHAPTER THINKING EXERCISE 7.1

The nurse is caring for a 26-year-old client in the Emergency Department.

History and Physical	Nurses Notes	Orders	Laboratory Results

1140: Brought to ED by friend; client has history of opioid addiction which developed following a severe back injury at a construction site. Has been struggling with clinical depression and attempted suicide a few months ago. Went to bar earlier this evening and had several alcoholic drinks; found "passed out" in the bathroom. Client currently very drowsy and barely responsive to verbal stimuli. Pupils small but not pinpoint; PERRLA. Breath sounds clear throughout lung fields. S_1 and S_2 present. Cap refill <3 seconds bilaterally. VS: T 98.4°F (36.9°C), HR 58 beats per minute and regular, RR 12 breaths per minute and regular but shallow; BP 90/42 mmHg; SpO_2 90% on RA.

1150: Peripheral IV access established and naloxone administered. Supplemental oxygen initiated.

1230: Client alert and oriented ×2 (person and place). PERRLA. Moves all extremities as requested. VS: T 98.6°F (37°C); HR 70 beats per minute and regular; RR 16 breaths per minute, regular, but shallow, BP 110/67 mmHg; SpO_2 99% on oxygen 4 L per minute.

Which of the following findings indicate that the client's condition has **improved**? **Select all that apply.**
- Temperature
- Heart rate
- Respiratory rate
- Blood pressure
- SpO_2
- Level of consciousness

⟩ END-OF-CHAPTER THINKING EXERCISE 7.2

The nurse is caring for a 69-year-old client in the family practice clinic.

History and Physical	Nurses Notes	Orders	Laboratory Results

1330: Follow-up clinic visit today for client with a long history of COPD, hypertension, and diabetes mellitus type 2. Positive for COVID-19 2 weeks ago with report of nasal congestion, headache, fever with chills, nonproductive cough, nausea and vomiting, muscle aches, and loss of taste and smell. Prescribed nirmatrelvir/ritonavir and corticosteroid inhaler after 3 days of illness onset. Follow-up visit scheduled today due to comorbidities and client's age. Currently alert and oriented ×4. Breath sounds clear throughout lung fields. S_1 and S_2 present. Bowel sounds present ×4. No headache, muscle aches, nausea and vomiting, or nasal congestion, but reports frequent episodes of dry cough and lack of taste and smell. VS: T 98.6°F (37°C), HR 78 beats per minute and regular, RR 18 breaths per minute and regular, BP 132/80 mmHg, SpO_2 95% on RA.

⚡ END-OF-CHAPTER THINKING EXERCISE 7.2—cont'd

For each current client finding, select whether the finding indicates that the client's condition has improved or not improved.

Client Findings	Improved	Not Improved
Cough		
Headache		
Nausea and vomiting		
Loss of taste and smell		
Temperature		
Nasal congestion		

⚡ END-OF-CHAPTER THINKING EXERCISE 7.3

The nurse is caring for an 11-year-old client in the pediatrician's office.

Nurses Notes	**History and Physical**	**Orders**	**Laboratory Results**

Office Visit 3 Weeks Ago

Medical History:

- Attention deficit/hyperactivity disorder (ADHD)
- Autism spectrum disorder (highly functional)
- Possible child abuse

Allergies: NKDA

Medications:

- Lisdexamfetamine 30 mg orally every morning
- Paroxetine 40 mg orally every morning

Social history: Father brought child to office with report of worsening defiance and disruptive behaviors in school and at home. Parents divorced; child spends weekends with mother and during the week with father. Physical exam showed healthy child except for old bruises in varying stages of healing on the chest and back. Father unable to explain cause of injuries. Chest X-ray ordered. Child denied physical abuse and stated that the bruising was from a fight with some kids at school last week. Informed father that the child's status will be reported to Child Protective Services (CPS) today.

History and Physical	**Nurses Notes**	**Orders**	**Laboratory Results**

Follow-Up Office Visit Today

1550:   Accompanied by mother for follow-up office visit today for preteen child who was seen 3 weeks ago for increased defiance and disruptive behaviors. During previous visit, father was instructed on techniques for managing disruptive behaviors; lisdexamfetamine dosage increased to 40 mg. CPS follow-up report inconclusive for child abuse. Mother states today that child did not have chest X-ray as requested without explanation of why procedure was not done. Mother reports disruptive behaviors have improved and child is less defiant. Still having some problems with impulse control. Tried to "run away from home" twice last week; but father found him at a friend's house. Physical exam shows no new bruising or other physical injuries; most old bruises faded.

Continued

END-OF-CHAPTER THINKING EXERCISE 7.3—cont'd

Complete the following sentence by selecting from the lists of options below.
The nurse determines that the client's condition has _____ **1 [Select]** _____ as evidenced by _____ **2 [Select]** _____ and
_____ **3 [Select]** _____ .

Options for 1	Options for 2	Options for 3
Improved	Not having a chest X-ray	Problem with impulse control
Not changed	No new bruising or injuries	Tried to run away from home
Worsened	Inconclusive CPS report	Less disruptive behaviors

END-OF-CHAPTER THINKING EXERCISE 7.4

The nurse is caring for a 38-year-old client in the postpartum unit.
Highlight the client findings that indicate the client's condition has **worsened**.

History and Physical	Nurses Notes	Orders	Laboratory Results

0225:   Client admitted to postpartum unit after being induced for normal vaginal delivery of twins. Breasts engorged without pain, redness, or warmth. Uterus firm at umbilicus level. Has not yet voided. Lochia bright red with a few small clots; no foul odor. No evidence of DVT. Acetaminophen given for mild discomfort. VS: T 98.2°F (36.9°C), HR 74 beats per minute and regular, RR 20 breaths per minute and regular, BP 114/66 mmHg; SpO$_2$ 98% on RA.

1940:   Breasts engorged without pain, redness, or warmth. States voiding large amounts ×3 since admission. Uterus boggy after massage. Lochia heavier with large clots; client states saturating two pads in the last hour. VS: T 98.2°F (36.9°C), HR 100 beats per minute and regular, RR 26 breaths per minute and regular, BP 88/46 mmHg; SpO$_2$ 96% on RA.

END-OF-CHAPTER THINKING EXERCISE 7.5

The nurse is caring for a 59-year-old client who had abdominal surgery.

History and Physical	Nurses Notes	Orders	Laboratory Results

Acute Surgical Unit

0745 (POD #1):   Obese client admitted 3 days ago for intestinal obstruction which was managed by IV fluids, nasogastric suction, and electrolyte replacement. Yesterday had colon resection and open laparotomy to remove malignant tumor. Alert and oriented ×4; breath sounds clear throughout lung fields. S$_1$ and S$_2$ present. Abdomen soft with diminished bowel sounds ×4. Surgical dressing dry and intact. Reports new-onset right calf pain of 7/10. Posterior right lower leg swelling, redness, and warmth. Cap refill <3 seconds bilaterally. VS: T 98.4°F (36.9°C), HR 74 beats per minute and regular, RR 20 breaths per minute and regular; BP 146/80 mmHg; SpO$_2$ 99% on 5 L per minute O$_2$ via NC.

0820:   Surgeon notified about possible right leg DVT. D-dimer and duplex ultrasound ordered.

1035:   Apixaban started; warm compresses and ambulation as tolerated ordered. Taught client about drug and need to avoid massaging the affected calf. Also told to report any signs and symptoms of pulmonary embolus.

Two Weeks Later in Surgeon's Office

1105:   Follow-up today for colon resection for malignant tumor. Alert and oriented ×4. Reports right leg feeling better with pain at 2/10. Minimal redness and warmth; no swelling present. No signs or symptoms of pulmonary embolus. Continues taking apixaban as prescribed. Breath sounds clear. Bowel sounds present ×4. Incision very reddened with yellowish-tan drainage at distal end. Client reports extreme tenderness near incision; states that all wound closure strips except two fell off. VS: T 100.4°F (38°C), HR 92 beats per minute and regular, RR 20 breaths per minute and regular; BP 122/74 mmHg; SpO$_2$ 95% on RA.

END-OF-CHAPTER THINKING EXERCISE 7.5—cont'd

For each current client finding, select whether the finding indicates that the client's condition has improved or worsened.

Client Findings	Improved	Worsened
Right calf redness and warmth		
Right calf swelling		
Right calf pain		
Abdominal incision		
Temperature		
Blood pressure		

END-OF-CHAPTER THINKING EXERCISE 7.6

The nurse is caring for a 2-year-old child with Kawasaki's disease.
Highlight the findings in the 1515 note that indicate the client's condition has **improved**.

History and Physical	Nurses Notes	Orders	Laboratory Results

Initial Pediatric Urgent Care Visit

0830:   Grandmother brought child to pediatric urgent care with concern about prolonged fever between 102°F (38.9°C) and 103°F (39.4°C) for the past 6 days with new onset of rash with reddened skin and mucous membranes. Skin on palms of hands and soles of feet started peeling yesterday. Child has been very irritable and having diarrhea 5–7 times a day. VS: T 103°F (39.4°C), HR 110 beats per minute and reg, RR 20 breaths per minute, BP 102/58 mmHg, SpO_2 96% on RA.

0945:   Transferred to acute care pediatric unit for suspected Kawasaki's disease (KD).

Acute Pediatric Unit 3 Days Later

1515:   Continuous cardiac monitoring shows no heart damage as a result of KD. No side or adverse effects of aspirin therapy. Rash evident on chest and abdomen. Skin less reddened and not peeling today. No diarrhea for 24 hours. VS: T 99°F (37.2°C), HR 94 beats per minute and reg, RR 18 breaths per minute, BP 98/54 mmHg, SpO_2 96% on RA.

END-OF-CHAPTER THINKING EXERCISE 7.7

The nurse is caring for an 83-year-old client with acute confusion and anxiety.

History and Physical	Nurses Notes	Orders	Laboratory Results

Initial Emergency Department Visit

1140: Brought to ED by family from home due to onset of acute confusion and anxiety. Client lives at home with family due to advanced age. Has been caring for self independently, is usually continent, and has no history of dementia or depression. Walks independently at home using a cane. Is well-groomed but very thin. Medical history includes hypertension, rheumatoid arthritis, osteoarthritis, and diverticulitis. Currently client is alert and oriented ×1 (person only). Withdraws arms and whimpers when touched by staff. Shaking during exam even though moving slowly to assess client and explaining each step. Breath sounds clear throughout lung fields. S_1 and S_2 present. Cap refill >3 seconds bilaterally. Can move all extremities but not on command. Abdomen soft and non-distended. Bowel sounds present ×4. Multiple bruises and skin tears on both arms. Bruises in various stages of healing on abdomen. Client yells out when abdomen touched. Family states that client falls frequently and skin is very thin from previous chronic steroid therapy. VS: T 98.4°F (36.9°C), HR 104 beats per minute and regular, RR 18 breaths per minute and regular, BP 98/60 mmHg, SpO$_2$ 94% on RA. Weight 110 lbs. (49.9 kg); BMI 16.2.

1255: Examined by nurse practitioner. Plan to admit client for possible urinary tract infection, malnutrition, and dehydration. Social work consult for potential elder abuse.

Assisted Living Center 2 Weeks Later

0900: Client admitted to center after hospital discharge; becoming acclimated to new environment. Alert and oriented ×4. Smiling and talking with residents during activity. Has gained 3 pounds since hospital admission several weeks ago. Skin tears and bruises slowly healing. No new injuries or falls. VS: T 98.6°F (37°C), HR 80 beats per minute and regular, RR 16 breaths per minute and regular, BP 116/74 mmHg, SpO$_2$ 94% on RA.

For each current client finding, select whether the finding indicates that the client's condition has improved or not changed.

Client Findings	Improved	Not Changed
Orientation		
Temperature		
Heart rate		
Blood pressure		
Mood and affect		

Answers and Rationales for Thinking Exercises

CHAPTER THINKING EXERCISES

THINKING EXERCISE 7.1

Answer:

History and Physical	Nurses Notes	Orders	Laboratory Results

2110: Family brought client to ED due to client's severe right back pain, fever, chills, and vomiting which started early this morning. No significant medical history. Client alert and oriented ×4, but wincing in severe pain rated at 10/10 on a 0–10 pain intensity scale. Breath sounds clear throughout lung fields; no dyspnea. S_1 and S_2 present. Bowel sounds present ×4; abdomen soft. VS: T 101.8°F (38.8°C); HR 112 beats per minute and regular; RR 28 breaths per minute and shallow; BP 148/92 mmHg; SpO_2 95% on RA.

2135: Voided urine with gross hematuria. Sample sent to lab. IV morphine administered.

2220: States feeling "a little better"; pain level now 6/10. VS: T 102°F (38.9°C); HR 94 beats per minute and regular; RR 20 breaths per minute and regular; BP 130/86 mmHg; SpO_2 96% on RA. Transferred for kidney ultrasound.

Rationale: The client initially reported severe right back (flank) pain at 10/10 which decreased to 6/10 after morphine was administered. Although a lower pain level is more desirable, the client's pain did improve, which demonstrated that care was effective. Client findings indicate that the pain is likely caused by urolithiasis (urinary tract or kidney stones) which typically causes extreme pain as stones move. The client's temperature worsened but other vital signs, including heart rate, respiratory rate, and blood pressure are improved as a result of analgesia. The SpO_2 remained about the same after morphine was given.

THINKING EXERCISE 7.2

Answer:

Client Findings	Improved	Worsened
Heart rate	X	
Pain intensity		X
Respiratory rate	X	
Blood pressure	X	
Bleeding from surgical site	X	

Rationale: The client had a BKA yesterday and is experiencing new-onset bleeding from the surgical site today. As a result, the client's blood pressure decreased; the heart and respiratory rate increased as compensation for decreased circulating blood volume. After interventions were implemented, the documentation in the 1440 note indicates that the client's vital signs improved and returned to baseline. The nurse noted no new bleeding on the reinforced surgical dressing which also indicates improvement. These findings demonstrate that nursing actions were effective. The client's pain, however, increased from 6/10 to 10/10 which worsened. The client's temperature and SpO_2 were essentially unchanged from earlier levels.

THINKING EXERCISE 7.3

Answer:
Select **4** client findings that indicate the client's condition has **improved** following surgery.
X Pulses
○ SpO₂
X Foot color
○ Foot temperature
X Right leg pain
X Capillary refill
○ Blood pressure

Rationale: The client experienced acute compartment syndrome as a result of lower extremity trauma with swelling and hypoperfusion. Before the fasciotomy to relieve pressure and restore perfusion, the client reported severe increasing pain, and had pallor, decreased temperature, prolonged capillary refill, and no palpable distal pulse in the affected leg. After surgery, the 1035 note indicates that the client's right distal pulse, skin color, and capillary refill had all improved. The client also reported right leg pain as 5/10, which was an improvement when compared to the earlier report of 10/10 pain intensity. The right foot continues to be cooler than the left, which shows no significant change. The client's SpO₂, blood pressure, heart rate, and respiratory rate all remained within normal ranges.

END-OF-CHAPTER THINKING EXERCISES

END-OF-CHAPTER THINKING EXERCISE 7.1

Answer:
Which of the following findings indicate that the client's condition has **improved**? **Select all that apply.**
○ Temperature
X Heart rate
X Respiratory rate
X Blood pressure
X SpO₂
X Level of consciousness

Rationale: The client likely experienced an overdose of opioids given the history of opioid addiction and the current assessment findings. As a result, the client was given a reversal agent, naloxone, which improved the client's level of consciousness from very drowsy to alert and oriented ×2, and increased the client's vital signs to normal ranges. The client was placed on supplemental oxygen which increased the SpO₂ to within the normal range of 95% or above. These findings indicate that interventions were effective for this client. The client's body temperature was not changed and remained within normal limits.

⚡ END-OF-CHAPTER THINKING EXERCISE 7.2

Answer:

Client Findings	Improved	Not Improved
Cough		X
Headache	X	
Nausea and vomiting	X	
Loss of taste and smell		X
Temperature	X	
Nasal congestion	X	

Rationale: The client was treated on an ambulatory basis for COVID-19 with an antiviral medication within 5 days of symptom onset. Because the client has several comorbidities that could cause COVID to worsen, a follow-up visit 2 weeks later was scheduled. During that visit, the client showed improvement in all signs and symptoms except for continued loss of taste and smell and frequent episodes of dry cough. These residual findings are common for many clients who have had this infection and may continue for weeks or months.

⚡ END-OF-CHAPTER THINKING EXERCISE 7.3

Answer:
The nurse determines that the client's condition has **improved** as evidenced by **no new bruising or injuries** and **less disruptive behaviors**.

Rationale: The child had been experiencing more disruptive and defiant behaviors as reported on the initial visit to the pediatrician. Nursing and collaborative actions, including teaching the parent about how to manage the child's behaviors and increasing the dosage of the child's medication, helped to decrease the incidence of disruptive behaviors. This finding indicates the client's condition has improved. During the initial visit, the office staff observed old bruising and injuries suggestive of child abuse. These allegations were reported and followed up, but Child Protective Services did not validate child abuse. The child had no new bruising or injuries on the follow-up visit, which also indicates improvement.

END-OF-CHAPTER THINKING EXERCISE 7.4

Answer:

History and Physical	**Nurses Notes**	Orders	Laboratory Results

0225:   Client admitted to postpartum unit after being induced for normal vaginal delivery of twins. Breasts engorged without pain, redness, or warmth. Uterus firm at umbilicus level. Has not yet voided. Lochia bright red with a few small clots; no foul odor. No evidence of DVT. Acetaminophen given for mild discomfort. VS: T 98.2°F (36.9°C), HR 74 beats per minute and regular, RR 20 breaths per minute and regular, BP 114/66 mmHg; SpO$_2$ 98% on RA.

1940:   Breasts engorged without pain, redness, or warmth. States voiding large amounts ×3 since admission. Uterus boggy after massage. Lochia heavier with large clots; client states saturating two pads in the last hour. VS: T 98.2°F (36.9°C), HR 100 beats per minute and regular, RR 26 breaths per minute and regular, BP 88/46 mmHg; SpO$_2$ 96% on RA.

Rationale: After childbirth, the client's uterine fundus needs to remain firm to prevent excessive bleeding. The client's fundus was firm at the umbilicus level at 0225 and vital signs were within normal ranges. However, at 1940, the nurse found the uterus to be boggy (soft) with a significant increase in vaginal bleeding with large clots. These findings are relevant cues that the client's condition has worsened. Additionally, the client's blood pressure decreased as a result of decreased fluid volume; the client also has tachycardia and tachypnea as compensatory responses to the loss of blood. These vital sign changes support the worsening of the client's condition which could become life-threatening. At this point, the client's SpO$_2$ has not changed significantly.

END-OF-CHAPTER THINKING EXERCISE 7.5

Answer:

Client Findings	Improved	Worsened
Right calf redness and warmth	X	
Right calf swelling	X	
Right calf pain	X	
Abdominal incision		X
Temperature		X
Blood pressure	X	

Rationale: The initial assessment findings indicated the client likely had a postoperative deep vein thrombosis (DVT) which was validated by diagnostic testing. The client's high BP could have been caused by anxiety and/or pain. As a result, nursing actions were taken and the client was placed on an anticoagulant to prevent the clot from becoming larger. Two weeks later, the client was followed up in the surgeon's office which showed major improvement when compared to initial findings related to the DVT, including minimal right calf redness and warmth, no right calf swelling, and less right calf pain. The client's blood pressure also decreased, which shows improvement rather than worsening of the client's condition. However, the client's abdominal incision was very tender, red, and draining, and the client's temperature was elevated. These findings indicate possible surgical wound infection, which indicates worsening of the client's condition related to the surgery.

END-OF-CHAPTER THINKING EXERCISE 7.6

Answer:

History and Physical	Nurses Notes	Orders	Laboratory Results

Initial Pediatric Urgent Care Visit

0830:   Grandmother brought child to pediatric urgent care with concern about prolonged fever between 102°F (38.9°C) and 103°F (39.4°C) for the past 6 days with new onset of rash with reddened skin and mucous membranes. Skin on palms of hands and soles of feet started peeling yesterday. Child has been very irritable and having diarrhea 5–7 times a day. VS: T 103°F (39.4°C), HR 110 beats per minute and reg, RR 20 breaths per minute, BP 102/58 mmHg, SpO$_2$ 96% on RA.

0945:   Transferred to acute care pediatric unit for suspected Kawasaki's disease (KD).

Acute Pediatric Unit 3 Days Later

1515:   Continuous cardiac monitoring shows no heart damage as a result of KD. No side or adverse effects of aspirin therapy. Rash evident on chest and abdomen. Skin less reddened and not peeling today. No diarrhea for 24 hours. VS: T 99°F (37.2°C), HR 94 beats per minute and reg, RR 18 breaths per minute, BP 98/54 mmHg, SpO$_2$ 96% on RA.

Rationale: The child had possible Kawasaki's disease with findings including diarrhea, fever, and reddened peeling skin. Vital signs other than body temperature remained within normal ranges for a child of this age. Three days later after interventions were started, the child's temperature decreased, diarrhea subsided, and skin was less reddened and peeling. These changes in assessment findings show improvement in the child's condition. The child's rash did not change, and vital signs other than temperature remained within normal limits.

END-OF-CHAPTER THINKING EXERCISE 7.7

Answer:

Client Findings	Improved	Not Changed
Orientation	X	
Temperature		X
Heart rate	X	
Blood pressure	X	
Mood and affect	X	

Rationale: This older client was living with family and developed possible UTI, malnutrition, and dehydration. Client findings resulting from these conditions were initially a low BMI, tachycardia, and hypotension. The client's acute confusion and anxiety support these conditions due to the client's advanced age. Additionally, the client had signs and symptoms associated with possible elder abuse, including being withdrawn, multiple bruises, and skin tears. Two weeks later the client was no longer living with family and improved as evidenced by normal vital signs (temperature was unchanged), no new injuries, and complete orientation. The client seemed content and happy as evidenced by smiling and interacting with other residents in the assisted living center. These behaviors support an improvement in the client's mood and affect.

REFERENCES

Alaseeri, R., Rajab, A., & Banakhar, M. (2021). Do personal differences and organizational factors influence nurses' decision making? A qualitative study. *Nursing Reports, 11*(3), 714–727.

American Nurses Association (ANA). (2021). *Nursing scope and standards of practice* (4th ed.). ANA.

Avlijas, T., Squires, J. E., Lalonde, M., & Backman, C. (2023). A concept analysis of the patient experience. *PXJ: Patient Experience Journal, 10*(1), 15–63.

Burdeu, G., Lowe, G., Rasmussen, B., & Consedine, J. (2021). Clinical cues used by nurses to recognize changes in patients' clinical states: A systematic review. *Nursing and Health Science, 23*(1), 9–28.

*Doyle, C., Lennox, L., & Bill, D. (2012). A systematic review of evidence in the links between patient experience and clinical safety and effectiveness. *BMJ Open, 3*(1).

*Koy, V., Yunibhand, J., & Angsuroch, Y. (2015). Nursing care quality: A concept analysis. *International Journal of Research in Medical Sciences, 3*(8), 1832–1838.

*Liu, Y., Avant, K. C., Aungsuroch, Y., Zhang, X.-Y., & Jiang, P. (2014). Patient outcomes in the field of nursing: A concept analysis. *International Journal of Nursing Sciences, 1*(1), 69–74.

Liyew, B., Tilahun, A., & Kassew, T. (2021). Practices and barriers towards physical assessment among nurses working in intensive care units. *BioMed Research International, 2021*.

Manetti, W. (2019). Sound clinical judgment in nursing: A concept analysis. *Nursing Forum, 54*(1), 102–110.

*Nibbelink, C. W., & Brewer, B. B. (2018). Decision-making in nursing practice: An integrative literature review. *Journal of Clinical Nursing, 27*(5–6), 917–928.

Orique, S. B., Despins, L., Wakefield, B. J., Erdelez, S., & Vogelsmeier, A. (2019). Perception of clinical deterioration cues among medical-surgical nurses. *Journal of Advanced Nursing, 75*(11), 2627–2637.

Patel, K. M., & Metersky, K. (2022). Reflective practice in nursing: A concept analysis. *International Journal of Nursing Knowledge, 33*(3), 180–187.

Potter, P. A., Perry, A. G., Stockert, P. A., & Hall, A. M. (2023). *Fundamentals of nursing* (11th ed.). Elsevier.

Touhy, T. A., & Jett, K. (2022). *Ebersole and Hess' Gerontological nursing and healthy aging* (6th ed.). Elsevier.

*Denotes classic reference.

How to Make Safe Clinical Judgments

THIS CHAPTER AT A GLANCE...

Readiness for Nursing Practice and Clinical Judgment Review
- Nurses' Responsibility for Making Safe, Appropriate Clinical Judgments
- Summary of Cognitive Skills Needed to Make Safe, Appropriate Clinical Judgments

Unfolding Case Study Examples
Stand-Alone Item Examples
- Bowtie Items
- Trend Items

LEARNING OUTCOMES

1. Identify the nurse's responsibility for making safe, appropriate clinical judgments.
2. Briefly summarize the process for using the six cognitive skills to make effective clinical judgments.
3. Correctly complete selected unfolding case studies to practice making safe, appropriate clinical judgments.
4. Correctly complete selected Stand-Alone items to practice making safe, appropriate clinical judgments.

Chapter 1 of this book introduced you to the clinical reasoning process to make safe, appropriate clinical judgments; this process is sometimes referred to as clinical decision-making. Chapters 2 through 7 provided detailed guidance to help you learn how to use each cognitive skill or step of the clinical reasoning process. This chapter provides the opportunity for you to practice putting those skills together using new test items similar to those you will encounter on the NCLEX®.

READINESS FOR NURSING PRACTICE AND CLINICAL JUDGMENT REVIEW

As discussed in Chapter 1, nurses must be able to care for clients competently and safely to be ready for professional practice. Nursing competencies require more than knowledge and skills; competencies should improve the quality of client care, ensure client safety, and reduce the incidence of near misses in care. Improving the quality of client care is dependent on your ability to develop strong clinical reasoning skills to make safe, appropriate clinical judgments. Recall that clinical reasoning is the *process* for nurse thinking, and clinical judgment is the result or *outcome* of that thinking (see Chapter 1).

Nurses' Responsibility for Making Safe, Appropriate Clinical Judgments

Unlike the role of other health care professionals, nurses are responsible for client care 24 hours a day and 7 days a week. In many health care settings, including home health, most clients need very complex care which requires nurses to be competent in making safe clinical judgments. As an essential component of that care, nurses have the responsibility and accountability to assess and accurately interpret relevant client findings, especially heart rate, blood pressure, oxygen saturation (SpO_2), and level of consciousness (LOC) (Burdeu et al., 2021).

Chapter 1 described a study of 5000 new RN graduates which found only 23% of the graduates could demonstrate basic clinical judgment competencies, including interpreting relevant client findings. Since those data were presented in 2015, the researchers measured clinical judgment competencies of graduates over the next 5 years. Unfortunately, the ability of new graduates to demonstrate basic clinical judgment competencies continued to decline over the 5-year study period as shown in Box 8.1.

BOX 8.1 Percentage of New Graduates with Basic Clinical Judgment Competencies

Year New Graduates Hired	% of New Graduates with Basic Clinical Judgment Competencies
2016	21%
2017	17%
2018	15%
2019	9%
2020	8%

From Kavanaugh, J.M., & Sharpnack, P.A. (2021). A crisis in competency: A defining moment in nursing education. *Online Journal of Issues in Nursing, 26*(1). https://doi.org/10.3912/OJIN.Vol26No01Man02

This book was developed to help you improve your basic clinical judgment skills, be ready for professional nursing practice, and be prepared to take the NCLEX®.

Summary of Cognitive Skills Needed to Make Safe, Appropriate Clinical Judgments

As defined by the NCBSN on the NCLEX-RN® Test Plan, clinical judgment is "the observed outcome of critical thinking and decision-making. It is an iterative process with multiple steps that uses nursing knowledge to observe and assess presenting situations, identify a prioritized client concern, and generate the best possible evidence-based solutions in order to deliver safe client care" (NCSBN, 2023). As shown in Box 8.2, six cognitive steps were identified by NCSBN as essential skills needed to make safe, appropriate clinical judgments.

Chapters 2 through 7 discussed each of these clinical judgment cognitive skills in detail. Each skill is briefly summarized here before you begin practice making clinical judgments using unfolding case studies and Stand-Alone items similar to what you will have on your licensure examination.

> ### BOX 8.2   Clinical Judgment Cognitive Skills/Steps with Definitions and Key Questions
>
> **Recognize Cues**: Identify relevant and important information from different sources (e.g., medical history, vital signs). *What matters most and now?*
> **Analyze Cues**: Organize and connect the recognized cues to the client's clinical presentation. *What could it mean?*
> **Prioritize Hypotheses**: Evaluate and prioritize hypotheses (urgency, likelihood, risk, difficulty, time constraints, etc.). *Where do I start?*
> **Generate Solutions**: Identify expected outcomes and use hypotheses to define a set of interventions for the expected outcomes. *What can I do?*
> **Take Action**: Implement the solution(s) that address the highest priority. *What will I do?*
> **Evaluate Outcomes**: Compare observed outcomes to expected outcomes. *Did it help?*

From National Council of State Boards of Nursing (NCSBN). (2023). *Next-Generation NCLEX®. NCLEX-RN® Test Plan.* NCSBN.

Recognize Cues: What Matters Most and Now?

Cue recognition can be defined as "the mental process involved in extracting and identifying *relevant* and important information from the presenting [client] situation" (Betts et al., 2019). As described in Chapter 2, this information includes both objective and subjective clinical cues. Test items that require you to recognize cues will ask you which client findings in a clinical situation require immediate follow-up.

To accurately recognize cues, remember to carefully review all client findings (both objective and subjective data) in the clinical situation. Anticipate common medical complications that are associated with or could occur as a result of the client's current condition. Determine which client findings are normal/usual or abnormal/unusual in the clinical situation. Be alert for findings that indicate possible clinical deterioration. Consider contextual factors that influence if client findings in the clinical situation are expected or unexpected. Finally, determine which client findings require **immediate** follow-up.

Analyze Cues: What Could It Mean?

As discussed in Chapter 3, analyzing cues is the ability to organize and link relevant assessment findings to the client's presenting clinical situation to determine probable client conditions. This clinical skill requires higher order thinking to interpret or make sense of relevant clinical cues and what they mean.

To begin analyzing cues, organize relevant client findings (that need immediate follow-up) to develop a pattern. Then compare these findings with your knowledge and determine if inconsistencies or gaps exist. On the NCLEX® you will be asked to determine which client findings are consistent with a variety of health conditions. Based on your interpretation of relevant findings, draw a conclusion or inference about the client's actual or potential condition(s).

Prioritize Hypotheses: Where Do I Start?

As discussed in Chapter 4, prioritizing hypotheses is a clinical judgment cognitive skill that helps you establish the best order for client care. This skill is particularly important when a client has multiple physical and mental client conditions and needs. To prioritize hypotheses, first review the list of client conditions (hypotheses) in the clinical situation that were generated from the analysis of relevant clinical cues. For actual conditions, evaluate hypotheses based on urgency and risk to client safety. For potential conditions, evaluate hypotheses based on the client's risk for potentially life-threatening complications or clinical deterioration.

Generate Solutions: What Can I Do?

To generate solutions, think about what potential nursing actions or interventions could be implemented for the client to meet the expected clinical outcomes for the priority health condition. Be sure to identify actions that are evidence-based and appropriate for the context of the clinical situation. Create a list of possible actions for the priority client condition based on your knowledge and experience. Finally, analyze each action for potential implementation. Chapter 5 discusses how to generate solutions in detail.

Take Actions: What Will I Do?

Nursing actions are interventions and assessments that are implemented to assist the client in improving health and attaining expected clinical outcomes. As discussed in Chapter 6, deciding which actions to take depends on the severity or urgency of the client's condition. Keep in mind that clients most at risk for medical complications or clinical deterioration require prompt nursing actions, including those who (Padilla & Mayo, 2018):

- Are emergency admissions
- Have acute or preexisting health conditions
- Have had recent surgeries
- Are recovering from critical illnesses

  Be sure to implement actions *immediately* for clients who have emergent Priority 1 conditions, such as:

- Absence of pulse or respirations
- Obstructed airway
- Potential harm to self or others
- Crushing chest pain with bradycardia
- Retractions with nasal flaring

Evaluate Outcomes: Did It Help?

After nursing actions have been implemented, determine if the expected clinical outcomes for the client have been met. As described in Chapter 7, to evaluate outcomes, first determine the parameters to monitor based on the expected outcome and nursing actions. Then collect and analyze client findings consistent with the priority client condition by comparing observed outcomes (based on collected relevant findings) with expected outcomes for managing the client condition. Make an inference (draw a conclusion) about the current status of the client condition to determine outcome achievement. Based on that inference, decide whether to continue, modify, or discontinue the plan of care. Throughout the entire evaluation process, be sure to reflect on your own practice related to the client situation.

UNFOLDING CASE STUDY EXAMPLES

As a reminder from Chapter 1, unfolding case studies are also called "evolving" cases because the client's clinical situation changes or evolves over time—usually minutes, hours, or days. Unfolding case studies as part of today's NCLEX® present realistic situations in which the client clinically deteriorates, develops a medical complication, or is at high risk for a complication during the case. Each unfolding case study consists of multiple client data and six test items that measure the six cognitive skills needed to make safe clinical judgments. As you practice answering test items for the unfolding case studies below, keep in mind what you learned about each cognitive skill, including the tips and strategies in each chapter! The answers and rationales for these unfolding case studies can be found at the end of this chapter.

UNFOLDING CASE STUDY 8.1

Thinking Exercise 8.1.1

The nurse is caring for an 87-year-old client in the skilled nursing unit. Highlight the client findings that require **immediate** follow-up.

History and Physical	Nurses Notes	Orders	Laboratory Results

0815: Unlicensed personnel states that client who is usually alert and oriented seems sleepy and very confused this AM. Tried twice to climb out of bed. Reports that client has not voided since last night before going to bed. Client's medical history includes two strokes, type 2 diabetes mellitus, hypertension, chronic heart failure, and osteoarthritis. Currently drowsy but easily awakened. No abnormal or adventitious breath sounds; skin warm and dry. Lips and mucous membranes dry. Abdomen soft and round. Cap refill 5 seconds; pedal pulses 1+ and equal. 2+ nonpitting edema in both feet. VS: T 100.6°F (38.1°C); HR 105 beats per minute and irregular; RR 20 breaths per minute; BP 88/52 mmHg; SpO$_2$ 89% on RA; FSBG 76 mg/dL (4.21 mmol/L).

Thinking Exercise 8.1.2

The nurse is caring for an 87-year-old client in the skilled nursing unit.

History and Physical	Nurses Notes	Orders	Laboratory Results

0815: Unlicensed personnel states that client who is usually alert and oriented seems sleepy and very confused this AM. Tried twice to climb out of bed. Reports that client has not voided since last night before going to bed. Client's medical history includes two strokes, type 2 diabetes mellitus, hypertension, chronic heart failure, and osteoarthritis. Currently drowsy but easily awakened. No abnormal or adventitious breath sounds; skin warm and dry. Lips and mucous membranes dry. Abdomen soft and round. Cap refill 5 seconds; pedal pulses 1+ and equal. 2+ nonpitting edema in both feet. VS: T 100.6°F (38.1°C); HR 105 beats per minute and irregular; RR 20 breaths per minute; BP 88/52 mmHg; SpO$_2$ 89% on RA; FSBG 76 mg/dL (4.21 mmol/L).

For each client finding listed below, determine if the finding is consistent with the health conditions of dehydration, chronic kidney disease, or heart failure. Some findings may be consistent with more than one condition.

Client Findings	Dehydration	Chronic Kidney Disease	Heart Failure
Has not voided since last night			
T 100.6°F (38.1°C);			
HR 105 beats per minute and irregular			
BP 88/52 mmHg			
2+ nonpitting edema in both feet			

Thinking Exercise 8.1.3

The nurse is caring for an 87-year-old client in the skilled nursing unit.

History and Physical	Nurses Notes	Orders	Laboratory Results

0815: Unlicensed personnel states that client who is usually alert and oriented seems sleepy and very confused this AM. Tried twice to climb out of bed. Reports that client has not voided since last night before going to bed. Client's medical history includes two strokes, type 2 diabetes mellitus, hypertension, chronic heart failure, and osteoarthritis. Currently drowsy but easily awakened. No abnormal or adventitious breath sounds; skin warm and dry. Lips and mucous membranes dry. Abdomen soft and round. Cap refill 5 seconds; pedal pulses 1+ and equal. 2+ nonpitting edema in both feet. VS: T 100.6°F (38.1°C); HR 105 beats per minute and irregular; RR 20 breaths per minute; BP 88/52 mmHg; SpO$_2$ 89% on RA; FSBG 76 mg/dL (4.21 mmol/L).

Complete the following sentence by selecting from the list of word choices below. The *priority* for nursing care at this time is to manage the client's [**Word Choice**].

Word Choices
Heart failure
Hypoglycemia
Dehydration
Chronic kidney disease
Dysrhythmia

Thinking Exercise 8.1.4

The nurse is caring for an 87-year-old client in the skilled nursing unit.

History and Physical	Nurses Notes	Orders	Laboratory Results

0815:   Unlicensed personnel states that client who is usually alert and oriented seems sleepy and very confused this AM. Tried twice to climb out of bed. Reports that client has not voided since last night before going to bed. Client's medical history includes two strokes, type 2 diabetes mellitus, hypertension, chronic heart failure, and osteoarthritis. Currently drowsy but easily awakened. No abnormal or adventitious breath sounds; skin warm and dry. Lips and mucous membranes dry. Abdomen soft and round. Cap refill 5 seconds; pedal pulses 1+ and equal. 2+ nonpitting edema present in both feet. VS: T 100.6°F (38.1°C); HR 105 beats per minute and irregular; RR 20 breaths per minute; BP 88/52 mmHg; SpO$_2$ 89% on RA; FSBG 76 mg/dL (4.21 mmol/L).

0840:   Notified nurse practitioner on call about changes in client's condition.

Select **3** orders the nurse would anticipate for the client at this time.
○ Begin supplemental oxygen via nasal cannula (NC).
○ Offer oral fluids every hour.
○ Transfer the client to the hospital.
○ Hold next insulin administration.
○ Take vital signs every 2 hours.

Thinking Exercise 8.1.5

The nurse is caring for an 87-year-old client in the skilled nursing unit.

History and Physical	Nurses Notes	Orders	Laboratory Results

0815:   Unlicensed personnel states that client who is usually alert and oriented seems sleepy and very confused this AM. Tried twice to climb out of bed. Reports that client has not voided since last night before going to bed. Client's medical history includes two strokes, type 2 diabetes mellitus, hypertension, chronic heart failure, and osteoarthritis. Currently drowsy but easily awakened. No abnormal or adventitious breath sounds; skin warm and dry. Lips and mucous membranes dry. Abdomen soft and round. Cap refill 5 seconds; pedal pulses 1+ and equal. 2+ nonpitting edema in both feet. VS: T 100.6°F (38.1°C); HR 105 beats per minute and irregular; RR 20 breaths per minute; BP 88/52 mmHg; SpO$_2$ 89% on RA; FSBG 76 mg/dL (4.21 mmol/L).

0840:   Notified nurse practitioner on call about changes in client's condition.

1230:   Client alert but remains disoriented and confused. Taking small amounts of fluids. VS: T 101°F (38.3°C); HR 110 beats per minute and irregular; RR 22 breaths per minute; BP 84/50 mmHg; SpO$_2$ 90% on oxygen 2 L per minute via NC. Voided 75 mL dark yellow amber urine in bedpan. Left message for NP about latest client findings.

1345:   Client admitted to the ED. Family notified.

Continued

↯ UNFOLDING CASE STUDY 8.1—cont'd

Which of the following actions are appropriate for the nurse to implement in the Emergency Department? **Select all that apply.**

○ Collect a urine sample for analysis.
○ Administer short-acting insulin per protocol.
○ Draw blood for lab testing.
○ Teach client the need to drink more fluids.
○ Establish peripheral venous access for IV fluids.
○ Insert an indwelling urinary catheter.
○ Increase oxygen flow to 3–4 L per minute via NC as needed.

Thinking Exercise 8.1.6

The nurse is caring for an 87-year-old client in the Emergency Department (ED).

History and Physical	Nurses Notes	Orders	Laboratory Results

Skilled Nursing Unit

0815:   Unlicensed personnel states that client who is usually alert and oriented seems sleepy and very confused this AM. Tried to climb out of bed. Reports that client has not voided since last night before going to bed. Client's medical history includes two strokes, type 2 diabetes mellitus, hypertension, chronic heart failure, and osteoarthritis. Currently drowsy but easily awakened. No abnormal or adventitious breath sounds; skin warm and dry. Lips and mucous membranes dry. Abdomen soft and round. Cap refill 5 seconds; pedal pulses 1+ and equal. 2+ nonpitting edema in both feet. VS: T 100.6°F (38.1°C); HR 105 beats per minute and irregular; RR 20 breaths per minute; BP 88/52 mmHg; SpO$_2$ 89% on RA; FSBG 76 mg/dL (4.21 mmol/L).

0840:   Notified nurse practitioner on call about changes in client's condition.

1230:   Client alert but remains disoriented and confused. Taking small amounts of fluids. VS: T 101°F (38.3°C); HR 110 beats per minute and irregular; RR 22 breaths per minute; BP 84/50 mmHg; SpO$_2$ 90% on oxygen 2 L per minute via NC. Voided 75 mL dark amber cloudy urine in bedpan. Left message for NP about latest client findings.

1345:   Client admitted to the ED. Family notified.

Emergency Department

1520:   Family at bedside. Normal saline infusing at 100 mL per hour. SpO$_2$ 94% on oxygen 3 L per minute via NC. Urinalysis showed numerous bacteria. Sample sent to lab for C&S for probable urinary tract infection. Waiting on other lab results. Occasionally sipping water. Alert and oriented to self; less confused. States feeling very tired and warm; dozing at times. VS: T 100.8°F (38.2°C); HR 102 beats per minute and irregular; RR 20 breaths per minute; BP 92/58 mmHg.

For each current finding listed below, select whether the client's condition has improved or not improved/worsened.

Client Findings	Improved	Not Improved/Worsened
SpO$_2$		
Level of consciousness		
Urine		
Blood pressure		

UNFOLDING CASE STUDY 8.2

Thinking Exercise 8.2.1
The nurse is caring for a 52-year-old client in the Urgent Care Center.

History and Physical	Nurses Notes	Progress Notes	Laboratory Results

1030: Client came to urgent care with partner and report of new-onset general weakness, palpitations, and lightheadedness. Alert and oriented ×4. Had frequent diarrheal stools for the past 24 hours likely due to eating tainted seafood, but diarrhea improving this morning. Medical history includes hypertension, COPD, hypothyroidism, GERD, and hypercholesterolemia. 62-pack-year smoking history. Reports drinking 2–3 beers most nights. Current medications:

*MVI with calcium tab once a day

*Amlodipine 10 mg orally once a day

*Levothyroxine sodium 112 µg orally once a day

*Famotidine OTC 20 mg before meals PRN

*Lovastatin 40 mg orally once a day

*Hydrochlorothiazide (HCTZ) 25 mg orally once a day (started 2 weeks ago)

Few crackles in lung bases; denies dyspnea or chest pain. Skin warm and dry. S_1 and S_2 present and irregular. Abdomen soft and round; hyperactive bowel sounds present ×4 quadrants. Cap refill <3 seconds; pulses 2+ and equal. VS: T 98.4°F (36.9°C); HR 94 beats per minute; RR 18 breaths per minute; BP 118/72 mmHg; SpO_2 94% on RA.

1055: Blood sent for stat lab testing; ECG shows flattened T waves, sustained ventricular tachycardia (SVT), and evidence of two previous myocardial infarctions. Troponins negative. Client denies having previous chest pain or dyspnea episodes.

History and Physical	Laboratory Results	Orders	Nurses Notes

Serum Laboratory Test/Reference Range	Current Results
Sodium (Na+) (136–145 mEq/L [136–145 mmol/L])	127 mEq/L (127 mmol/L)
Potassium (K+) (3.5–5.0 mEq/L [3.5–5.0 mmol/L])	2.8 mEq/L (2.8 mmol/L)
Thyroid stimulating hormone (TSH) (0.3–5.0 µU/mL [0.3–5.0 mU/L])	2.4 µU/mL (2.4 mU/L)
Blood urea nitrogen (BUN) (10–20 mg/dL [3.6–7.1 mmol/L])	23 mg/dL (8.2 mmol/L)
Creatinine (0.5–1.1 mg/dL [44.2–97.3 µmol/L])	1.1 mg/dL (97.3 µmol/L)

Select **4** client findings that require **immediate** follow-up.
○ Smoking history
○ Crackles in lung bases
○ Alcohol intake
○ Ventricular tachycardia
○ Palpitations
○ Flattened T waves
○ Serum sodium level
○ Serum potassium level
○ BUN level

Continued

UNFOLDING CASE STUDY 8.2—cont'd

Thinking Exercise 8.2.2

The nurse is caring for a 52-year-old client in the Urgent Care Center.

History and Physical	Nurses Notes	Progress Notes	Laboratory Results

1030:   Client came to urgent care with partner and report of new-onset general weakness, palpitations, and lightheadedness. Alert and oriented ×4. Had frequent diarrheal stools for the past 24 hours likely due to eating tainted seafood, but diarrhea improving this morning. Medical history includes hypertension, COPD, hypothyroidism, GERD, and hypercholesterolemia. 62-pack-year smoking history. Reports drinking 2–3 beers most nights. Current medications:

*MVI with calcium tab once a day

*Amlodipine 10 mg orally once a day

*Levothyroxine sodium 112 µg orally once a day

*Famotidine OTC

*Lovastatin 20 mg orally once a day

*Hydrochlorothiazide (HCTZ) 25 mg orally once a day (started 2 weeks ago)

Few crackles in lung bases; denies dyspnea or chest pain. Skin warm and dry. S_1 and S_2 present and irregular. Abdomen soft and round; hyperactive bowel sounds present ×4 quadrants. Cap refill <3 seconds; pulses 2+ and equal. VS: T 98.4°F (36.9°C); HR 94 beats per minute; RR 18 breaths per minute; BP 118/72 mmHg; SpO_2 94% on RA.

1055:   Blood sent for stat lab testing; ECG shows flattened T waves, sustained ventricular tachycardia (SVT), and evidence of two previous myocardial infarctions. Troponins negative. Client denies having previous chest pain or dyspnea episodes.

History and Physical	Laboratory Results	Progress Notes	Nurses Notes

Serum Laboratory Test/Reference Range	Current Results
Sodium (Na⁺) (136–145 mEq/L [136–145 mmol/L])	127 mEq/L (127 mmol/L)
Potassium (K⁺) (3.5–5.0 mEq/L [3.5–5.0 mmol/L])	2.8 mEq/L (2.8 mmol/L)
Thyroid stimulating hormone (TSH) (0.3–5.0 µU/mL [0.3–5.0 mU/L])	2.4 µU/mL (2.4 mU/L)
Blood urea nitrogen (BUN) (10–20 mg/dL [3.6–7.1 mmol/L])	23 mg/dL (8.2 mmol/L)
Creatinine (0.5–1.1 mg/dL [44.2–97.3 µmol/L])	1.1 mg/dL (97.3 µmol/L)

Complete the following sentence by selecting from the lists of options below. The nurse analyzes client data and determines that the client is most at risk for **1 [Select]** because the client has **2 [Select]** and **3 [Select]**.

Options for 1	Options for 2	Options for 3
Chest pain	Hyponatremia	Hypertension
Respiratory failure	Hypokalemia	Tachycardia
Cardiac dysrhythmias	COPD	Flattened T waves

UNFOLDING CASE STUDY 8.2—cont'd

Thinking Exercise 8.2.3

The nurse is caring for a 52-year-old client in the Urgent Care Center.

History and Physical	Nurses Notes	Progress Notes	Laboratory Results

1030: Client came to urgent care with partner and report of new-onset general weakness, palpitations, and lightheadedness. Alert and oriented ×4. Had frequent diarrheal stools for the past 24 hours likely due to eating tainted seafood, but diarrhea improving this morning. Medical history includes hypertension, COPD, hypothyroidism, GERD, and hypercholesterolemia. 62-pack-year smoking history. Reports drinking 2–3 beers most nights. Current medications:

*MVI with calcium tab once a day

*Amlodipine 10 mg orally once a day

*Levothyroxine sodium 112 µg orally once a day

*Famotidine OTC

*Lovastatin 20 mg orally once a day

*Hydrochlorothiazide (HCTZ) 25 mg orally once a day (started 2 weeks ago)

Few crackles in lung bases; denies dyspnea or chest pain. Skin warm and dry. S_1 and S_2 present and irregular. Abdomen soft and round; hyperactive bowel sounds present ×4 quadrants. Cap refill <3 seconds; pulses 2+ and equal. VS: T 98.4°F (36.9°C); HR 94 beats per minute; RR 18 breaths per minute; BP 118/72 mmHg; SpO_2 94% on RA.

1055: Blood sent for stat lab testing; ECG shows flattened T waves, sustained ventricular tachycardia (SVT), and evidence of two previous myocardial infarctions. Troponins negative. Client denies having previous chest pain or dyspnea episodes.

History and Physical	Laboratory Results	Progress Notes	Nurses Notes

Serum Laboratory Test/Reference Range	Current Results
Sodium (Na⁺) (136–145 mEq/L [136–145 mmol/L])	127 mEq/L (127 mmol/L)
Potassium (K⁺) (3.5–5.0 mEq/L [3.5–5.0 mmol/L])	2.8 mEq/L (2.8 mmol/L)
Thyroid stimulating hormone (TSH) (0.3–5.0 µU/mL [0.3–5.0 mU/L])	2.4 µU/mL (2.4 mU/L)
Blood urea nitrogen (BUN) (10–20 mg/dL [3.6–7.1 mmol/L])	23 mg/dL (8.2 mmol/L)
Creatinine (0.5–1.1 mg/dL [44.2–97.3 µmol/L])	1.1 mg/dL (97.3 µmol/L)

Complete the following sentence by selecting from the list of word choices below. The **priority** for client care at this time is to manage the **[Word Choice]**.

Word Choices	
Hypokalemia	Elevated BUN
Hyponatremia	ECG abnormalities

Continued

UNFOLDING CASE STUDY 8.2—cont'd

Thinking Exercise 8.2.4

The nurse prepares for a 52-year-old client in the Urgent Care Center to be directly admitted to the acute cardiac unit.

History and Physical	Nurses Notes	Progress Notes	Laboratory Results

1030: Client came to urgent care with partner and report of new-onset general weakness, palpitations, and lightheadedness. Alert and oriented ×4. Had frequent diarrheal stools for the past 24 hours likely due to eating tainted seafood, but diarrhea improving this morning. Medical history includes hypertension, COPD, hypothyroidism, GERD, and hypercholesterolemia. 62-pack-year smoking history. Reports drinking 2–3 beers most nights. Current medications:

*MVI with calcium tab once a day

*Amlodipine 10 mg orally once a day

*Levothyroxine sodium 112 µg orally once a day

*Famotidine OTC

*Lovastatin 20 mg orally once a day

*Hydrochlorothiazide (HCTZ) 25 mg orally once a day (started 2 weeks ago)

Few crackles in lung bases; denies dyspnea or chest pain. Skin warm and dry. S_1 and S_2 present and irregular. Abdomen soft and round; hyperactive bowel sounds present ×4 quadrants. Cap refill <3 seconds; pulses 2+ and equal. VS: T 98.6°F (38.1°C); HR 94 beats per minute; RR 18 breaths per minute; BP 118/72 mmHg; SpO_2 94% on RA.

1055: Blood sent for stat lab testing; ECG shows flattened T waves, sustained ventricular tachycardia (SVT), and evidence of two previous myocardial infarctions. Troponins negative. Client denies having previous chest pain or dyspnea episodes. Plan to transfer client for direct admission to acute cardiac unit.

History and Physical	Laboratory Results	Progress Notes	Nurses Notes

Serum Laboratory Test/Reference Range	Current Results
Sodium (Na^+) (136–145 mEq/L [136–145 mmol/L])	127 mEq/L (127 mmol/L)
Potassium (K^+) (3.5–5.0 mEq/L [3.5–5.0 mmol/L])	2.8 mEq/L (2.8 mmol/L)
Thyroid stimulating hormone (TSH) (0.3–5.0 µU/mL [0.3–5.0 mU/L])	2.4 µU/mL (2.4 mU/L)
Blood urea nitrogen (BUN) (10–20 mg/dL [3.6–7.1 mmol/L])	23 mg/dL (8.2 mmol/L)
Creatinine (0.5–1.1 mg/dL [44.2–97.3 µmol/L])	1.1 mg/dL (97.3 µmol/L)

Which of the following potential nursing actions in the acute cardiac unit would be appropriate based on the client's priority need? **Select all that apply.**

- Discontinue the client's HCTZ.
- Provide continuous cardiac monitoring.
- Initiate oxygen via high-flow nasal cannula.
- Establish peripheral venous access.
- Administer potassium infusion per agency protocol.
- Prepare client for cardiac catheterization.
- Administer sodium polystyrene sulfonate.
- Administer morphine IV per agency protocol.

Thinking Exercise 8.2.5

The nurse is caring for a 52-year-old client admitted to the acute cardiac unit from the Urgent Care Center.

History and Physical	Nurses Notes	Progress Notes	Laboratory Results

Urgent Care Center

1030: Client came to urgent care with partner and report of new-onset general weakness, palpitations, and lightheadedness. Alert and oriented ×4. Had frequent diarrheal stools for the past 24 hours likely due to eating tainted seafood, but diarrhea improving this morning. Medical history includes hypertension, COPD, hypothyroidism, GERD, and hypercholesterolemia. 62-pack-year smoking history. Reports drinking 2–3 beers most nights. Current medications:

*MVI with calcium tab once a day

*Amlodipine 10 mg orally once a day

*Levothyroxine sodium 112 µg orally once a day

*Famotidine OTC

*Lovastatin 20 mg orally once a day

*Hydrochlorothiazide (HCTZ) 25 mg orally once a day (started 2 weeks ago)

Few crackles in lower lung bases; denies dyspnea or chest pain. Skin warm and dry. S_1 and S_2 present and irregular. Abdomen soft and round; hyperactive bowel sounds present ×4 quadrants. Cap refill <3 seconds; pulses 2+ and equal. VS: T 98.6°F (38.1°C); HR 94 beats per minute; RR 18 breaths per minute; BP 118/72 mmHg; SpO$_2$ 94% on RA.

1055: Blood sent for stat lab testing; ECG shows flattened T waves, sustained ventricular tachycardia (SVT), and evidence of two previous myocardial infarctions. Troponins negative. Client denies having previous chest pain or dyspnea episodes. Plan to transfer client for direct admission to acute cardiac unit.

Acute Cardiac Unit

1310: Peripheral IV started in right forearm. IV of 5%D/0.45%NS infusing at 100 mL per hour. Supplemental potassium administered per cardiac protocol. Labs to be redrawn in 4 hours. Oxygen started at 2 L per minute via NC. Orders received; hold HCTZ. VS: T 98.6°F (38.1°C); HR 94 beats per min; RR 18 breaths per min; BP 116/68 mmHg; SpO$_2$ 99% on O$_2$ at 2 L per minute via NC. BMI 30.4.

History and Physical	Laboratory Results	Progress Notes	Nurses Notes

Serum Laboratory Test/Reference Range	Urgent Care Results
Sodium (Na$^+$) (136–145 mEq/L [136–145 mmol/L])	127 mEq/L (127 mmol/L)
Potassium (K$^+$) (3.5–5.0 mEq/L [3.5–5.0 mmol/L])	2.8 mEq/L (2.8 mmol/L)
Thyroid stimulating hormone (TSH) (0.3–5.0 µU/mL [0.3–5.0 mU/L])	2.4 µU/mL (2.4 mU/L)
Blood urea nitrogen (BUN) (10–20 mg/dL [3.6–7.1 mmol/L])	23 mg/dL (8.2 mmol/L)
Creatinine (0.5–1.1 mg/dL [44.2–97.3 µmol/L])	1.1 mg/dL (97.3 µmol/L)

The nurse provides teaching to help the client promote health and prevent further illness. Which of the following statements should be included in the client teaching? **Select all that apply.**

- ○ "The social worker is going to provide you with information about smoking and alcohol cessation programs."
- ○ "Be sure to include potassium-rich foods in your diet such as bananas, potatoes, and oranges."
- ○ "Avoid eating foods that are high in sodium, including ham, bacon, and salty snacks."
- ○ "Regular exercise and healthy eating habits will help you lose weight."
- ○ "Consuming beer every night can cause weight gain and other health problems."

Continued

Thinking Exercise 8.2.6

The nurse is caring for a 52-year-old client admitted to the acute cardiac unit from the Urgent Care Center.

Highlight the findings in the 1310 nurses notes and 1730 laboratory results that demonstrate the client's condition is **improving**.

History and Physical	Nurses Notes	Progress Notes	Laboratory Results

Urgent Care Center

1030: Client came to urgent care with partner and report of new-onset general weakness, palpitations, and lightheadedness. Alert and oriented ×4. Had frequent diarrheal stools for the past 24 hours likely due to eating tainted seafood, but diarrhea improving this morning. Medical history includes hypertension, COPD, hypothyroidism, GERD, and hypercholesterolemia. 62-pack-year smoking history. Reports drinking 2–3 beers most nights. Current medications:

*MVI with calcium tab once a day

*Amlodipine 10 mg orally once a day

*Levothyroxine sodium 112 µg orally once a day

*Famotidine OTC

*Lovastatin 20 mg orally once a day

*Hydrochlorothiazide (HCTZ) 25 mg orally once a day (started 2 weeks ago)

Few crackles in lower lung bases; denies dyspnea or chest pain. Skin warm and dry. S_1 and S_2 present and irregular. Abdomen soft and round; hyperactive bowel sounds present × 4 quadrants. Cap refill <3 seconds; pulses 2+ and equal. VS: T 98.6°F (38.1°C); HR 94 beats per minute; RR 18 breaths per minute; BP 118/72 mmHg; SpO$_2$ 94% on RA.

1055: Blood sent for stat lab testing; ECG shows flattened T waves, sustained ventricular tachycardia (SVT), and evidence of two previous myocardial infarctions. Troponins negative. Client denies having previous chest pain or dyspnea episodes. Plan to transfer client for direct admission to acute cardiac unit.

Acute Cardiac Unit

1310: Peripheral IV started in right forearm. IV of 5%D/0.45%NS infusing at 100 mL per hour. Supplemental potassium administered per cardiac protocol. Labs to be redrawn in 4 hours. Oxygen started at 2 L per minute via NC. Orders received; hold HCTZ. VS: T 98.6°F (38.1°C); HR 94 beats per minute; RR 18 breaths per minute; BP 116/68 mmHg; SpO$_2$ 99% on O$_2$ at 2 L per minute via NC. BMI 30.4.

History and Physical	Laboratory Results	Progress Notes	Nurses Notes

Serum Laboratory Test/ Reference Range	Urgent Care Results	1730 Results
Sodium (Na$^+$) (136–145 mEq/L [136–145 mmol/L])	127 mEq/L (127 mmol/L)	133 mEq/L (133 mmol/L)
Potassium (K$^+$) (3.5–5.0 mEq/L [3.5–5.0 mmol/L])	2.8 mEq/L (2.8 mmol/L)	3.4 mEq/L (3.4 mmol/L)
Thyroid stimulating hormone (TSH) (0.3–5.0 µU/mL [0.3–5.0 mU/L])	3 µU/mL (3 mU/L)	3 µU/mL (3 mU/L)
Blood urea nitrogen (BUN) (10–20 mg/dL [3.6–7.1 mmol/L])	23 mg/dL (8.2 mmol/L)	16 mg/dL (5.7 mmol/L)
Creatinine (0.5–1.1 mg/dL [44.2–97.3 µmol/L])	1.1 mg/dL (97.3 µmol/L)	1.1 mg/dL (97.3 µmol/L)

UNFOLDING CASE STUDY 8.3

Thinking Exercise 8.3.1

The nurse is caring for a 73-year-old client in the Emergency Department (ED).

History and Physical	Nurses Notes	Orders	Laboratory Results

2025: Client accompanied by wife with report of frequent vomiting for the past 3 days, shortness of breath that started today, anorexia, and generalized weakness. Vomited large amount of dark brown emesis twice today. Client has been generally healthy and never admitted to the ED or acute care. Medical history includes well-controlled hypertension and chronic gout. Alert and oriented ×4. Denies pain or nausea. Skin warm and dry. Lips and mucous membranes dry. Diminished breath sounds in lower lung bases bilaterally. Abdomen grossly distended. Faint bowel sounds in upper abdomen; absent bowel sounds in lower abdomen. Cap refill <3 seconds; pedal pulses 1+ and equal. VS: T 99°F (37.2°C); HR 151 beats per minute and irregular; RR 48 breaths per minute and shallow; BP 139/88 mmHg; SpO$_2$ 88% on RA.

Which of the following client findings requires **immediate** follow-up? **Select all that apply.**

- Temperature
- Heart rate
- Respiratory rate
- Blood pressure
- SpO$_2$
- Pedal pulses
- Diminished breath sounds
- Absent bowel sounds

Thinking Exercise 8.3.2

The nurse is caring for a 73-year-old client in the Emergency Department (ED).

History and Physical	Nurses Notes	Orders	Laboratory Results

2025: Client accompanied by wife with report of frequent vomiting for the past 3 days, shortness of breath that started today, anorexia, and generalized weakness. Vomited large amount of dark brown emesis twice today. Client has been generally healthy and never admitted to the ED or acute care. Medical history includes well-controlled hypertension and chronic gout. Alert and oriented ×4. Denies pain or nausea. Skin warm and dry. Lips and mucous membranes dry. Diminished breath sounds in lower lung bases bilaterally. Abdomen grossly distended. Faint bowel sounds in upper abdomen; absent bowel sounds in lower abdomen. Cap refill <3 seconds; pedal pulses 1+ and equal. VS: T 99.2°F (37.3°C); HR 151 beats per minute and irregular; RR 48 breaths per minute and shallow; BP 139/88 mmHg; SpO$_2$ 88% on RA.

For each client finding listed below, select whether the finding is consistent with the health conditions of dehydration, bowel obstruction, or pneumonia. Some findings may be consistent with more than one condition.

Client Findings	Dehydration	Bowel Obstruction	Pneumonia
Diminished breath sounds			
HR 151 beats per minute and irregular			
RR 48 breaths per minute and shallow			
SpO$_2$ 88% on RA			
Absent bowel sounds			

Continued

Thinking Exercise 8.3.3

The nurse is caring for a 73-year-old client in the Emergency Department (ED).

History and Physical	Nurses Notes	Orders	Laboratory Results

2025: Client accompanied by wife with report of frequent vomiting for the past 3 days, shortness of breath that started today, anorexia, and generalized weakness. Vomited large amount of dark brown emesis twice today. Client has been generally healthy and never admitted to the ED or acute care. Medical history includes well-controlled hypertension and chronic gout. Alert and oriented ×4. Denies pain or nausea. Skin warm and dry. Lips and mucous membranes dry. Diminished breath sounds in lower lung bases bilaterally. Abdomen grossly distended. Faint bowel sounds in upper abdomen; absent bowel sounds in lower abdomen. Cap refill <3 seconds; pedal pulses 1+ and equal. VS: T 99.2°F (37.3°C); HR 151 beats per minute and irregular; RR 48 breaths per minute and shallow; BP 139/88 mmHg; SpO$_2$ 88% on RA.

Complete the following sentence by selecting from the list of word choices below. The **priority** for care at this time is to manage the client's **[Word Choice]**.

Word Choices
SpO$_2$
Fever
Tachycardia
Tachypnea
Blood pressure

Thinking Exercise 8.3.4

The nurse is caring for a 73-year-old client in the Emergency Department (ED).

History and Physical	Nurses Notes	Orders	Laboratory Results

2025: Client accompanied by wife with report of frequent vomiting for the past 3 days, shortness of breath that started today, anorexia, and generalized weakness. Vomited large amount of dark brown emesis twice today. Client has been generally healthy and never admitted to the ED or acute care. Medical history includes well-controlled hypertension and chronic gout. Alert and oriented ×4. Denies pain or nausea. Skin warm and dry. Lips and mucous membranes dry. Diminished breath sounds in lower lung bases bilaterally. Abdomen grossly distended. Faint bowel sounds in upper abdomen; absent bowel sounds in lower abdomen. Cap refill <3 seconds; pedal pulses 1+ and equal. VS: T 99.2°F (37.3°C); HR 151 beats per minute and irregular; RR 48 breaths per minute and shallow; BP 139/88 mmHg; SpO$_2$ 88% on RA.

2110: ECG completed; blood drawn for stat blood work. Chest X-ray and cardiac ultrasound at bedside. Voiding very dark yellow urine using urinal. No nausea or vomiting.

Select whether the following potential nursing actions are indicated or not indicated.

Potential Nursing Actions	Indicated	Not Indicated
Start supplemental oxygen via NC		
Obtain peripheral venous access		
Administer 0.9% NS at 80 mL per hour		
Apply continuous cardiac monitoring		
Keep client in supine flat position		

UNFOLDING CASE STUDY 8.3—cont'd

Thinking Exercise 8.3.5
The nurse is caring for a 73-year-old client in the Post-Anesthesia Care Unit (PACU).

History and Physical	Nurses Notes	Orders	Laboratory Results

Emergency Department

2025:   Client accompanied by wife with report of frequent vomiting for the past 3 days, shortness of breath that started today, anorexia, and generalized weakness. Vomited large amount of dark brown emesis twice today. Client has been generally healthy and never admitted to the ED or acute care. Medical history includes well-controlled hypertension and chronic gout. Alert and oriented ×4. Denies pain or nausea. Skin warm and dry. Lips and mucous membranes dry. Diminished breath sounds in lower lung bases bilaterally. Abdomen grossly distended. Faint bowel sounds in upper abdomen; absent bowel sounds in lower abdomen. Cap refill <3 seconds; pedal pulses 1+ and equal. VS: T 99.2°F (37.3°C); HR 151 beats per minute and irregular; RR 48 breaths per minute and shallow; BP 139/88 mmHg; SpO_2 88% on RA.

2110:   ECG completed; blood drawn for stat blood work. Chest X-ray and cardiac ultrasound at bedside. Voiding very dark yellow urine using urinal. No nausea or vomiting.

2345:   Results from chest X-ray show small amount of fluid or infection in lung bases. No cardiac abnormalities. Planning chest and abdominal CT scans without contrast. VS: T 98.6°F (37°C); HR 132 beats per minute and irregular; RR 36 breaths per minute and shallow; BP 142/90 mmHg; SpO_2 91% on 3 L per minute via NC.

0305:   Results from CT scans show small amount of fluid in lung bases and probable small bowel obstruction. Client to be admitted when acute bed available. Abdominal CT with contrast scheduled in the next hour. VS: T 98.6°F (37°C); HR 138 beats per minute and irregular; RR 40 breaths per minute and shallow; BP 144/92 mmHg; SpO_2 90% on 3 L per minute via NC. Increased O_2 to 4 L per minute.

0700:   Transferred to operating suite for emergent abdominal surgery. Most recent abdominal scan shows complete small bowel obstruction caused by possible external mass in lower abdomen.

PACU the Next Day

1050:   Admitted to PACU with IV infusing at 150 mL per hour, O_2 at 4 L per minute via NC, and NG tube to low continuous suction draining copious amount of dark brown drainage. Alert and oriented ×4. Large abdominal surgical dressing dry and intact. No drain present. Surgeon reports removal of scar tissue as cause of obstruction. VS: T 100.8°F (38.2°C); HR 146 beats per minute and irregular; RR 24 breaths per minute and shallow; BP 86/40 mmHg; SpO_2 88%. Surgeon notified about VS.

Select **6** nursing actions that would be appropriate and essential for the client at this time.
○ Call a sepsis alert code immediately.
○ Draw lactate (lactic acid) level stat.
○ Place indwelling urinary catheter.
○ Increase oxygen to 6 L per minute via NC.
○ Clamp NG tube immediately.
○ Place client in sitting position.
○ Decrease IV fluid rate to 100 mL per hour.
○ Start IV broad-spectrum antibiotic therapy.
○ Administer norepinephrine (NE) per protocol.
○ Plan transfer to critical care unit.

Continued

UNFOLDING CASE STUDY 8.3—cont'd

Thinking Exercise 8.3.6
This nurse is caring for a 73-year-old client in the acute surgical unit. Highlight the client findings in the acute surgical unit note (POD #7) that demonstrate the client's condition has **improved**.

History and Physical	Nurses Notes	Orders	Laboratory Results

Emergency Department

2025: Client accompanied by wife with report of frequent vomiting for the past 3 days, shortness of breath that started today, anorexia, and generalized weakness. Vomited large amount of dark brown emesis twice today. Client has been generally healthy and never admitted to the ED or acute care. Medical history includes well-controlled hypertension and chronic gout. Alert and oriented ×4. Denies pain or nausea. Skin warm and dry. Lips and mucous membranes dry. Diminished breath sounds in lower lung bases bilaterally. Abdomen grossly distended. Faint bowel sounds in upper abdomen; absent bowel sounds in lower abdomen. Cap refill <3 seconds; pedal pulses 1+ and equal. VS: T 99.2°F (37.3°C); HR 151 beats per minute and irregular; RR 48 breaths per minute and shallow; BP 139/88 mmHg; SpO$_2$ 88% on RA.

2110: ECG completed; blood drawn for stat blood work. Chest X-ray and cardiac ultrasound at bedside. Voiding very dark yellow urine using urinal. No nausea or vomiting.

2345: Results from chest X-ray show small amount of fluid or infection in lung bases. No cardiac abnormalities. Planning chest and abdominal CT scans without contrast. VS: T 98.6°F (37°C); HR 132 beats per minute and irregular; RR 36 breaths per minute and shallow; BP 142/90 mmHg; SpO$_2$ 91% on 3 L per minute via NC.

0305: Results from CT scans show small amount of fluid in lung bases and probable small bowel obstruction. Client to be admitted when acute bed available. Abdominal CT with contrast scheduled in the next hour. VS: T 98.6°F (37°C); HR 138 beats per minute and irregular; RR 40 breaths per minute and shallow; BP 144/92 mmHg; SpO$_2$ 90% on 3 L per minute via NC. Increased O$_2$ to 4 L per minute.

0700: Transferred to operating suite for emergent abdominal surgery. Most recent abdominal scan shows complete small bowel obstruction caused by possible external mass in lower abdomen.

PACU the Next Day

1050: Admitted to PACU with IV infusing at 150 mL per hour, O$_2$ at 4 L per minute via NC, and NG tube to low continuous suction draining copious amount of dark brown drainage. Alert and oriented ×4. Large abdominal surgical dressing dry and intact. No drain present. Surgeon reports removal of scar tissue as cause of obstruction. VS: T 100.8°F (38.2°C); HR 146 beats per minute and irregular; RR 24 breaths per minute and shallow; BP 86/40 mmHg; SpO$_2$ 88%. Surgeon notified about VS.

Acute Surgical Unit POD #7

1630: Client and wife discussing discharge plans for tomorrow with case manager. Client receiving IV antibiotic therapy for bilateral diffuse pneumonia for the past 4 days. Will be discharged on oral antibiotic therapy but likely will not require home oxygen. Client alert and oriented ×4. No adventitious breath sounds auscultated. Abdomen soft and round. Surgical incision slightly reddened with small amount of tannish drainage; surgical resident removed half of staples. Wound culture obtained. Able to walk from the bed to bathroom without assistance. Denies pain or nausea. Eating small amounts of solid food. VS: T 98.8°F (37.1°C); HR 98 beats per minute and irregular; RR 20 breaths per minute and shallow; BP 124/78 mmHg; SpO$_2$ 95% on RA.

Thinking Exercise 8.4.1

The nurse is caring for a 45-year-old client in the neuroscience unit. Highlight the client findings that require **immediate** follow-up.

History and Physical	Nurses Notes	Orders	Laboratory Results

0830:   Client admitted yesterday from the ED with closed head injury following a motor vehicle crash. History of type 1 diabetes mellitus (DM). Alert and oriented ×2 (person and place). PERRLA; cranial nerves and reflexes intact. Reports headache at 3/10. Moves all extremities freely. Muscle strength 5/5. Saline lock in place in left forearm. Skin warm and dry. Lung sounds clear throughout; S_1 and S_2 present. Abdomen soft and round; bowel sounds present ×4. Cap refill <3 seconds; pulses 2+ and equal. VS: T 98.6°F (37°C); HR 82 beats per minute and regular; RR 18 breaths per minute; BP 116/66 mmHg; SpO_2 96% on RA. FSBG 147 mg/dL (8.2 mmol/L).

1300:   Reports feeling unusually sleepy; oriented ×1 (person only). PERRLA; states vision is getting blurry. Cranial nerves and reflexes intact. Reports headache at 8/10 and new-onset nausea. Slowly moves all extremities. Muscle strength 4/5. VS: T 98.6°F (37°C); HR 67 beats per minute and regular; RR 24 breaths per minute and irregular; BP 152/58 mmHg; SpO_2 94% on RA. FSBG 81 mg/dL (4.5 mmol/L).

Complete the following sentence by selecting from the list of word choices below. The client findings that require **immediate** follow-up include **[Word Choice]**, **[Word Choice]**, and **[Word Choice]**.

Word Choices
Bradycardia
Blurry vision
Severe headache
Muscle weakness
Elevated blood pressure
Decreased level of consciousness (LOC)

Thinking Exercise 8.4.2

History and Physical	Nurses Notes	Orders	Laboratory Results

0830:   Client admitted yesterday from the ED with closed head injury following a motor vehicle crash. History of type 1 diabetes mellitus (DM). Alert and oriented ×2 (person and place). PERRLA; cranial nerves and reflexes intact. Reports headache at 3/10. Moves all extremities freely. Muscle strength 5/5. Saline lock in place in left forearm. Skin warm and dry. Lung sounds clear throughout; S_1 and S_2 present. Abdomen soft and round; bowel sounds present ×4. Cap refill <3 seconds; pulses 2+ and equal. VS: T 98.6°F (37°C); HR 82 beats per minute and regular; RR 18 breaths per minute; BP 116/66 mmHg; SpO_2 96% on RA. FSBG 147 mg/dL (8.2 mmol/L).

1300:   Reports feeling unusually sleepy; oriented ×1 (person only). PERRLA; states vision is getting blurry. Cranial nerves and reflexes intact. Reports headache at 8/10 and new-onset nausea. Slowly moving all extremities. Muscle strength 4/5. VS: T 98.6°F (37°C); HR 67 beats per minute and regular; RR 24 breaths per minute; BP 152/58 mmHg; SpO_2 94% on RA. Denies dyspnea. FSBG 81 mg/dL (4.5 mmol/L).

Complete the following sentence by selecting from the lists of options below. The nurse analyzes the assessment findings and determines that the client is experiencing **1 [Select]** as evidenced by **2 [Select]** and **3 [Select]**.

Options for 1	Options for 2	Options for 3
Hypoglycemia	Severe headache	Increased respiratory rate
Increasing intracranial pressure (ICP)	Decreased blood glucose	Bradycardia
Respiratory distress	Decreased SpO_2	Decreased level of consciousness

UNFOLDING CASE STUDY 8.4—cont'd

Thinking Exercise 8.4.3

History and Physical	Nurses Notes	Orders	Laboratory Results

0830: Client admitted yesterday from the ED with closed head injury following a motor vehicle crash. History of type 1 diabetes mellitus (DM). Alert and oriented ×2 (person and place). PERRLA; cranial nerves and reflexes intact. Reports headache at 3/10. Moves all extremities freely. Muscle strength 5/5. Saline lock in place in left forearm. Skin warm and dry. Lung sounds clear throughout; S_1 and S_2 present. Abdomen soft and round; bowel sounds present ×4. Cap refill <3 seconds; pulses 2+ and equal. VS: T 98.6°F (37°C); HR 82 beats per minute and regular; RR 18 breaths per minute; BP 116/66 mmHg; SpO_2 96% on RA. FSBG 147 mg/dL (8.2 mmol/L).

1300: Reports feeling unusually sleepy; oriented ×1 (person only). PERRLA; states vision is getting blurry. Cranial nerves and reflexes intact. Reports headache at 8/10 and new-onset nausea. Slowly moving all extremities. Muscle strength 4/5. VS: T 98.6°F (37°C); HR 67 beats per minute and regular; RR 24 breaths per minute; BP 152/58 mmHg; SpO_2 94% on RA. Denies dyspnea. FSBG 81 mg/dL (4.5 mmol/L).

Select the **1** priority for client care at this time.
○ Increase the client's blood glucose.
○ Manage the client's hypertension.
○ Reduce the pressure on the client's brain.
○ Manage the client's severe headache pain.
○ Improve the client's oxygenation.
○ Manage the client's new-onset nausea.

Thinking Exercise 8.4.4

History and Physical	Nurses Notes	Orders	Laboratory Results

0830: Client admitted yesterday from the ED with closed head injury following a motor vehicle crash. History of type 1 diabetes mellitus (DM). Alert and oriented ×2 (person and place). PERRLA; cranial nerves and reflexes intact. Reports headache at 3/10. Moves all extremities freely. Muscle strength 5/5. Saline lock in place in left forearm. Skin warm and dry. Lung sounds clear throughout; S_1 and S_2 present. Abdomen soft and round; bowel sounds present ×4. Cap refill <3 seconds; pulses 2+ and equal. VS: T 98.6°F (37°C); HR 82 beats per minute and regular; RR 18 breaths per minute; BP 116/66 mmHg; SpO_2 96% on RA. FSBG 147 mg/dL (8.2 mmol/L).

1300: Reports feeling unusually sleepy; oriented ×1 (person only). PERRLA; states vision is getting blurry. Cranial nerves and reflexes intact. Reports headache at 8/10 and new-onset nausea. Slowly moving all extremities. Muscle strength 4/5. VS: T 98.6°F (37°C); HR 67 beats per minute and regular; RR 24 breaths per minute; BP 152/58 mmHg; SpO_2 94% on RA. Denies dyspnea. FSBG 81 mg/dL (4.5 mmol/L).

Select whether the following potential orders are appropriate or not appropriate for the client at this time.

Potential Orders	Appropriate	Not Appropriate
Keep the client sitting in a 30 degrees reclining position		
Administer IV furosemide per protocol		
Begin supplemental oxygen via NC		
Keep client's head in a neutral position		

Thinking Exercise 8.4.5

History and Physical	Nurses Notes	Orders	Laboratory Results

Neuroscience Unit Day #2

0830: Client admitted yesterday from the ED with closed head injury following a motor vehicle crash. History of type 1 diabetes mellitus (DM). Alert and oriented ×2 (person and place). PERRLA; cranial nerves and reflexes intact. Reports headache at 3/10. Moves all extremities freely. Muscle strength 5/5. Saline lock in place in left forearm. Skin warm and dry. Lung sounds clear throughout; S_1 and S_2 present. Abdomen soft and round; bowel sounds present ×4. Cap refill <3 seconds; pulses 2+ and equal. VS: T 98.6°F (37°C); HR 82 beats per minute and regular; RR 18 breaths per minute; BP 116/66 mmHg; SpO_2 96% on RA. FSBG 147 mg/dL (8.2 mmol/L).

1300: Reports feeling unusually sleepy; oriented ×1 (person only). PERRLA; states vision is getting blurry. Cranial nerves and reflexes intact. Reports headache at 8/10 and new-onset nausea. Slowly moving all extremities. Muscle strength 4/5. VS: T 98.6°F (37°C); HR 67 beats per minute and regular; RR 24 breaths per minute; BP 152/58 mmHg; SpO_2 94% on RA. Denies dyspnea. FSBG 81 mg/dL (4.5 mmol/L). Transfer to Neuroscience ICU.

Neuroscience ICU Day of Admission

1325: Hypertonic saline (HS) solution with furosemide infusion started at 25 mL per hour to deliver 2 mg per hour furosemide. Client's head in neutral position while at 30 degrees in bed. VS: T 98.4°F (36.9°C); HR 74 beats per minute and regular; RR 20 breaths per minute; BP 136/64 mmHg; SpO_2 98% on oxygen at 2 L per minute via NC.

Which of the following nursing actions are appropriate for the client at this time? **Select all that apply.**
- ○ Monitor sodium level during hypertonic saline infusion.
- ○ Document fluid intake and urinary output.
- ○ Place client on high-flow oxygen.
- ○ Take vital signs every hour ×4, then every 2 hours.
- ○ Document FSBG level every hour.
- ○ Monitor for signs and symptoms of fluid overload.

Thinking Exercise 8.4.6

History and Physical	Nurses Notes	Orders	Laboratory Results

Neuroscience Unit Day #2

0830: Client admitted yesterday from the ED with closed head injury following a motor vehicle crash. History of type 1 diabetes mellitus (DM). Alert and oriented ×2 (person and place). PERRLA; cranial nerves and reflexes intact. Reports headache at 3/10. Moves all extremities freely. Muscle strength 5/5. Saline lock in place in left forearm. Skin warm and dry. Lung sounds clear throughout; S_1 and S_2 present. Abdomen soft and round; bowel sounds present ×4. Cap refill <3 seconds; pulses 2+ and equal. VS: T 98.6°F (37°C); HR 82 beats per minute and regular; RR 18 breaths per minute; BP 116/66 mmHg; SpO_2 96% on RA. FSBG 147 mg/dL (8.2 mmol/L).

1300: Reports feeling unusually sleepy; oriented ×1 (person only). PERRLA; states vision is getting blurry. Cranial nerves and reflexes intact. Reports headache at 8/10 and new-onset nausea. Slowly moving all extremities. Muscle strength 4/5. VS: T 98.6°F (37°C); HR 67 beats per minute and regular; RR 24 breaths per minute; BP 152/58 mmHg; SpO_2 94% on RA. Denies dyspnea. FSBG 81 mg/dL (4.5 mmol/L).

Neuroscience ICU Day of Admission

1325: Hypertonic saline (HS) solution with furosemide infusion started at 25 mL per hour to deliver 2 mg per hour furosemide. Client's head in neutral position while at 30 degrees in bed. VS: T 98.4°F (36.9°C); HR 74 beats per minute and regular; RR 20 breaths per minute; BP 136/64 mmHg; SpO_2 98% on oxygen at 2 L per minute via NC. Seizure precautions initiated.

Neuroscience ICU Day #2

0740: Alert and oriented ×4. PERRLA; cranial nerves and reflexes intact. Reports headache pain at 2/10. Moves all extremities freely. No evidence of seizure. Muscle strength 4/5. VS: T 98.4°F (36.9°C); HR 78 beats per minute and regular; RR 18 breaths per minute; BP 120/70 mmHg; SpO_2 99% on oxygen at 2 L per minute via NC.

> **UNFOLDING CASE STUDY 8.4—cont'd**

Based on the most recent nurses note, select whether the following findings demonstrate the client is progressing or not progressing.

Client Findings	Progressing	Not Progressing
Alert and oriented ×4		
Headache pain at 2/10		
Muscle strength 4/5		
BP 120/70 mmHg		

> **UNFOLDING CASE STUDY 8.5**

Thinking Exercise 8.5.1
The nurse is caring for a 21-year-old client in the Emergency Department (ED).

History and Physical	Nurses Notes	Orders	Laboratory Results

1530:   Client admitted to ED with worsening signs and symptoms of anorexia nervosa (AN). Parents report client eats almost no solid food except lettuce and drinks large amounts of water. Client has "passed out" several times over the last 2 days including a fall down the steps. Has history of clinical depression, severe anxiety, and substance use disorder. Currently alert and oriented ×4. States feeling more fatigued and weaker than usual; started having palpitations this morning. Reports feeling hopeless about the client's "situation." No abnormal or adventitious breath sounds; skin cool, clammy, but very dry. Several healing bruises on arms and legs. Lips and mucous membranes dry. Several teeth missing and other teeth are eroded and discolored. Client's bones, especially ribs and pelvis, very prominent. Fingertips bluish and cold; hands slightly swollen. Cap refill >3 seconds; peripheral pulses 1+. 2+ pitting edema in both feet and lower legs. VS: T 97.6°F (36.4°C); HR 76 beats per minute and irregular; RR 22 breaths per minute and regular; BP 82/46 mmHg; SpO$_2$ 94% on RA; FSBG 48 mg/dL (2.7 mmol/L). BMI 16.1.

Select **3** client findings that require **immediate** follow-up.
- BMI 16.1
- Cool, dry skin
- Increased fatigue and weakness
- Bluish swollen hands
- Peripheral pulses 1+
- BP 82/46 mmHg
- SpO$_2$ 94% on RA
- RR 22 breaths per minute
- FSBG 48 mg/dL (2.7 mmol/L)
- Feeling of hopelessness

Thinking Exercise 8.5.2

The nurse is caring for a 21-year-old client in the Emergency Department (ED).

History and Physical	Nurses Notes	Orders	Laboratory Results

1530: Client admitted to ED with worsening signs and symptoms of anorexia nervosa (AN). Parents report client eats almost no solid food except lettuce and drinks large amounts of water. Client has "passed out" several times over the last 2 days including a fall down the steps. Has history of clinical depression, severe anxiety, and substance use disorder. Currently alert and oriented ×4. States feeling more fatigued and weaker than usual; started having palpitations this morning. Reports feeling hopeless about the client's "situation." No abnormal or adventitious breath sounds; skin cool, clammy, but very dry. Several healing bruises on arms and legs. Lips and mucous membranes dry. Several teeth missing and other teeth are eroded and discolored. Client's bones, especially ribs and pelvis, very prominent. Fingertips bluish and cold; hands slightly swollen. Cap refill >3 seconds; pedal pulses 1+ and equal. 2+ pitting edema in both feet and lower legs. VS: T 97.6°F (36.4°C); HR 76 beats per minute and irregular; RR 22 breaths per minute and regular; BP 84/46 mmHg; SpO_2 94% on RA; FSBG 48 mg/dL (2.7 mmol/L). BMI 16.1.

1625: ECG completed and blood drawn for labs.

Complete the following sentence by selecting from the list of word choices below. The nurse analyzes assessment findings and determines that the client likely has **[Word Choice]**.

Word Choices	
Fluid overload	Diabetes mellitus
Electrolyte imbalances	Respiratory distress

Thinking Exercise 8.5.3

The nurse is caring for a 21-year-old client in the Emergency Department (ED).

History and Physical	Nurses Notes	Orders	Laboratory Results

1530: Client admitted to ED with worsening signs and symptoms of anorexia nervosa (AN). Parents report client eats almost no solid food except lettuce and drinks large amounts of water. Client has "passed out" several times over the last 2 days including a fall down the steps. Has history of clinical depression, severe anxiety, and substance use disorder. Currently alert and oriented ×4. States feeling more fatigued and weaker than usual; started having palpitations this morning. Reports feeling hopeless about the client's "situation." No abnormal or adventitious breath sounds; skin cool, clammy, but very dry. Several healing bruises on arms and legs. Lips and mucous membranes dry. Several teeth missing and other teeth are eroded and discolored. Client's bones, especially ribs and pelvis, very prominent. Fingertips bluish and cold; hands slightly swollen. Cap refill >3 seconds; pedal pulses 1+ and equal. 2+ pitting edema in both feet and lower legs. VS: T 97.6°F (36.4°C); HR 76 beats per minute and irregular; RR 22 breaths per minute and regular; BP 84/46 mmHg; SpO_2 94% on RA; FSBG 48 mg/dL (2.7 mmol/L). BMI 16.1.

1625: ECG completed and blood drawn for labs.

History and Physical	Laboratory Results	Orders	Nurses Notes

Serum Laboratory Test/Reference Range	ED Results
Sodium (Na+) (136–145 mEq/L [136–145 mmol/L])	128 mEq/L (128 mmol/L)
Potassium (K+) (3.5–5.0 mEq/L [3.5–5.0 mmol/L])	2.4 mEq/L (2.4 mmol/L)
Blood urea nitrogen (BUN) (10–20 mg/dL [3.6–7.1 mmol/L])	37 mg/dL (13.2 mmol/L)
Creatinine (0.5–1.1 mg/dL [44.2–97.3 µmol/L])	1.3 mg/dL (114.9 µmol/L)

Continued

UNFOLDING CASE STUDY 8.5—cont'd

Complete the following sentence by selecting from the list of options below. The *priority* for care at this time is to manage **1 [Select]** because the client could develop **2 [Select]**.

Options for 1	Options for 2
Hypokalemia	Fluid overload
Hyponatremia	Cardiac dysrhythmias
Elevated creatinine	Acute kidney injury

Thinking Exercise 8.5.4

The nurse is caring for a 21-year-old client in the Emergency Department (ED).

History and Physical	Nurses Notes	Orders	Laboratory Results

1530:   Client admitted to ED with worsening signs and symptoms of anorexia nervosa (AN). Parents report client eats almost no solid food except lettuce and drinks large amounts of water. Client has "passed out" several times over the last 2 days including a fall down the steps. Has history of clinical depression, severe anxiety, and substance use disorder. Currently alert and oriented ×4. States feeling more fatigued and weaker than usual; started having palpitations this morning. Reports feeling hopeless about the client's "situation." No abnormal or adventitious breath sounds; skin cool, clammy, but very dry. Several healing bruises on arms and legs. Lips and mucous membranes dry. Several teeth missing and other teeth are eroded and discolored. Client's bones, especially ribs and pelvis, very prominent. Fingertips bluish and cold; hands slightly swollen. Cap refill >3 seconds; pedal pulses 1+ and equal. 2+ pitting edema in both feet and lower legs. VS: T 97.6°F (36.4°C); HR 76 beats per minute and irregular; RR 22 breaths per minute and regular; BP 84/46 mmHg; SpO$_2$ 94% on RA; FSBG 48 mg/dL (2.7 mmol/L). BMI 16.1.

1625:   ECG completed and blood drawn for labs.

History and Physical	Laboratory Results	Orders	Nurses Notes

Serum Laboratory Test/Reference Range	ED Results
Sodium (Na$^+$) (136–145 mEq/L [136–145 mmol/L])	128 mEq/L (128 mmol/L)
Potassium (K$^+$) (3.5–5.0 mEq/L [3.5–5.0 mmol/L])	2.4 mEq/L (2.4 mmol/L)
Blood urea nitrogen (BUN) (10–20 mg/dL [3.6–7.1 mmol/L])	37 mg/dL (13.2 mmol/L)
Creatinine (0.5–1.1 mg/dL [44.2–97.3 µmol/L])	1.3 mg/dL (114.9 µmol/L)

Select whether the following potential nursing actions are indicated or not indicated for the client at this time.

Potential Nursing Actions	Indicated	Not Indicated
Start supplemental oxygen via NC		
Obtain peripheral venous access		
Apply continuous cardiac monitoring		
Prepare to provide supplemental potassium		

UNFOLDING CASE STUDY 8.5—cont'd

Thinking Exercise 8.5.5

The nurse is caring for a 21-year-old client in the Emergency Department (ED).

History and Physical	Nurses Notes	Orders	Laboratory Results

1530: Client admitted to ED with worsening signs and symptoms of anorexia nervosa (AN). Parents report client eats almost no solid food except lettuce and drinks large amounts of water. Client has "passed out" several times over the last 2 days including a fall down the steps. Has history of clinical depression, severe anxiety, and substance use disorder. Currently alert and oriented ×4. States feeling more fatigued and weaker than usual; started having palpitations this morning. Reports feeling hopeless about the client's "situation." No abnormal or adventitious breath sounds; skin cool, clammy, but very dry. Several healing bruises on arms and legs. Lips and mucous membranes dry. Several teeth missing and other teeth are eroded and discolored. Client's bones, especially ribs and pelvis, very prominent. Fingertips bluish and cold; hands slightly swollen. Cap refill >3 seconds; pedal pulses 1+ and equal. 2+ pitting edema in both feet and lower legs. VS: T 97.6°F (36.4°C); HR 76 beats per minute and irregular; RR 22 breaths per minute and regular; BP 84/46 mmHg; SpO$_2$ 94% on RA; FSBG 48 mg/dL (2.7 mmol/L). BMI 16.1.

1625: ECG completed and blood drawn for labs. Cardiac monitor applied. NSR with occasional PVCs.

1640: Peripheral IV started in left forearm infusing 5%D/0.45%NS at 125 mL per hour. Potassium infusion started per protocol. Psychiatrist in to examine client.

History and Physical	Laboratory Results	Orders	Nurses Notes

Serum Laboratory Test/Reference Range	ED Results
Sodium (Na$^+$) (136–145 mEq/L [136–145 mmol/L])	128 mEq/L (128 mmol/L)
Potassium (K$^+$) (3.5–5.0 mEq/L [3.5–5.0 mmol/L])	2.4 mEq/L (2.4 mmol/L)
Blood urea nitrogen (BUN) (10–20 mg/dL [3.6–7.1 mmol/L])	37 mg/dL (13.2 mmol/L)
Creatinine (0.5–1.1 mg/dL [44.2–97.3 µmol/L])	1.3 mg/dL (114.9 µmol/L)

Which of the following actions would the nurse implement for the client at this time? **Select all that apply.**

○ Monitor serum electrolyte values.
○ Assess for cardiac dysrhythmias.
○ Screen for suicidal ideation.
○ Consult with registered dietitian nutritionist
○ Consult with social worker or mental health professional.

Continued

UNFOLDING CASE STUDY 8.5—cont'd

Thinking Exercise 8.5.6
The nurse is caring for a 21-year-old client in the Emergency Department (ED). Highlight the assessment findings in the 1810 nurses note that indicate client care has been **effective**.

History and Physical	Nurses Notes	Orders	Laboratory Results

1530: Client admitted to ED with worsening signs and symptoms of anorexia nervosa (AN). Parents report client eats almost no solid food except lettuce and drinks large amounts of water. Client has "passed out" several times over the last 2 days including a fall down the steps. Has history of clinical depression, severe anxiety, and substance use disorder. Currently alert and oriented ×4. States feeling more fatigued and weaker than usual; started having palpitations this morning. Reports feeling hopeless about the client's "situation." No abnormal or adventitious breath sounds; skin cool, clammy, but very dry. Several healing bruises on arms and legs. Lips and mucous membranes dry. Several teeth missing and other teeth are eroded and discolored. Client's bones, especially ribs and pelvis, very prominent. Fingertips bluish and cold; hands slightly swollen. Cap refill >3 seconds; pedal pulses 1+ and equal. 2+ pitting edema in both feet and lower legs. VS: T 97.6°F (36.4°C); HR 76 beats per minute and irregular; RR 22 breaths per minute and regular; BP 84/46 mmHg; SpO$_2$ 94% on RA; FSBG 48 mg/dL (2.7 mmol/L). BMI 16.1.

1625: ECG completed and blood drawn for labs. Cardiac monitor applied. NSR with occasional PVCs.

1640: Peripheral IV started in left forearm infusing 5%D/0.45%NS at 125 mL per hour. Potassium infusion started per protocol. Social worker consult initiated. Psychiatrist in to examine client.

1810: Plan to transfer client to cardiac unit for monitoring overnight; client is not at risk for self-harm or harm to others. Stat potassium: 2.9 mEq/L (2.9 mmol/L). VS: T 97.8°F (36.5°C); HR 82 beats per minute and irregular; RR 20 breaths per minute and regular; BP 98/46 mmHg; SpO$_2$ 94% on RA; FSBG 75 mg/dL (4.2 mmol/L).

History and Physical	Laboratory Results	Orders	Nurses Notes

Serum Laboratory Test/Reference Range	ED Results
Sodium (Na$^+$) (136–145 mEq/L [136–145 mmol/L])	128 mEq/L (128 mmol/L)
Potassium (K$^+$) (3.5–5.0 mEq/L [3.5–5.0 mmol/L])	2.4 mEq/L (2.4 mmol/L)
Blood urea nitrogen (BUN) (10–20 mg/dL [3.6–7.1 mmol/L])	37 mg/dL (13.2 mmol/L)
Creatinine (0.5–1.1 mg/dL [44.2–97.3 µmol/L])	1.3 mg/dL (114.9 µmol/L)

UNFOLDING CASE STUDY 8.6

Thinking Exercise 8.6.1

The nurse is caring for a 38-year-old pregnant client in the obstetrician's office.

History and Physical	Nurses Notes	Orders	Laboratory Results

Obstetrician Visit at 32-Weeks' Pregnancy

1115:   Client visit for follow-up on weight gain and high blood pressure. Last week client had gained 7 lb (3.2 kg) since visit 4 weeks before. Today client has 2+ pitting edema both feet. BP elevated to 144/89 mmHg last week. Current VS: T 98.6°F (37°C); HR 84 beats per minute and regular; RR 18 breaths per minute and regular; BP 152/90 mmHg; SpO$_2$ 96% on RA. Trace protein in urine. Denies any headaches, visual changes, or seizure activity. Sent to hospital OB department for fetal and maternal monitoring.

Obstetrician Visit at 33-Weeks' Pregnancy

0900:   Client visit for follow-up on weight gain and high blood pressure. Spent 3 hours in hospital OB department for monitoring but sent home with daily BP monitoring via telehealth. Goal is to have cesarean section at 37 weeks if BP can be managed until that time. Client has reduced salt and stopped working to increase rest since last week. Gain of 2.2 lb (1 kg) this past week. 2+ pitting edema both feet. BP 140/88 mmHg. Trace protein in urine. Denies any headaches, visual changes, or seizure activity.

Obstetrician Visit at 34-Weeks' Pregnancy

1030:   Client visit for follow-up on weight gain and high blood pressure. BP 158/94 mmHg. SpO$_2$ 94% on RA. Has had occasional headaches over the past week. 1+ urinary protein. 3+ pitting edema both feet. Plan to admit client to hospital OB department.

Complete the following sentence by selecting from the list of word choices below. The assessment finding that requires **immediate** follow-up is the client's **[Word Choice]**.

Word Choices	
Headache	Foot edema
High blood pressure	Weight gain

Continued

UNFOLDING CASE STUDY 8.6—cont'd

Thinking Exercise 8.6.2
The nurse is caring for a 38-year-old pregnant client in the obstetrician's office.

History and Physical	Nurses Notes	Orders	Laboratory Results

Obstetrician Visit at 32-Weeks' Pregnancy

1115:   Client visit for follow-up on weight gain and high blood pressure. Last week client had gained 7 lb (3.2 kg) since visit 4 weeks before. Today client has 2+ pitting edema both feet. BP elevated to 144/89 mmHg last week. Current VS: T 98.6°F (37°C); HR 84 beats per minute and regular; RR 18 breaths per minute and regular; BP 152/90 mmHg; SpO$_2$ 96% on RA. Trace protein in urine. Denies any headaches, visual changes, or seizure activity. Sent to hospital OB department for fetal and maternal monitoring.

Obstetrician Visit at 33-Weeks' Pregnancy

0900:   Client visit for follow-up on weight gain and high blood pressure. Spent 3 hours in hospital OB department for monitoring but sent home with daily BP monitoring via telehealth. Goal is to have cesarean section at 37 weeks if BP can be managed until that time. Client has reduced salt and stopped working to increase rest since last week. Gain of 2.2 lb (1 kg) this past week. 2+ pitting edema both feet. BP 140/88 mmHg. Trace protein in urine. Denies any headaches, visual changes, or seizure activity.

Obstetrician Visit at 34-Weeks' Pregnancy

1030:   Client visit for follow-up on weight gain and high blood pressure. BP 158/94 mmHg. SpO$_2$ 94% on RA. Has had occasional headaches over the past week. 1+ urinary protein. 3+ pitting edema both feet. SpO$_2$ 94% on RA. Plan to admit client to hospital OB department.

Complete the following sentence by selecting from the lists of options below. The client is most at risk for **1 [Select]** as evidenced by **2 [Select]** and **3 [Select]**.

Options for 1	Options for 2	Options for 3
Heart failure	Weight gain	Proteinuria
Preeclampsia	Pitting edema	Headaches
Migraines	High blood pressure	SpO$_2$

Thinking Exercise 8.6.3
The nurse is caring for a 38-year-old pregnant client in the obstetrician's office.

History and Physical	Nurses Notes	Orders	Laboratory Results

Obstetrician Visit at 32-Weeks' Pregnancy

1115:   Client visit for follow-up on weight gain and high blood pressure. Last week client had gained 7 lb (3.2 kg) since visit 4 weeks before. Today client has 2+ pitting edema both feet. BP elevated to 144/89 mmHg last week. Current VS: T 98.6°F (37°C); HR 84 beats per minute and regular; RR 18 breaths per minute and regular; BP 152/90 mmHg; SpO$_2$ 96% on RA. Trace protein in urine. Denies any headaches, visual changes, or seizure activity. Sent to hospital OB department for fetal and maternal monitoring.

Obstetrician Visit at 33-Weeks' Pregnancy

0900:   Client visit for follow-up on weight gain and high blood pressure. Spent 3 hours in hospital OB department for monitoring but sent home with daily BP monitoring via telehealth. Goal is to have cesarean section at 37 weeks if BP can be managed until that time. Client has reduced salt and stopped working to increase rest since last week. Gain of 2.2 lb (1 kg) this past week. 2+ pitting edema both feet. BP 140/88 mmHg. Trace protein in urine. Denies any headaches, visual changes, or seizure activity.

Obstetrician Visit at 34-Weeks' Pregnancy

1030:   Client visit for follow-up on weight gain and high blood pressure. BP 158/94 mmHg. SpO$_2$ 94% on RA. Has had occasional headaches over the past week. 1+ urinary protein. 3+ pitting edema both feet. Plan to admit client to hospital OB department.

UNFOLDING CASE STUDY 8.6—cont'd

Select the **1 priority** for client and baby care at this time.
- Decrease pitting edema.
- Decrease client's blood pressure.
- Manage the client's headache pain.
- Administer supplemental oxygen.
- Prepare for delivery of the baby.

Thinking Exercise 8.6.4

The nurse is caring for a 38-year-old pregnant client in the inpatient birthing suite.

History and Physical	Nurses Notes	Orders	Laboratory Results

Obstetrician Visit at 32-Weeks' Pregnancy

1115: Client visit for follow-up on weight gain and high blood pressure. Last week client had gained 7 lb (3.2 kg) since visit 4 weeks before. Today client has 2+ pitting edema both feet. BP elevated to 144/89 mmHg last week. Current VS: T 98.6°F (37°C); HR 84 beats per minute and regular; RR 18 breaths per minute and regular; BP 152/90 mmHg; SpO$_2$ 96% on RA. Trace protein in urine. Denies any headaches, visual changes, or seizure activity. Sent to hospital OB department for fetal and maternal monitoring.

Obstetrician Visit at 33-Weeks' Pregnancy

0900: Client visit for follow-up on weight gain and high blood pressure. Spent 3 hours in hospital OB department for monitoring but sent home with daily BP monitoring via telehealth. Goal is to have cesarean section at 37 weeks if BP can be managed until that time. Client has reduced salt and stopped working to increase rest since last week. Gain of 2.2 lb (1 kg) this past week. 2+ pitting edema both feet. BP 140/88 mmHg. Trace protein in urine. Denies any headaches, visual changes, or seizure activity.

Obstetrician Visit at 34-Weeks' Pregnancy

1030: Client visit for follow-up on weight gain and high blood pressure. BP 158/94 mmHg. SpO$_2$ 94% on RA. Has had occasional headaches over the past week. 1+ urinary protein. 3+ pitting edema both feet. Plan to admit client to hospital OB department.

Hospital OB Department (Day of Admission)

1205: Client at 34 weeks, 2 days; admitted for evaluation of high blood pressure and proteinuria. BP 162/98 mmHg. Denies headache, nausea, or visual changes. Peripheral venous access established for IV fluids; client NPO. Indwelling urinary catheter placed. Discussed with client and partner the possibility of C-section today or tomorrow.

Select whether the following potential nursing actions are indicated or not indicated for the client at this time.

Potential Nursing Actions	Indicated	Not Indicated
Administer IV antihypertensive drug per protocol		
Apply continuous cardiac monitoring		
Administer IV magnesium sulfate per protocol		
Administer IV corticosteroid per protocol		
Provide preoperative teaching related to expectations for mother and baby		

Continued

UNFOLDING CASE STUDY 8.6—cont'd

Thinking Exercise 8.6.5
The nurse is caring for a 38-year-old pregnant client in the obstetrician's office.

History and Physical	Nurses Notes	Orders	Laboratory Results

Obstetrician Visit at 32-Weeks' Pregnancy

1115:   Client visit for follow-up on weight gain and high blood pressure. Last week client had gained 7 lb (3.2 kg) since visit 4 weeks before. Today client has 2+ pitting edema both feet. BP elevated to 144/89 mmHg last week. Current VS: T 98.6°F (37°C); HR 84 beats per minute and regular; RR 18 breaths per minute and regular; BP 152/90 mmHg; SpO$_2$ 96% on RA. Trace protein in urine. Denies any headaches, visual changes, or seizure activity. Sent to hospital OB department for fetal and maternal monitoring.

Obstetrician Visit at 33-Weeks' Pregnancy

0900:   Client visit for follow-up on weight gain and high blood pressure. Spent 3 hours in hospital OB department for monitoring but sent home with daily BP monitoring via telehealth. Goal is to have cesarean section at 37 weeks if BP can be managed until that time. Client has reduced salt and stopped working to increase rest since last week. Gain of 2.2 lb (1 kg) this past week. 2+ pitting edema both feet. BP 140/88 mmHg. Trace protein in urine. Denies any headaches, visual changes, or seizure activity.

Obstetrician Visit at 34-Weeks' Pregnancy

1030:   Client visit for follow-up on weight gain and high blood pressure. BP 158/94. SpO$_2$ 94% on RA. Has had occasional headaches over the past week. 1+ urinary protein. 3+ pitting edema both feet. Plan to admit client to hospital OB department.

Hospital OB Department (Day of Admission)

1205:   Client at 34 weeks, 2 days, admitted for evaluation of high blood pressure and proteinuria. BP 162/98 mmHg. Denies headache, nausea, or visual changes. Peripheral venous access established for IV fluids; client NPO. Indwelling urinary catheter placed. Discussed with client and partner the possibility of C-section today or tomorrow.

1620:   C-section performed. Baby boy delivered at 4 lb (1.8), 17 in (43.2 cm). Apgar 1 min: 6; Apgar 5 min: 8. Placed on mother's chest for few minutes before preparing to admit to NICU. Explained the expectations for newborn care in NICU.

Which of the following actions will the nurse likely implement in NICU for this 34-week-old newborn? **Select all that apply.**

○ Place baby on mechanical ventilator.
○ Insert nasogastric tube for feeding.
○ Maintain quiet environment.
○ Apply continuous cardiac monitoring.
○ Ask mother to bring breast milk for baby.
○ Insert indwelling urinary catheter.

UNFOLDING CASE STUDY 8.6—cont'd

Thinking Exercise 8.6.6

The nurse is caring for a baby born at 34 weeks. Highlight the findings in the NICU note that indicate the baby is **improving**.

History and Physical	Nurses Notes	Orders	Laboratory Results

Obstetrician Visit at 32-Weeks' Pregnancy

1115:   Client visit for follow-up on weight gain and high blood pressure. Last week client had gained 7 lb (3.2 kg) since visit 4 weeks before. Today client has 2+ pitting edema both feet. BP elevated to 144/89 mmHg last week. Current VS: T 98.6°F (37°C); HR 84 beats per minute and regular; RR 18 breaths per minute and regular; BP 152/90 mmHg; SpO$_2$ 96% on RA. Trace protein in urine. Denies any headaches, visual changes, or seizure activity. Sent to hospital OB department for fetal and maternal monitoring.

Obstetrician Visit at 33-Weeks' Pregnancy

0900:   Client visit for follow-up on weight gain and high blood pressure. Spent 3 hours in hospital OB department for monitoring but sent home with daily BP monitoring via telehealth. Goal is to have cesarean section at 37 weeks if BP can be managed until that time. Client has reduced salt and stopped working to increase rest since last week. Gain of 2.2 lb (1 kg) this past week. 2+ pitting edema both feet. BP 140/88 mmHg. Trace protein in urine. Denies any headaches, visual changes, or seizure activity.

Obstetrician Visit at 34-Weeks' Pregnancy

1030:   Client visit for follow-up on weight gain and high blood pressure. BP 158/94. SpO$_2$ 94% on RA. Has had occasional headaches over the past week. 1+ urinary protein. 3+ pitting edema both feet. Plan to admit client to hospital OB department. Discussed with client and partner the possibility of C-section today or tomorrow.

Hospital OB Department (Day of Admission)

1205:   Client at 34 weeks, 2 days, admitted for evaluation of high blood pressure and proteinuria. BP 162/98 mmHg. Denies headache, nausea, or visual changes. Peripheral venous access established for IV fluids; client NPO. Indwelling urinary catheter placed. Obstetrician to examine client to determine plan of care for preeclampsia.

1620:   C-section performed. Baby boy delivered at 4 lb (1.8), 17 in (43.2 cm). Apgar 1 min: 7; Apgar 5 min: 8. Placed on mother's chest for few minutes before preparing to admit to NICU. Nurse explained expectations for newborn care in NICU.

NICU 2 Weeks Later

1000:   Parents in to visit baby and assist with morning care. Newborn on high-flow oxygen after 10 days on CPAP since birth. NG tube removed yesterday; baby on bottle-feeding using mother's breast milk, but not always consuming minimum required to meet nutritional needs. Gained 8 ounces since birth 2 weeks ago with goal weight of 5 lb (2.3 kg) prior to discharge. Voiding and stools adequate.

UNFOLDING CASE STUDY 8.7

Thinking Exercise 8.7.1

The nurse is caring for a 12-year-old child in the acute pediatric unit following surgical repair of a right tibial fracture. Highlight the client findings in the 1630 nurses note that require **immediate** follow-up.

History and Physical	Nurses Notes	Orders	Laboratory Results

1215:   Client drowsy after surgery but easily awakened. Able to communicate. States pain is not too bad, "maybe a 4/10." Reports feeling nauseated and refusing water. Family at bedside. Breath sounds clear throughout lung fields. Abdomen soft and flat; diminished bowel sounds ×4. Splint with elastic wrap over surgical dressing dry and in place on right leg from ankle to groin. Right foot slightly cooler than left. Pedal pulses 2+ and equal. Skin color equal in both feet. Able to slightly move right toes. Cap refill <3 seconds. IV infusing at 80 mL per hour. VS: T 98.1°F (36.7°C); HR 88 beats per minute and regular; RR 18 breaths per minute and regular; BP 100/66 mmHg; SpO$_2$ 99% on RA.

1630:   Family reports that client's pain has markedly increased even though analgesic given less than an hour ago, but nausea has lessened. Taking small amounts of fluids; voided 180 mL ×1. Client describes pain now as 9/10; states the affected leg and foot are throbbing. Splint with elastic wrap over surgical dressing dry and in place on right leg from ankle to groin. Right foot much colder than left. Right pedal pulse nonpalpable; right foot paler than left. Unable to move right toes or foot. Cap refill >3 seconds. IV infusing at 80 mL per hour. VS: T 98.1°F (36.7°C); HR 94 beats per minute and regular; RR 20 breaths per minute and regular; BP 122/74 mmHg; SpO$_2$ 98% on RA.

Thinking Exercise 8.7.2

The nurse is caring for a 12-year-old child in the acute pediatric unit following surgical repair of a right tibial fracture.

History and Physical	Nurses Notes	Orders	Laboratory Results

1215:   Client drowsy after surgery but easily awakened. Able to communicate. States pain is not too bad, "maybe a 4/10." Reports feeling nauseated and refusing water. Family at bedside. Breath sounds clear throughout lung fields. Abdomen soft and flat; diminished bowel sounds ×4. Splint with elastic wrap over surgical dressing dry and in place on right leg from ankle to groin. Right foot slightly cooler than left. Pedal pulses 2+ and equal. Skin color equal in both feet. Able to slightly move right toes. Cap refill <3 seconds. IV infusing at 80 mL per hour. VS: T 98.1°F (36.7°C); HR 88 beats per minute and regular; RR 18 breaths per minute and regular; BP 100/66 mmHg; SpO$_2$ 99% on RA.

1630:   Family reports that client's pain has markedly increased even though analgesic given less than an hour ago, but nausea has lessened. Taking small amounts of fluids; voided 180 mL ×1. Client describes pain now as 9/10; states the affected leg and foot are throbbing. Splint with elastic wrap over surgical dressing dry and in place on right leg from ankle to groin. Right foot much colder than left. Right pedal pulse nonpalpable; right foot paler than left. Unable to move right toes or foot. Cap refill >3 seconds. IV infusing at 80 mL per hour. VS: T 98.1°F (36.7°C); HR 94 beats per minute and regular; RR 20 breaths per minute and regular; BP 122/74 mmHg; SpO$_2$ 98% on RA.

UNFOLDING CASE STUDY 8.7—cont'd

For each client finding listed below, determine if the finding is consistent with the health conditions of deep vein thrombosis or acute compartment syndrome. Some findings may be consistent with more than one condition.

Client Findings	Deep Vein Thrombosis	Acute Compartment Syndrome
Severe pain in affected leg		
Right foot colder and paler than left		
Unable to palpate right pedal pulse		
Capillary refill >3 seconds		

Thinking Exercise 8.7.3

The nurse is caring for a 12-year-old child in the acute pediatric unit following surgical repair of a right tibial fracture.

History and Physical	Nurses Notes	Orders	Laboratory Results

1215: Client drowsy after surgery but easily awakened. Able to communicate. States pain is not too bad, "maybe a 4/10." Reports feeling nauseated and refusing water. Family at bedside. Breath sounds clear throughout lung fields. Abdomen soft and flat; diminished bowel sounds ×4. Splint with elastic wrap over surgical dressing dry and in place on right leg from ankle to groin. Right foot slightly cooler than left. Pedal pulses 2+ and equal. Skin color equal in both feet. Able to slightly move right toes. Cap refill <3 seconds. IV infusing at 80 mL per hour. VS: T 98.1°F (36.7°C); HR 88 beats per minute and regular; RR 18 breaths per minute and regular; BP 100/66 mmHg; SpO$_2$ 99% on RA.

1630: Family reports that client's pain has markedly increased even though analgesic given less than an hour ago, but nausea has lessened. Taking small amounts of fluids; voided 180 mL ×1. Client describes pain now as 9/10; states the affected leg and foot are throbbing. Splint with elastic wrap over surgical dressing dry and in place on right leg from ankle to groin. Right foot much colder than left. Right pedal pulse nonpalpable; right foot paler than left. Unable to move right toes or foot. Cap refill >3 seconds. IV infusing at 80 mL per hour. VS: T 98.1°F (36.7°C); HR 94 beats per minute and regular; RR 20 breaths per minute and regular; BP 122/74 mmHg; SpO$_2$ 98% on RA.

Complete the following sentence by selecting from the lists of options below. The ***priority*** for care at this time is to manage the client's **1 [Select]** because this condition can cause **2 [Select]**.

Options for 1	Options for 2
Compartment syndrome	Malnutrition
Nausea	Shock
Severe pain	Tissue necrosis

Continued

UNFOLDING CASE STUDY 8.7—cont'd

Thinking Exercise 8.7.4

The nurse is caring for a 12-year-old child in the acute pediatric unit following surgical repair of a right tibial fracture.

History and Physical	Nurses Notes	Orders	Laboratory Results

1215:   Client drowsy after surgery but easily awakened. Able to communicate. States pain is not too bad, "maybe a 4/10." Reports feeling nauseated and refusing water. Family at bedside. Breath sounds clear throughout lung fields. Abdomen soft and flat; diminished bowel sounds ×4. Splint with elastic wrap over surgical dressing dry and in place on right leg from ankle to groin. Right foot slightly cooler than left. Pedal pulses 2+ and equal. Skin color equal in both feet. Able to slightly move right toes. Cap refill <3 seconds. IV infusing at 80 mL per hour. VS: T 98.1°F (36.7°C); HR 88 beats per minute and regular; RR 18 breaths per minute and regular; BP 100/66 mmHg; SpO$_2$ 99% on RA.

1630:   Family reports that client's pain has markedly increased even though analgesic given less than an hour ago, but nausea has lessened. Taking small amounts of fluids; voided 180 mL ×1. Client describes pain now as 9/10; states the affected leg and foot are throbbing. Splint with elastic wrap over surgical dressing dry and in place on right leg from ankle to groin. Right foot much colder than left. Right pedal pulse nonpalpable; right foot paler than left. Unable to move right toes or foot. Cap refill >3 seconds. IV infusing at 80 mL per hour. VS: T 98.1°F (36.7°C); HR 94 beats per minute and regular; RR 20 breaths per minute and regular; BP 122/74 mmHg; SpO$_2$ 98% on RA.

Which of the following potential nursing actions would be appropriate for the client at this time? **Select all that apply.**

○ Obtain surgical consent for a fasciotomy.
○ Make the client NPO in preparation for possible surgery.
○ Prepare for skeletal traction application.
○ Notify the surgeon immediately.
○ Elevate the affected leg.
○ Perform frequent neurovascular checks.

Thinking Exercise 8.7.5

The nurse is caring for a 12-year-old child in the acute pediatric unit following surgical repair of a right tibial fracture and open fasciotomy.

History and Physical	Nurses Notes	Orders	Laboratory Results

1215:   Client drowsy after surgery but easily awakened. Able to communicate. States pain is not too bad, "maybe a 4/10." Reports feeling nauseated and refusing water. Family at bedside. Breath sounds clear throughout lung fields. Abdomen soft and flat; diminished bowel sounds ×4. Splint with elastic wrap over surgical dressing dry and in place on right leg from ankle to groin. Right foot slightly cooler than left. Pedal pulses 2+ and equal. Skin color equal in both feet. Able to slightly move right toes. Cap refill <3 seconds. IV infusing at 80 mL per hour. VS: T 98.1°F (36.7°C); HR 88 beats per minute and regular; RR 18 breaths per minute and regular; BP 100/66 mmHg; SpO$_2$ 99% on RA.

1630:   Family reports that client's pain has markedly increased even though analgesic given less than an hour ago, but nausea has lessened. Taking small amounts of fluids; voided 180 mL ×1. Client describes pain now as 9/10; states the affected leg and foot are throbbing. Splint with elastic wrap over surgical dressing dry and in place on right leg from ankle to groin. Right foot much colder than left. Right pedal pulse nonpalpable; right foot paler than left. Unable to move right toes or foot. Cap refill >3 seconds. IV infusing at 80 mL per hour. VS: T 98.1°F (36.7°C); HR 94 beats per minute and regular; RR 20 breaths per minute and regular; BP 122/74 mmHg; SpO$_2$ 98% on RA.

1710:   Surgeon explained to client and family about the need to relieve the pressure on the lower leg to prevent tissue necrosis and potential loss of part of the right leg. Client made NPO for open fasciotomy of lower right leg later this evening. Obtained consent from family for surgery.

2045:   Returned from PACU after open right lower leg fasciotomy; wound covered with bulky dressing that is dry and intact. Right foot remains somewhat cooler and paler than left. Left pedal pulse 2+; right pedal pulse 1+. Client reports pain at 5/10 and receiving analgesics as needed. Nausea and vomiting ×2 in PACU. Breath sounds clear throughout lung fields. Abdomen soft and flat; diminished bowel sounds ×4. IV infusing in right forearm at 100 mL per hour. VS: T 99.2°F (37.3°C); HR 70 beats per minute and regular; RR 20 breaths per minute and regular; BP 102/56 mmHg; SpO$_2$ 96% on RA.

> **UNFOLDING CASE STUDY 8.7—cont'd**

Select the **3** actions that the nurse should implement as part of postoperative care.

○ Keep the client NPO for the next 2 days.
○ Perform frequent neurovascular assessments ("circ checks").
○ Request antiemetic drug for nausea and vomiting.
○ Elevate the surgical leg on two or more pillows.
○ Clarify wound care orders.

Thinking Exercise 8.7.6

The nurse is caring for a 12-year-old child in the acute pediatric unit following surgical repair of a right tibial fracture and open fasciotomy. Highlight the client findings in the 2045 nurses note that indicates the client's condition is **improving**.

History and Physical	Nurses Notes	Orders	Laboratory Results

1215: Client drowsy after surgery but easily awakened. Able to communicate. States pain is not too bad, "maybe a 4/10." Reports feeling nauseated and refusing water. Family at bedside. Breath sounds clear throughout lung fields. Abdomen soft and flat; diminished bowel sounds ×4. Splint with elastic wrap over surgical dressing dry and in place on right leg from ankle to groin. Right foot slightly cooler than left. Pedal pulses 2+ and equal. Skin color equal in both feet. Able to slightly move right toes. Cap refill <3 seconds. IV infusing at 80 mL per hour. VS: T 98.1°F (36.7°C); HR 88 beats per minute and regular; RR 18 breaths per minute and regular; BP 100/66 mmHg; SpO$_2$ 99% on RA.

1630: Family reports that client's pain has markedly increased even though analgesic given less than an hour ago, but nausea has lessened. Taking small amounts of fluids; voided 180 mL ×1. Client describes pain now as 9/10; states the affected leg and foot are throbbing. Splint with elastic wrap over surgical dressing dry and in place on right leg from ankle to groin. Right foot much colder than left. Right pedal pulse nonpalpable; right foot paler than left. Unable to move right toes or foot. Cap refill >3 seconds. IV infusing at 80 mL per hour. VS: T 98.1°F (36.7°C); HR 94 beats per minute and regular; RR 20 breaths per minute and regular; BP 122/74 mmHg; SpO$_2$ 98% on RA.

1710: Surgeon explained to client and family about the need to relieve the pressure on the lower leg to prevent tissue necrosis and potential loss of part of the right leg. Client made NPO for open fasciotomy of lower right leg later this evening. Obtained consent from family for surgery.

2045: Returned from PACU after open right lower leg fasciotomy; wound covered with bulky dressing that is dry and intact. Right foot remains somewhat cooler and paler than left. Left pedal pulse 2+; right pedal pulse 1+. Client reports pain at 5/10 and receiving analgesics as needed. Nausea and vomiting ×2 in PACU. Breath sounds clear throughout lung fields. Abdomen soft and flat; diminished bowel sounds ×4. IV infusing in right forearm at 100 mL per hour. VS: T 99.2°F (37.3°C); HR 70 beats per minute and regular; RR 20 breaths per minute and regular; BP 102/56 mmHg; SpO$_2$ 96% on RA.

STAND-ALONE ITEM EXAMPLES

In addition to new item types used as part of unfolding cases, the current NCLEX® includes two types of Stand-Alone test items—the Bowtie and Trend items. For both types of items, the client information is presented within one or more medical record tabs and does *not* unfold or evolve over time. The Bowtie item requires you to use each of the six cognitive skills to make good clinical judgments. When answering a Bowtie item, first recognize and analyze relevant clinical findings to determine the priority condition the client is most likely experiencing. Then decide on the most appropriate nursing actions that would help manage the condition. Finally, consider the parameters you would want to monitor to determine if expected outcomes to improve the client's condition were met.

By contrast, the Trend item requires you to use one or more of the six clinical judgment cognitive skills. Trend items present client data over time—minutes, hours, days, or weeks. Any test item that measures any of the cognitive skills may be part of a Trend question.

As you practice each of the Stand-Alone test items below, keep in mind what you learned about each clinical judgment skill, including the strategies outlined at the end of each chapter! The answers and rationales for these Stand-Alone items can be found at the end of this chapter.

Bowtie Items

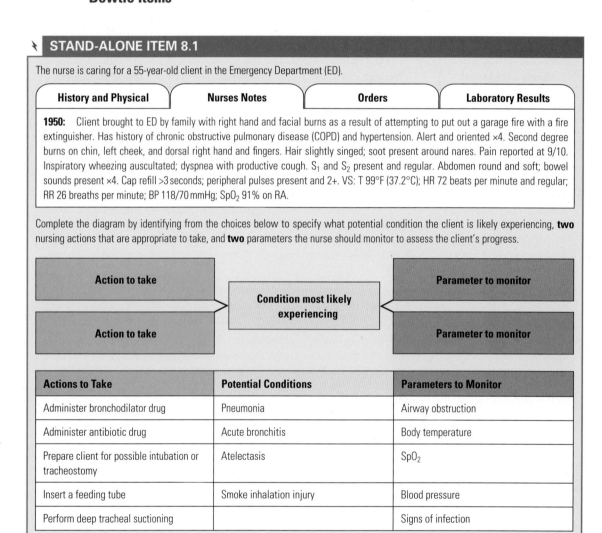

STAND-ALONE ITEM 8.1

The nurse is caring for a 55-year-old client in the Emergency Department (ED).

History and Physical	Nurses Notes	Orders	Laboratory Results

1950:   Client brought to ED by family with right hand and facial burns as a result of attempting to put out a garage fire with a fire extinguisher. Has history of chronic obstructive pulmonary disease (COPD) and hypertension. Alert and oriented ×4. Second degree burns on chin, left cheek, and dorsal right hand and fingers. Hair slightly singed; soot present around nares. Pain reported at 9/10. Inspiratory wheezing auscultated; dyspnea with productive cough. S_1 and S_2 present and regular. Abdomen round and soft; bowel sounds present ×4. Cap refill >3 seconds; peripheral pulses present and 2+. VS: T 99°F (37.2°C); HR 72 beats per minute and regular; RR 26 breaths per minute; BP 118/70 mmHg; SpO_2 91% on RA.

Complete the diagram by identifying from the choices below to specify what potential condition the client is likely experiencing, **two** nursing actions that are appropriate to take, and **two** parameters the nurse should monitor to assess the client's progress.

Action to take		Parameter to monitor
	Condition most likely experiencing	
Action to take		Parameter to monitor

Actions to Take	Potential Conditions	Parameters to Monitor
Administer bronchodilator drug	Pneumonia	Airway obstruction
Administer antibiotic drug	Acute bronchitis	Body temperature
Prepare client for possible intubation or tracheostomy	Atelectasis	SpO_2
Insert a feeding tube	Smoke inhalation injury	Blood pressure
Perform deep tracheal suctioning		Signs of infection

STAND-ALONE ITEM 8.2

The nurse is caring for a 22-year-old client in the Emergency Department (ED).

History and Physical	Nurses Notes	Orders	Laboratory Results

0635:   Client brought to ED by family with report of severe headache, fever, stiff neck, photophobia, and nausea. Has had symptoms for the past 2 days but today headache pain increased to 9/10. Attends local college and lives in apartment with five other students. States that family does not believe in getting vaccines because "God watches over us." No significant health history. Alert and oriented ×4. PERRLA. Breath sounds clear throughout lung fields; no adventitious sounds. S_1 and S_2 present and regular. Abdomen flat and soft; bowel sounds present ×4. Able to move all extremities but weak and lethargic. Cap refill >3 seconds; peripheral pulses present and 2+. VS: T 103°F (39.4°C); HR 95 beats per minute and regular; RR 20 breaths per minute; BP 126/64 mmHg; SpO_2 95% on RA.

Complete the diagram by identifying from the choices below to specify what potential condition the client is likely experiencing, **two** nursing actions that are appropriate to take, and **two** parameters the nurse should monitor to assess the client's progress.

Action to take	→	Condition most likely experiencing	←	Parameter to monitor
Action to take				Parameter to monitor

Actions to Take	Potential Conditions	Parameters to Monitor
Consult with physical therapist	Meningioma	Respiratory status
Establish peripheral venous access for antibiotics and corticosteroids	Meningitis	Body temperature
Prepare client for possible lumbar puncture	Migraine headache	SpO_2
Administer an analgesic for headache	West Nile encephalitis	Neurologic status
Prepare client for possible surgery		Blood pressure

STAND-ALONE ITEM 8.3

The nurse is caring for a 40-year-old client in the postpartum unit.

History and Physical	Nurses Notes	Orders	Laboratory Results

0810:   PPD #1. G2P2 had normal spontaneous vaginal delivery (NSVD) at 39 weeks. Breath sounds clear throughout lung fields; no adventitious sounds. S_1 and S_2 present and regular. Abdomen nontender with firm fundus at umbilicus; bowel sounds present ×4. Lochia increasing to one saturated pad every 1–1 ½ hours. Voiding as usual. Lactation specialist in to check on client. Breastfeeding without difficulty. States feeling very nervous about taking care of a baby and toddler when going home. VS: T 98.6°F (37°C); HR 84 beats per minute and regular; RR 18 breaths per minute; BP 116/60 mmHg; SpO_2 98% on RA.

1625:   Client reports increasing bleeding saturating almost two pads per hour. States feels a little lightheaded when getting up to the BR. Voiding clear yellow urine. Fundus slightly boggy and massaged. HR 96 beats per minute; BP 100/52 mmHg; SpO_2 98% on RA. Will recheck in 30–60 minute.

1730:   Client has stayed in bed for the past hour. Reports feeling very thirsty even though consuming fluids. Abdomen nontender with firm fundus at umbilicus. Continues to saturate almost two pads an hour. VS: T 99°F (37.2°C) HR 104 beats per minute; RR 22 breaths per minute; BP 92/50 mmHg; SpO_2 96% on RA.

Complete the diagram by identifying from the choices below to specify what potential condition the client is likely experiencing, **two** nursing actions that are appropriate to take, and **two** parameters the nurse should monitor to assess the client's progress.

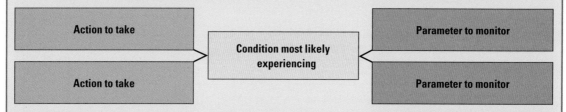

Actions to Take	Potential Conditions	Parameters to Monitor
Consult with social worker	Preeclampsia	Urinary output
Establish peripheral venous access for fluids	Hypovolemia	Lochia amount
Monitor vital signs every 30–60 minutes	Fluid overload	SpO_2
Place client in sitting position	Postpartum depression	Respiratory rate
Administer an IV diuretic		Blood pressure

Trend Items

STAND-ALONE ITEM 8.4

The nurse is caring for a 20-year-old client in the critical care unit with probable fentanyl overdose who is breathing without the assistance of mechanical ventilation.

History and Physical	Nursing Flow Sheet	Orders	Laboratory Results

Parameters	Admission 0345	0445	0545	0645
Temperature	98.2°F (36.8°C)	98°F (36.7°C)	98°F (36.7°C)	97.8°F (36.6°C)
Heart Rate	70 beats per minute	68 beats per minute	62 beats per minute	62 beats per minute
Respiratory Rate	16 breaths per minute	14 breaths per minute	14 breaths per minute	14 breaths per minute
Blood Pressure	108/50 mmHg	104/50 mmHg	100/48 mmHg	94/46 mmHg
Glasgow Coma Scale (GCS) Score	8	8	7	7
SpO_2	97% on high-flow oxygen	97% on high-flow oxygen	95% on high-flow oxygen	94% on high-flow oxygen

Complete the following sentence by selecting from the lists of options below. The nurse determines that the client is experiencing **1 [Select]** as evidenced by **2 [Select]**.

Options for 1	Options for 2
Coma	Low heart rate
Hypoxia	Low GCS score
Bradycardia	Low SpO_2

STAND-ALONE ITEM 8.5

The nurse is caring for a 49-year-old client in the Urgent Care Center with a history of type 1 diabetes mellitus, and receives the following laboratory results.

History and Physical	Laboratory Results	Progress Notes	Nurses Notes

Serum Laboratory Test/ Reference Range	Results 6 months Ago	Current Results
Blood urea nitrogen (10–20 mg/dL [3.6–7.1 mmol/L])	20 mg/dL (7.1 mmol/L)	38 mg/dL (13.8 mmol/L)
Creatinine (0.6–1.3 mg/dL [53.05–114.95 µmol/L])	1.7 mg/dL (150.3 mmol/L)	3.2 mg/dL (282.9 mmol/L)
Sodium (136–145 mEq/L [136–145 mmol/L])	139 mEq/L (139 mmol/L)	148 mEq/L (148 mmol/L)
Potassium (3.5–5 mEq/L [3.5–5 mmol/L])	4.4 mEq/L (4.4 mmol/L)	5.3 mEq/L (5.3 mmol/L)
Blood glucose (74–106 mg/dL [4.1–5.9 mmol/L])	154 mg/dL (8.6 mmol/L)	201 mg/dL (11.2 mmol/L)

Complete the following sentence by selecting from the list of word choices below. The nurse analyzes laboratory findings to determine that the client is most likely experiencing **[Word Choice]**.

Word Choices
Diabetic ketoacidosis
Chronic kidney disease
Hyperglycemic hyperosmolar syndrome

Answers and Rationales for Unfolding Case Studies and Stand-Alone Items

UNFOLDING CASE STUDY 8.1

Thinking Exercise 8.1.1
Answer:

History and Physical	Nurses Notes	Orders	Laboratory Results

0815:   Unlicensed personnel states that client who is usually alert and oriented seems sleepy and very confused this AM. Tried twice to climb out of bed. Reports that client has not voided since last night before going to bed. Client's medical history includes two strokes, type 2 diabetes mellitus, hypertension, chronic heart failure, and osteoarthritis. Currently drowsy but easily awakened. No abnormal or adventitious breath sounds; skin warm and dry. Lips and mucous membranes dry. Abdomen soft and round. Cap refill 5 seconds; pedal pulses 1+ and equal. 2+ nonpitting edema in both feet. VS: T 100.6°F (38.1°C); HR 105 beats per minute and irregular; RR 20 breaths per minute; BP 88/52 mmHg; SpO$_2$ 89% on RA; FSBG 76 mg/dL (4.21 mmol/L).

UNFOLDING CASE STUDY 8.1—cont'd

Rationale: The client's level of consciousness (LOC) and cognitive status changed from being alert and oriented to drowsy and confused. This sudden neurologic change requires immediate follow-up and continued monitoring for possible decreasing LOC which could become potentially life-threatening. The client has also not voided since bedtime the night before. The nurse would follow-up on this finding to determine if the client is making urine (indicating kidney dysfunction) or retaining urine in the bladder. The client has a fever which could indicate infection or inflammation. An older adult who has a fever can become quickly dehydrated which can lead to hypovolemic shock, a potentially life-threatening complication. The client's blood pressure is low (systolic BP is below 90 mmHg) which would suggest possible decreased blood volume needing immediate follow-up. The client is slightly tachycardic most likely to compensate for hypotension and consistent with dehydration. The client could also be experiencing tachycardia because the client's SpO_2 is below 90%, indicating hypoxia. This low SpO_2 requires immediate follow-up to ensure the client's major organs are adequately perfused. The client's dry skin and mucous membranes, slowed capillary refill, weak pedal pulses, and nonpitting foot edema are commonly seen in older adults due to physiologic changes associated with aging and are not life-threatening. All other client findings are within normal or usual parameters.

Thinking Exercise 8.1.2
Answer:

Client Findings	Dehydration	Chronic Kidney Disease	Heart Failure
Has not voided since last night	X	X	
T 100.6°F (38.1°C);	X		
HR 105 beats per minute and irregular	X	X	X
BP 88/52 mmHg	X		X
2+ nonpitting edema in both feet	X	X	X

Rationale: All of the listed client findings are consistent with dehydration in which clients typically are hypovolemic. Having less fluid in the body can cause temperature elevation, tachycardia, and low blood pressure, especially in older adults. To conserve fluid, the kidneys retain water and sodium in the body, preventing normal urinary output and causing edema. In addition, hypotension can lead to vasoconstriction which forces fluid from the intravascular compartment into the interstitial spaces causing edema. Clients who have chronic kidney disease (CKD) experience fluid retention and edema with oliguria or anuria. Fluid excess increases blood volume, which causes high blood pressure rather than hypotension. Tachycardia in clients who have CKD is usually the result of increased potassium levels. Neither CKD nor heart failure cause temperature elevation, but tachycardia and blood pressure changes are common in clients who have heart failure. Foot and ankle edema occurs if the client has fluid excess associated with cardiac dysfunction.

Thinking Exercise 8.1.3
Answer:
The *priority* for nursing care at this time is to manage the client's **dehydration**.

Rationale: The client's findings are consistent with dehydration (fluid deficit or hypovolemia) which can lead to hypovolemic shock, a life-threatening condition. Therefore, this condition is the priority for nursing and collaborative care. The client's blood glucose is within normal limits and, therefore, the client does not have hypoglycemia. The current client findings are not completely consistent with heart failure or chronic kidney disease. Although tachycardia is a cardiac dysrhythmia, an irregular HR of 105 is not likely life-threatening and may be caused by dehydration.

Continued

UNFOLDING CASE STUDY 8.1—cont'd

Thinking Exercise 8.1.4
Answer:
X Begin supplemental oxygen via nasal cannula (NC).
X Offer oral fluids every hour.
o Transfer the client to the hospital.
o Hold next insulin administration.
X Take vital signs every 2 hours.

Rationale: To meet the priority goal of managing dehydration, the client requires fluid replacement. In the skilled nursing unit, the nursing staff would offer oral fluids frequently if the client is able to take them. If the client does not consume adequate oral fluids to become hydrated, then IV fluids would be needed. The nurse in the skilled unit would monitor vital signs frequently, which could realistically be documented every 2 hours. Because the client has a low SpO_2, the nurse would also begin supplemental oxygen via NC at a low flow rate. The client is a type 2 diabetic client but it is unknown if the client has been on insulin therapy. However, the current blood glucose level is within usual parameters and there would be no reason for insulin to be held. If the client's condition does not improve after implementing these three orders, then the client may be considered for transfer to the acute care hospital.

Thinking Exercise 8.1.5
Answer:
X Collect a urine sample for analysis.
o Administer short-acting insulin per protocol.
X Draw blood for lab testing.
o Teach client the need to drink more fluids.
X Establish peripheral venous access for IV fluids.
o Insert an indwelling urinary catheter.
X Increase oxygen flow to 3–4 L per minute via NC as needed.

Rationale: The client in the ED needs immediate interventions, with careful monitoring of the client's condition. Given that the client voided only a small amount of dark amber cloudy urine, the nurse would collect a urine sample for analysis, including determining the presence of bacteria. Laboratory testing to assess kidney function and confirm dehydration would also be needed. Venous access for infusing IV fluids is necessary to replace fluid volume and correct any electrolyte imbalances. Oxygen therapy was initiated in the skilled nursing unit but the client's SpO_2 is still at 90%. Therefore, the oxygen flow rate should be increased. The client remains disoriented and would not likely understand the need to drink more fluids. At this time, there is no indication that the client requires insulin administration. An indwelling urinary catheter would be avoided unless the client retains urine in the bladder due to possibly causing a catheter-associated urinary tract infection (CAUTI).

Thinking Exercise 8.1.6
Answer:

Client Findings	Improved	Not Improved/Worsened
SpO_2	X	
Level of consciousness	X	
Urinalysis		X
Blood pressure	X	

Rationale: The client's condition is beginning to improve as evidenced by an increased SpO_2, increased LOC from drowsy to alert, and a normal blood pressure. However, the client has a confirmed urinary tract infection that requires prompt treatment to prevent urosepsis, a life-threatening condition.

UNFOLDING CASE STUDY 8.2

Thinking Exercise 8.2.1
Answer:
- ○ Smoking history
- ○ Crackles in lung bases
- ○ Alcohol intake
- **X** Ventricular tachycardia
- ○ Palpitations
- **X** Flattened T waves
- **X** Serum sodium level
- **X** Serum potassium level
- ○ BUN level

Rationale: The client has ventricular tachycardia which if sustained can be life-threatening, leading to ventricular fibrillation or asystole. Therefore, this dysrhythmia needs immediate follow-up. While uncomfortable, palpitations are not life-threatening. The T-wave represents ventricular repolarization; T-wave changes, such as flattening, can be benign or indicate myocardial ischemia. This condition can be life-threatening and should be immediately followed up. Both the serum sodium and potassium are very low and could be life-threatening. Sodium is needed for muscle integrity and neurologic function; potassium is also needed for muscle integrity, including myocardial function. Although the client denies chest pain or dyspnea, these findings need immediate follow-up. Only a few crackles are present in the lung bases and the client is not in respiratory distress. Therefore, this finding can be followed up later. The BUN level is only slightly elevated and could indicate a variety of conditions, including dehydration, increased catabolism, high protein intake, and kidney dysfunction. Therefore, this finding does not need immediate follow-up. The client's history of smoking and alcohol intake can be followed up later.

Thinking Exercise 8.2.2
Answer:
The nurse analyzes client data and determines that the client is most at risk for **cardiac dysrhythmias** because the client has **hypokalemia** and **flattened T waves**.

Rationale: The client's sustained ventricular tachycardia (SVT) was likely caused by potassium loss from diarrhea. The intestinal contents are high in potassium content. If not treated or if not responsive to treatment, SVT can evolve into life-threatening dysrhythmias including ventricular fibrillation or asystole. Flattened T waves could indicate myocardial ischemia or infarction, which often causes life-threatening cardiac dysrhythmias.

Thinking Exercise 8.2.3
Answer:
The *priority* for client care at this time is to manage the **hypokalemia**.

Rationale: The client's low potassium level needs to be corrected to possibly reverse the client's dysrhythmias. Although the sodium level is also low, it is not at the critical level and the client can likely tolerate this imbalance due to being young. The BUN is only slightly elevated, which is not a priority. The ECG abnormalities can only change by managing their cause, in this case, hypokalemia.

Thinking Exercise 8.2.4
Answer:
- **X** Discontinue the client's HCTZ.
- **X** Provide continuous cardiac monitoring.
- ○ Initiate oxygen via high-flow nasal cannula.
- **X** Establish peripheral venous access.
- **X** Administer potassium infusion per agency protocol.
- ○ Prepare client for cardiac catheterization.
- ○ Administer sodium polystyrene sulfonate.
- ○ Administer morphine IV per agency protocol.

Continued

Rationale: Given the priority for client care, potential nursing actions include preventing additional loss of potassium by discontinuing HCTZ and administering IV potassium replacement. HCTZ is a diuretic that eliminates excess fluid but also causes loss of sodium and potassium. The client should have continuous cardiac monitoring to observe the status of the SVT and the onset of any additional dysrhythmias. At this time, oxygen via high-flow method is not needed. However, a low flow rate via a nasal cannula may increase perfusion to major body organs. A cardiac catheterization or morphine are not indicated at this time. Sodium polystyrene sulfonate is a medication used for clients who have hyperkalemia. Potassium is lost from the body because the client has extensive diarrhea caused by the drug. This client has a low potassium and should not take this drug.

Thinking Exercise 8.2.5
Answer:
X "The social worker is going to provide you with information about smoking and alcohol cessation programs."
X "Be sure to include potassium-rich foods in your diet such as bananas, potatoes, and oranges."
○ "Avoid eating foods that are high in sodium, including ham, bacon, and salty snacks."
X "Regular exercise and healthy eating habits will help you lose weight."
X "Consuming beer every night can cause weight gain and other health problems."

Rationale: All of these statements could be included in health teaching for the client's health promotion except for avoiding high-sodium foods. The client's sodium level has been low and needs to be stabilized. Therefore, dietary restrictions are not appropriate at this time.

Thinking Exercise 8.2.6
Answer:

History and Physical	Nurses Notes	Progress Notes	Laboratory Results

Urgent Care Center

1030: Client came to urgent care with partner and report of new-onset general weakness, palpitations, and lightheadedness. Alert and oriented ×4. Had frequent diarrheal stools for the past 24 hours likely due to eating tainted seafood, but diarrhea improving this morning. Medical history includes hypertension, COPD, hypothyroidism, GERD, and hypercholesterolemia. 62-pack-year smoking history. Reports drinking 2–3 beers most nights. Current medications:

*MVI with calcium tab once a day

*Amlodipine 10 mg orally once a day

*Levothyroxine sodium 112 µg orally once a day

*Famotidine OTC

*Lovastatin 20 mg orally once a day

*Hydrochlorothiazide (HCTZ) 25 mg orally once a day (started 2 weeks ago)

Few crackles in lower lung bases; denies dyspnea or chest pain. Skin warm and dry. S_1 and S_2 present and irregular. Abdomen soft and round; hyperactive bowel sounds present ×4 quadrants. Cap refill <3 seconds; pulses 2+ and equal. VS: T 98.6°F (38.1°C); HR 94 beats per minute; RR 18 breaths per minute; BP 118/72 mmHg; SpO_2 94% on RA.

1055: Blood sent for stat lab testing; ECG shows flattened T waves, ventricular tachycardia, and evidence of two previous myocardial infarctions. Troponins negative. Client denies having previous chest pain or dyspnea episodes. Plan to transfer client for direct admission to acute cardiac unit.

Acute Cardiac Unit

1310: Peripheral IV started in right forearm. IV of 5%D/0.45%NS infusing at 100 mL per hour. Supplemental potassium administered per cardiac protocol. Labs to be redrawn in 4 hours. Oxygen started at 2 L per minute via NC. Orders received; hold HCTZ. VS: T 98.6°F (38.1°C); HR 94 beats per minute; RR 18 breaths per minute; BP 116/68 mmHg; SpO_2 99% on O_2 at 2 L per minute via NC. BMI 30.4.

UNFOLDING CASE STUDY 8.2—cont'd

History and Physical	Laboratory Results	Progress Notes	Nurses Notes

Serum Laboratory Test/ Reference Range	Urgent Care Results	1730 Results
Sodium (Na⁺) (136–145 mEq/L [136–145 mmol/L])	127 mEq/L (127 mmol/L)	133 mEq/L (133 mmol/L)
Potassium (K⁺) (3.5–5.0 mEq/L [3.5–5.0 mmol/L])	2.8 mEq/L (2.8 mmol/L)	3.4 mEq/L (3.4 mmol/L)
Thyroid stimulating hormone (TSH) (0.3–5.0 μU/mL [0.3–5.0 mU/L])	3 μU/mL (3 mU/L)	3 μU/mL (3 mU/L)
Blood urea nitrogen (BUN) (10–20 mg/dL [3.6–7.1 mmol/L])	23 mg/dL (8.2 mmol/L)	16 mg/dL (5.7 mmol/L)
Creatinine (0.5–1.1 mg/dL [44.2–97.3 μmol/L])	1.1 mg/dL (97.3 μmol/L)	1.1 mg/dL (97.3 μmol/L)

Rationale: The client is beginning to improve as evidenced by a heart rate within normal limits and a high SpO$_2$ even though the client is receiving oxygen. The client's sodium, potassium, and BUN values have improved but are not necessarily within normal limits. Other client findings are within usual parameters.

UNFOLDING CASE STUDY 8.3

Thinking Exercise 8.3.1
Answer:
- ○ Temperature
- **X** Heart rate
- **X** Respiratory rate
- ○ Blood pressure
- **X** SpO$_2$
- ○ Pedal pulses
- **X** Diminished breath sounds
- ○ Absent bowel sounds

Rationale: The client has potentially life-threatening ventricular tachycardia that could lead to ventricular fibrillation. Therefore, this finding needs immediate, emergent follow-up. The client also has respiratory distress, including shortness of breath, tachypnea, diminished breath sounds, and a below-normal SpO$_2$. These findings are also potentially life-threatening and require immediate follow-up. Having absent bowel sounds would be addressed later after evaluating the client for possible cardiopulmonary condition(s). While the client's temperature and blood pressure are elevated, they are not urgent or emergent and do not require immediate follow-up. Having 1+ pedal pulses is not unusual for older adults who often have arteriosclerosis and decreased perfusion in the lower extremities.

Thinking Exercise 8.3.2
Answer:

Client Findings	Dehydration	Bowel Obstruction	Pneumonia
Diminished breath sounds		X	X
HR 151 beats per minute and irregular	X	X	
RR 48 breaths per minute and shallow		X	X
SpO$_2$ 88% on RA	X		X
Absent bowel sounds		X	

Rationale: Dehydration is a fluid volume deficit that occurs most often in older adults and infants. With less circulating blood volume, the heart compensates by increasing its rate to ensure that oxygen is delivered throughout the body, especially major organs. Therefore, tachycardia and a low peripheral oxygen saturation level are common in clients who are dehydrated. Pneumonia is a respiratory infection that interferes with gas exchange in the alveoli of the lungs due to accumulation of exudate and/or fluid. As a result, the client often has diminished breath sounds, tachypnea, low SpO_2, fatigue, fever, and a productive cough. The client who has a bowel obstruction has decreased or absent bowel sounds, abdominal pain and distention, and vomiting. These findings can cause fluid and electrolyte imbalances, including dehydration and hypokalemia; both of these conditions can result in tachycardia. Severe abdominal distention can elevate the diaphragm to prevent complete lung expansion, causing findings such as tachypnea and diminished breath sounds.

Thinking Exercise 8.3.3
Answer:
The *priority* for care at this time is to manage the client's **tachycardia**.

Rationale: Because the client has potentially life-threatening tachycardia, the priority for care is to prevent lethal dysrhythmias that could develop. The client's tachypnea, low SpO_2, and elevated blood pressure are not at life-threatening levels. The client does not have a fever.

Thinking Exercise 8.3.4
Answer:

Potential Nursing Actions	Indicated	Not Indicated
Start supplemental oxygen via NC	X	
Obtain peripheral venous access	X	
Administer 0.9% NS at 80 mL per hour		X
Apply continuous cardiac monitoring	X	
Keep client in supine flat position		X

Rationale: The client has cardiopulmonary findings including severe tachycardia and tachypnea and would therefore need to sit upright to facilitate lung expansion rather than lie flat in a supine position. Supplemental oxygen would help increase the SpO_2 and possibly decrease the RR. Continuous cardiac monitoring would be essential to monitor the heart for additional or potentially lethal dysrhythmias. IV access is important for fluid resuscitation and medications to decrease the heart rate. A low IV fluid rate of 80 mL/hour is not adequate to replace lost fluids from vomiting.

Thinking Exercise 8.3.5
Answer:
X Call a sepsis alert code immediately.
X Draw lactate (lactic acid) level stat.
X Place indwelling urinary catheter.
○ Increase oxygen to 6 L per minute via NC.
○ Clamp NG tube immediately.
X Place client in sitting position.
○ Decrease IV fluid rate to 100 mL per hour.
X Start IV broad-spectrum antibiotic therapy.
○ Administer norepinephrine (NE) per protocol.
X Plan transfer to critical care unit.

Rationale: The client has a fever, tachycardia, and hypotension. These findings are consistent with early sepsis, which is the body's unusual response to infection. If not detected and managed early, the client can progress to septic shock, causing major body organ failure and even death. The nurse would call a sepsis code alert and draw a stat lactate (lactic acid) level. An elevation in lactate (lactic acid) (normal

⚡ UNFOLDING CASE STUDY 8.3—cont'd

is below 2 mmol/L) is called lactic acidosis and occurs when the client's oxygen level becomes low in spite of fluid replacement and oxygen therapy. To assess kidney function, the nurse would insert an indwelling urinary catheter. The client should be placed in a sitting position to assist with respiratory function and a transfer to a critical care unit should be planned. Broad-spectrum antibiotic therapy is essential to treat the underlying infection. Increasing the oxygen to 6 L per minute using a traditional nasal cannula would not be useful. A high-flow nasal cannula can deliver this increase in oxygen flow and may help improve the SpO_2 level. At this point, the client's IV fluid rate would be increased to determine if the blood pressure would return to a normal level. If not, norepinephrine or other vasopressor may be needed.

Thinking Exercise 8.3.6
Answer:

History and Physical	Nurses Notes	Orders	Laboratory Results

Emergency Department

2025: Client accompanied by wife with report of frequent vomiting for the past 3 days, shortness of breath that started today, anorexia, and generalized weakness. Vomited large amount of dark brown emesis twice today. Client has been generally healthy and never admitted to the ED or acute care. Medical history includes well-controlled hypertension and chronic gout. Alert and oriented ×4. Denies pain or nausea. Skin warm and dry. Lips and mucous membranes dry. Diminished breath sounds in lower lung bases bilaterally. Abdomen grossly distended. Faint bowel sounds in upper abdomen; absent bowel sounds in lower abdomen. Cap refill <3 seconds; pedal pulses 1+ and equal. VS: T 99.2°F (37.3°C); HR 151 beats per minute and irregular; RR 48 breaths per minute and shallow; BP 139/88 mmHg; SpO_2 88% on RA.

2110: ECG completed; blood drawn for stat blood work. Chest X-ray and cardiac ultrasound at bedside. Voiding very dark yellow urine using urinal. No nausea or vomiting.

2345: Results from chest X-ray show small amount of fluid or infection in lung bases. No cardiac abnormalities. Planning chest and abdominal CT scans without contrast. VS: T 98.6°F (37°C); HR 132 beats per minute and irregular; RR 36 breaths per minute and shallow; BP 142/90 mmHg; SpO_2 91% on 3 L per minute via NC.

0305: Results from CT scans show small amount of fluid in lung bases and probable small bowel obstruction. Client to be admitted when acute bed available. Abdominal CT with contrast scheduled in the next hour. VS: T 98.6°F (37°C); HR 138 beats per minute and irregular; RR 40 breaths per minute and shallow; BP 144/92 mmHg; SpO_2 90% on 3 L per minute via NC. Increased O_2 to 4 L per minute.

0700: Transferred to operating suite for emergent abdominal surgery. Most recent abdominal scan shows complete small bowel obstruction caused by possible external mass in lower abdomen.

PACU the Next Day

1050: Admitted to PACU with IV infusing at 150 mL per hour, O_2 at 4 L per minute via NC, and NG tube to low continuous suction draining copious amount of dark brown drainage. Alert and oriented ×4. Large abdominal surgical dressing dry and intact. No drain present. Surgeon reports removal of scar tissue as cause of obstruction. VS: T 100.8°F (38.2°C); HR 146 beats per minute and irregular; RR 24 breaths per minute and shallow; BP 86/40 mmHg; SpO_2 92%. Surgeon notified about VS.

Acute Surgical Unit POD #7

1630: Client and wife discussing discharge plans for tomorrow with case manager. Client receiving IV antibiotic therapy for bilateral diffuse pneumonia for the past 4 days. Will be discharged on oral antibiotic therapy but likely will not require home oxygen. Client alert and oriented ×4. No adventitious breath sounds auscultated. Abdomen soft and round. Surgical incision slightly reddened with small amount of tannish drainage; surgical resident removed half of staples. Wound culture obtained. Able to walk from the bed to bathroom without assistance. Denies pain or nausea. Eating small amounts of solid food. VS: T 98.8°F (37.1°C); HR 98 beats per minute and irregular; RR 20 breaths per minute and shallow; BP 124/78 mmHg; SpO_2 95% on RA.

Rationale: The client is able to ambulate and eat small amounts of solid food without vomiting. All vital signs are near or at normal limits even without supplemental oxygen. The client's abdomen is not grossly distended but is soft and round. These findings show major improvement in the client's condition.

UNFOLDING CASE STUDY 8.4

Thinking Exercise 8.4.1
Answer:
The client findings that require *immediate* follow-up include **severe headache, elevated blood pressure**, and **decreased level of consciousness (LOC)**.

Rationale: In this case, the client's findings changed significantly between 0830 and 1300 following a motor vehicle crash. The most concerning change is the decrease in level of consciousness (LOC) from alert and oriented ×2 to sleepy and oriented ×1. A continuing decline in LOC can be life-threatening and, therefore, this client finding requires immediate follow-up. The client's vital signs were within normal parameters earlier in the day, but several hours later the blood pressure increased significantly and the heart rate decreased. However, the heart rate remains within normal limits. The client's headache pain increased from 3/10 to 8/10 when the blood pressure increased. Although pain is an isolated finding, it is not usually life-threatening. The increase in pain occurring with changes in LOC and BP requires immediate follow-up. Early muscle weakness and blurry vision are not potentially life-threatening and can be addressed at a later time.

Thinking Exercise 8.4.2
Answer:
The nurse analyzes the assessment findings and determines that the client is experiencing **increasing intracranial pressure (ICP)** as evidenced by **severe headache** and **decreased level of consciousness**.

Rationale: Based on analysis of client findings, especially those that changed over a 4 ½-hour period, the nurse would determine that the client experienced a traumatic brain injury which has caused increasing intracranial pressure (ICP) as evidenced by the decreased LOC and severe headache. Even though the client's RR increased from 18 breaths per minute to 24 breaths per minute, the client is not experiencing respiratory distress. The client denies dyspnea and the SpO_2 is not markedly decreased. The client's FSBG is within the normal range and, therefore, the client is not hypoglycemic.

Thinking Exercise 8.4.3
Answer:
- ○ Increase the client's blood glucose.
- ○ Manage the client's hypertension.
- **X** Reduce the pressure on the client's brain.
- ○ Manage the client's severe headache pain.
- ○ Improve the client's oxygenation.
- ○ Manage the client's new-onset nausea.

Rationale: Because the client is experiencing increasing ICP, the priority is to reduce this pressure. If the ICP continues to increase, the client's brain could experience secondary brain injury. The client's blood pressure level, pain, and nausea are not priorities for management at this time. Both the blood glucose and SpO_2 are within the normal range.

Thinking Exercise 8.4.4
Answer:

Potential Orders	Appropriate	Not Appropriate
Keep the client sitting in a 30 degrees reclining position	X	
Administer IV furosemide per protocol	X	
Begin supplemental oxygen via NC	X	
Keep client's head in a neutral position	X	

UNFOLDING CASE STUDY 8.4—cont'd

Rationale: All of the potential orders are appropriate and should be anticipated by the nurse. Furosemide is a diuretic which can help reduce fluid pressing on the brain. Supplemental oxygen is needed to increase perfusion to the brain which can help reduce secondary brain injury. A semireclining position (at least 30 degrees) and the client's head in a neutral position help to facilitate venous drainage from the cranium, which helps prevent the buildup of additional fluid.

Thinking Exercise 8.4.5
Answer:
X Monitor sodium level during hypertonic saline infusion.
X Document fluid intake and urinary output.
○ Place client on high-flow oxygen.
X Take vital signs every hour ×4, then every 2 hours.
○ Document FSBG level every hour.
○ Monitor for signs and symptoms of fluid overload.

Rationale: A hypertonic saline infusion delivers a large amount of sodium to the body, but is helpful in reducing fluid producing pressure on the brain. Therefore, the nurse would monitor the serum sodium level during the implementation of this infusion. Intake and output should also be monitored to ensure increased urinary output. Vital signs are an excellent indicator of increasing ICP and should be monitored frequently for significant changes that demonstrate effectiveness of treatment or worsening of the client's condition. There is no need to change to high-flow oxygen because the client is not in respiratory distress. The client's blood glucose is within the normal range. Administering hypertonic IV fluids should reduce body fluid, not cause an excess or overload.

Thinking Exercise 8.4.6
Answer:

Client Findings	Progressing	Not Progressing
Alert and oriented ×4	X	
Headache pain at 2/10	X	
Muscle strength 4/5		X
BP 120/70 mmHg	X	

Rationale: As a result of treatment, the client has progressed from being sleepy and oriented ×1 to being alert and oriented ×4. The client's headache pain has drastically reduced from 8/10 to 2/10, which also shows improvement or progression, and the client's blood pressure has also returned to a normal level. However, the client continues to have mild muscle weakness at 4/5 instead of the baseline of 5/5, demonstrating that the weakness is not improving at this time.

⚡ UNFOLDING CASE STUDY 8.5

Thinking Exercise 8.5.1
Answer:
- ○ BMI 16.1
- ○ Cool, dry skin
- ○ Increased fatigue and weakness
- ○ Bluish swollen hands
- ○ Peripheral pulses 1+
- **X** BP 82/46 mmHg
- ○ SpO$_2$ 94% on RA
- ○ RR 22 breaths per minute
- **X** FSBG 48 mg/dL (2.7 mmol/L)
- ○ Feeling of hopelessness

Rationale: The client has a history of having an eating disorder and, therefore, many of the findings are expected even though they are abnormal. The physical findings that are significant and require immediate follow-up are the client's low blood pressure and low blood glucose. Both of these findings are potentially life-threatening. The client's feeling of hopelessness is common in individuals who have clinical depression, but would be followed up later after the physiologic findings are addressed. The client is in a safe environment where the client can be observed by multiple health care professionals.

Thinking Exercise 8.5.2
Answer:
The nurse analyzes assessment findings and determines that the client likely has **electrolyte imbalances**.

Rationale: Given the client had syncope, is experiencing palpitations, and has an irregular pulse, the client likely has electrolyte imbalances. Additionally, the client is grossly underweight and does not consume adequate nutrients needed for proper organ functioning. There are no client findings that support the conditions of diabetes mellitus, fluid overload, or respiratory distress.

Thinking Exercise 8.5.3
Answer:
The *priority* for care at this time is to manage **hypokalemia** because the client could develop **cardiac dysrhythmias**.

Rationale: The laboratory results show that the client's potassium is at a critically low value which can result in cardiac dysrhythmias. Potassium is needed to ensure adequate function of all three types of muscle—skeletal, smooth, and cardiac. The creatinine level is only slightly elevated and is not the priority for care. The client's serum sodium is low, but it is not at a critical value level.

Thinking Exercise 8.5.4
Answer:

Potential Nursing Actions	Indicated	Not Indicated
Start supplemental oxygen via NC	X	
Obtain peripheral venous access	X	
Apply continuous cardiac monitoring	X	
Prepare to provide supplemental potassium	X	

UNFOLDING CASE STUDY 8.5—cont'd

Rationale: All of the listed potential nursing actions are indicated to manage hypokalemia to prevent cardiac dysrhythmias. The client requires supplemental IV potassium rather than waiting for the effect of oral replacement. Continuous cardiac monitoring is needed to assess for potentially life-threatening changes. Although the client is not experiencing respiratory distress, the client could benefit from supplemental oxygen to increase oxygen supply to major organs, especially the heart.

Thinking Exercise 8.5.5
Answer:
X Monitor serum electrolyte values.
X Assess for cardiac dysrhythmias.
X Screen for suicidal ideation.
○ Consult with registered dietitian nutritionist.
X Consult with social worker or mental health professional.

Rationale: During implementation of the plan of care, the nurse would carefully monitor for cardiac dysrhythmias and assess serum electrolyte values, especially potassium levels. Because the client expressed feelings of hopelessness and based on the mental health history, the client should be screened for suicidal ideation. A specially trained social worker or mental health professional usually performs the screening and may provide counseling if needed. It would not be helpful to contact the registered dietitian nutritionist to teach the client about nutrition because the client has an eating disorder which is considered a mental health condition.

Thinking Exercise 8.5.6
Answer:

History and Physical	Nurses Notes	Orders	Laboratory Results

1530:   Client admitted to ED with worsening signs and symptoms of anorexia nervosa (AN). Parents report client eats almost no solid food except lettuce and drinks large amounts of water. Client has "passed out" several times over the last 2 days including a fall down the steps. Has history of clinical depression, severe anxiety, and substance use disorder. Currently alert and oriented ×4. States feeling more fatigued and weaker than usual; started having palpitations this morning. Reports feeling hopeless about the client's "situation." No abnormal or adventitious breath sounds; skin cool, clammy, but very dry. Several healing bruises on arms and legs. Lips and mucous membranes dry. Several teeth missing and other teeth are eroded and discolored. Client's bones, especially ribs and pelvis, very prominent. Fingertips bluish and cold; hands slightly swollen. Cap refill >3 seconds; pedal pulses 1+ and equal. 2+ pitting edema in both feet and lower legs. VS: T 97.6°F (36.4°C); HR 76 beats per minute and irregular; RR 22 breaths per minute and regular; BP 84/46 mmHg; SpO$_2$ 94% on RA; FSBG 48 mg/dL (2.7 mmol/L). BMI 16.1.

1625:   ECG completed and blood drawn for labs. Cardiac monitor applied. NSR with occasional PVCs.

1640:   Peripheral IV started in left forearm infusing 5%D/0.45%NS at 125 mL per hour. Potassium infusion started per protocol. Social worker consult initiated. Psychiatrist in to examine client.

1810:   Plan to transfer client to cardiac unit for monitoring overnight; client is not at risk for self-harm or harm to others. Stat potassium: 2.9 mEq/L (2.9 mmol/L). VS: T 97.8°F (36.5°C); HR 82 beats per minute and irregular; RR 20 breaths per minute and regular; BP 98/46 mmHg; SpO$_2$ 94% on RA; FSBG 75 mg/dL (4.2 mmol/L).

Rationale: As a result of providing IV fluids with potassium replacement, the client's serum potassium level increased. Although it is not within the normal range, the level is no longer at a critical life-threatening level. The client's blood pressure and blood glucose also increased most likely due to the administration of IV fluids that contain dextrose. The other client findings have not changed significantly.

↓ UNFOLDING CASE STUDY 8.6

Thinking Exercise 8.6.1

Answer:

The assessment finding that requires *immediate* follow-up is the client's **high blood pressure**.

Rationale: The client's blood pressure is higher than 150/90 mmHg, which requires immediate follow-up. Hypertension during pregnancy can decrease blood flow to the placenta, depriving the fetus of vital oxygen and nutrients and resulting in possible intrauterine growth restriction, premature birth, preeclampsia, and/or placental abruption. Weight gain, foot edema, and occasional headaches do not place the fetus at the same level of risk when compared to high blood pressure.

Thinking Exercise 8.6.2

Answer:

The client is most at risk for **preeclampsia** as evidenced by **high blood pressure** and **proteinuria**.

Rationale: This client is at high risk for preeclampsia, a multisystem progressive complication during pregnancy after 20 weeks. This complication is manifested by high blood pressure, proteinuria, and fluid retention which can progress to major organ dysfunction. There is no evidence that the client is at risk for migraine headaches. Clients with heart failure often retain fluid but do not have proteinuria.

Thinking Exercise 8.6.3

Answer:

- ○ Decrease pitting edema.
- ○ Decrease client's blood pressure.
- ○ Manage the client's headache pain.
- ○ Administer supplemental oxygen.
- **X** Prepare for delivery of the baby.

Rationale: The client's blood pressure continues to increase and needs to be managed as quickly as possible. However, managing the blood pressure, the client's headache pain, or pitting edema does not guarantee the safety of the baby and client. Instead, the priority for care is to deliver the baby to prevent negative outcomes for both the fetus and client. Applying supplemental oxygen is part of the plan of care but not the priority to ensure safety of the client and fetus.

Thinking Exercise 8.6.4

Answer:

Potential Nursing Actions	Indicated	Not Indicated
Administer IV antihypertensive drug per protocol	X	
Apply continuous cardiac monitoring	X	
Administer IV magnesium sulfate per protocol	X	
Administer IV corticosteroid per protocol	X	
Provide preoperative teaching related to expectations for mother and baby	X	

Rationale: All of these actions are indicated for a pregnant client who has preeclampsia with high blood pressure. To prevent complications like placenta abruption, the nurse would expect to administer IV antihypertensive medication. Magnesium sulfate is indicated to help prevent seizures as preeclampsia progresses. Because the fetus is under 37 weeks and does not have completely mature lungs, an IV corticosteroid would likely be given to the client to prevent newborn respiratory complications and improve newborn breathing. The client is expected to have an emergent C-section to manage complications and would need preoperative teaching about expectations for the client and baby.

UNFOLDING CASE STUDY 8.6—cont'd

Thinking Exercise 8.6.5

Answer:

- ○ Place baby on mechanical ventilator.
- **X** Insert nasogastric tube for feeding.
- **X** Maintain quiet environment.
- **X** Apply continuous cardiac monitoring.
- **X** Ask mother to bring breast milk for baby.
- ○ Insert indwelling urinary catheter.

Rationale: A 34-week newborn may have respiratory distress needing mechanical ventilation, continuous positive airway pressure (CPAP), or supplemental oxygen. This newborn's Apgar score suggests the baby can breathe independently but likely may need partial respiratory support. Premature newborns tend to become easily overstimulated and, therefore, a quiet environment with minimal handling is required. Premature newborns also become fatigued quickly when feeding using a bottle or breasts. Therefore, the baby would have a nasogastric tube for feeding but could be fed the client's breast milk. An indwelling urinary catheter would be avoided as long as the newborn is voiding regularly.

Thinking Exercise 8.6.6

Answer:

History and Physical	Nurses Notes	Orders	Laboratory Results

Obstetrician Visit at 32-Weeks' Pregnancy

1115:   Client visit for follow-up on weight gain and high blood pressure. Last week client had gained 7 lb (3.2 kg) since visit 4 weeks before. Today client has 2+ pitting edema both feet. BP elevated to 144/89 mmHg last week. Current VS: T 98.6°F (37°C); HR 84 beats per minute and regular; RR 18 breaths per minute and regular; BP 152/90 mmHg; SpO$_2$ 96% on RA. Trace protein in urine. Denies any headaches, visual changes, or seizure activity. Sent to hospital OB department for fetal and maternal monitoring.

Obstetrician Visit at 33-Weeks' Pregnancy

0900:   Client visit for follow-up on weight gain and high blood pressure. Spent 3 hours in hospital OB department for monitoring but sent home with daily BP monitoring via telehealth. Goal is to have cesarean section at 37 weeks if BP can be managed until that time. Client has reduced salt and stopped working to increase rest since last week. Gain of 2.2 lb (1 kg) this past week. 2+ pitting edema both feet. BP 140/88 mmHg. Trace protein in urine. Denies any headaches, visual changes, or seizure activity.

Obstetrician Visit at 34-Weeks' Pregnancy

1030:   Client visit for follow-up on weight gain and high blood pressure. BP 158/94. SpO$_2$ 94% on RA. Has had occasional headaches over the past week. 1+ urinary protein. 3+ pitting edema both feet. Plan to admit client to hospital OB department. Discussed with client and partner the need for emergent C-section today or tomorrow.

Hospital OB Department (Day of Admission)

1205:   Client at 34 weeks admitted for evaluation of high blood pressure and proteinuria. Denies headache, nausea, or visual changes. Peripheral venous access established for IV fluids; client NPO. Indwelling urinary catheter placed. Obstetrician to examine client to determine plan of care for preeclampsia.

1620:   C-section performed. Baby boy delivered at 4 lb (1.8), 17 in (43.2 cm). Apgar 1 min: 7; Apgar 5 min: 8. Placed on mother's chest for few minutes before preparing to admit to NICU. Nurse explained expectations for newborn care in NICU.

NICU 2 Weeks Later

1000:   Parents in to visit baby and assist with morning care. Newborn on high-flow oxygen after 10 days on CPAP since birth. NG tube removed yesterday; baby on bottle-feeding using mother's breast milk, but not always consuming minimum required to meet nutritional needs. Gained 8 ounces since birth 2 weeks ago with goal weight of 5 lb (2.3 kg) prior to discharge. Voiding and stools adequate.

Continued

UNFOLDING CASE STUDY 8.6—cont'd

Rationale: The baby's respiratory status has improved because high-flow oxygen is less supportive than CPAP. Although the baby is not always consuming adequate nutrients, the baby is gaining weight and is able to bottle feed. These findings show that the newborn's condition is improving.

UNFOLDING CASE STUDY 8.7

Thinking Exercise 8.7.1
Answer:

History and Physical	Nurses Notes	Orders	Laboratory Results

1215:   Client drowsy after surgery but easily awakened. Able to communicate. States pain is not too bad, "maybe a 4/10." Reports feeling nauseated and refusing water. Family at bedside. Breath sounds clear throughout lung fields. Abdomen soft and flat; diminished bowel sounds ×4. Splint with elastic wrap over surgical dressing dry and in place on right leg from ankle to groin. Right foot slightly cooler than left. Pedal pulses 2+ and equal. Skin color equal in both feet. Able to slightly move right toes. Cap refill <3 seconds. IV infusing at 80 mL per hour. VS: T 98.1°F (36.7°C); HR 88 beats per minute and regular; RR 18 breaths per minute and regular; BP 100/66 mmHg; SpO$_2$ 99% on RA.

1630:   Family reports that client's pain has markedly increased even though analgesic given less than an hour ago, but nausea has lessened. Taking small amounts of fluids; voided 180 mL ×1. Client describes pain now as 9/10; states the affected leg and foot are throbbing. Splint with elastic wrap over surgical dressing dry and in place on right leg from ankle to groin. Right foot much colder than left. Right pedal pulse nonpalpable; right foot paler than left. Unable to move right toes or foot. Cap refill >3 seconds. IV infusing at 80 mL per hour. VS: T 98.1°F (36.7°C); HR 94 beats per minute and regular; RR 20 breaths per minute and regular; BP 122/74 mmHg; SpO$_2$ 98% on RA.

Rationale: The client findings changed over a 4-hour period of time, including a marked increase in pain to 9/10 even after an analgesic was given. The client's affected right foot became pale and cooler than earlier, with an inability to move the foot. In addition, the client's capillary refill slowed to >3 seconds. Vital signs are relatively stable although the child's blood pressure and pulse increased. These increases may be an autonomic response to severe pain and probable anxiety.

Thinking Exercise 8.7.2
Answer:

Client Findings	Deep Vein Thrombosis	Acute Compartment Syndrome
Severe pain in affected leg	X	X
Right foot colder and paler than left		X
Unable to palpate right pedal pulse		X
Capillary refill >3 seconds		X

Rationale: A deep vein thrombus is a blood clot that usually develops in the lower extremities as a result of surgery or decreased mobility. Client findings typically include redness, warmth, swelling, and pain. The client is experiencing pain in the affected leg. Acute compartment syndrome is the result of increased pressure on blood vessels (especially arteries), nerves, and muscle tissue within compartments of fascia located in the lower leg. The swelling that occurs after orthopedic surgery or trauma may cause this rather uncommon complication. The result of increased pressure and swelling is severe pain, coolness, pallor (in light-skinned clients), and paresthesias due to impaired perfusion. If not identified early, the client may also have pulselessness in the distal foot and ankle.

UNFOLDING CASE STUDY 8.7—cont'd

Thinking Exercise 8.7.3
Answer:
The *priority* for care at this time is to manage the client's **compartment syndrome** because this condition can cause **tissue necrosis**.

Rationale: The client likely has acute compartment syndrome which, if not treated, can cause tissue necrosis, which is limb-threatening. Nausea and severe pain as isolated conditions are not limb- or life-threatening.

Thinking Exercise 8.7.4
Answer:
- ○ Obtain surgical consent for a fasciotomy.
- **X** Make the client NPO in preparation for possible surgery.
- ○ Prepare for skeletal traction application.
- **X** Notify the surgeon immediately.
- ○ Elevate the affected leg.
- **X** Perform frequent neurovascular checks.

Rationale: The nurse would notify the surgeon immediately because additional surgery may be needed to relieve the compartment pressure. The surgeon is responsible for obtaining consent for surgery—not the nurse. To help prepare for possible surgery, the nurse would make the client NPO and continue to monitor the neurovascular status of the affected leg and foot. Elevating the affected leg would increase venous blood flow back to the heart, but slow essential arterial blood flow to the foot. Skeletal traction is a treatment for stabilizing fractures and other deformities, and would not be appropriate for this client.

Thinking Exercise 8.7.5
Answer:
- ○ Keep the client NPO for the next 2 days.
- **X** Perform frequent neurovascular assessments ("circ checks").
- **X** Request antiemetic drug for nausea and vomiting.
- ○ Elevate the surgical leg on two or more pillows.
- **X** Clarify wound care orders.

Rationale: After the fasciotomy to relieve pressure in the affected leg, the nurse would clarify wound care instructions by the surgeon. The incision remains open to heal from the inside out, but surgeons vary regarding their preferred wound care. The nurse would continue to frequently assess the neurovascular status of the affected leg and compare those findings with the other leg. The leg should not be highly elevated to prevent a decrease in the arterial blood flow to the affected foot. However, some surgeons prefer a short period of elevation on one pillow to help prevent swelling after the fasciotomy. The nurse would obtain an order for an antiemetic drug because the child needs to be able to have adequate nutrition for wound healing; the client should not remain NPO for 2 days.

Continued

UNFOLDING CASE STUDY 8.7—cont'd

Thinking Exercise 8.7.6
Answer:

History and Physical	Nurses Notes	Orders	Laboratory Results

1215: Client drowsy after surgery but easily awakened. Able to communicate. States pain is not too bad, "maybe a 4/10." Reports feeling nauseated and refusing water. Family at bedside. Breath sounds clear throughout lung fields. Abdomen soft and flat; diminished bowel sounds ×4. Splint with elastic wrap over surgical dressing dry and in place on right leg from ankle to groin. Right foot slightly cooler than left. Pedal pulses 2+ and equal. Skin color equal in both feet. Able to slightly move right toes. Cap refill <3 seconds. IV infusing at 80 mL/hour. VS: T 98.1°F (36.7°C); HR 88 beats per minute and regular; RR 18 breaths per minute and regular; BP 100/66 mmHg; SpO$_2$ 99% on RA.

1630: Family reports that client's pain has markedly increased even though analgesic given less than an hour ago, but nausea has lessened. Taking small amounts of fluids; voided 180 mL ×1. Client describes pain now as 9/10; states the affected leg and foot are throbbing. Splint with elastic wrap over surgical dressing dry and in place on right leg from ankle to groin. Right foot much colder than left. Right pedal pulse nonpalpable; right foot paler than left. Unable to move right toes or foot. Cap refill >3 seconds. IV infusing at 80 mL per hour. VS: T 98.1°F (36.7°C); HR 94 beats per minute and regular; RR 20 breaths per minute and regular; BP 122/74 mmHg; SpO$_2$ 98% on RA.

1710: Surgeon explained to client and family about the need to relieve the pressure on the lower leg to prevent tissue necrosis and potential loss of part of the right leg. Client made NPO for open fasciotomy of lower right leg later this evening. Obtained consent from family for surgery.

2045: Returned from PACU after open right lower leg fasciotomy; wound covered with bulky dressing that is dry and intact. Right foot remains somewhat cooler and paler than left. Left pedal pulse 2+; right pedal pulse 1+. Client reports pain at 5/10 and receiving analgesics as needed. Nausea and vomiting ×2 in PACU. Breath sounds clear throughout lung fields. Abdomen soft and flat; diminished bowel sounds ×4. IV infusing in right forearm at 100 mL per hour. VS: T 99.2°F (37.3°C); HR 70 beats per minute and regular; RR 20 breaths per minute and regular; BP 102/56 mmHg; SpO$_2$ 96% on RA.

Rationale: After surgery, the child's foot is better perfused but is still somewhat cooler and paler than the left foot. The pedal pulse in the affected foot is now palpable at 1+, which shows improvement compared to an absent pulse. The client's pain level has decreased from a 9/10 to a 5/10 showing improvement in the client's condition. The other findings are either the same and within normal limits or worsened.

STAND-ALONE ITEM 8.1

Answer:

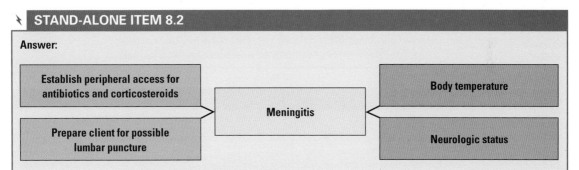

| Administer bronchodilator drug | → | Smoke inhalation injury | ← | Airway obstruction |
| Prepare client for possible intubation or tracheostomy | | | | SpO$_2$ |

Rationale: The client was exposed to a fire which caused burns on the face and hands. In addition, the client's hair is singed and there is soot around the nares. These findings are consistent with probable smoke inhalation injury. The client has respiratory findings (wheezing, dyspnea, productive cough) which could be due to COPD or smoke inhalation. It is unlikely that the client has atelectasis or pneumonia because breath sounds would be diminished. Pneumonia and acute bronchitis are infections that usually cause a fever, which this client does not have. The client could possibly have asthma but this condition is a chronic condition like COPD with exacerbations. The client has no history of asthma. Smoke inhalation injury can progress as inflammation increases to obstruct the airway. Therefore, the nurse would prepare the client for the possibility of intubation or a tracheostomy and possible mechanical ventilation. However, administering bronchodilator and antiinflammatory drugs should help to prevent airway obstruction. Antibiotic therapy is not appropriate because the client does not have an infection. Suctioning does not prevent airway obstruction or hypoxia. A feeding tube is not indicated for the client at this time but may be needed later. After implementing the appropriate actions, the nurse would frequently assess the client for airway obstruction and monitor SpO$_2$ levels to assess for hypoxia. Monitoring blood pressure, temperature, and indications of infection would not demonstrate whether the plan of care was effective.

STAND-ALONE ITEM 8.2

Answer:

| Establish peripheral access for antibiotics and corticosteroids | → | Meningitis | ← | Body temperature |
| Prepare client for possible lumbar puncture | | | | Neurologic status |

Rationale: The client has classic findings consistent with meningitis: stiff neck, severe headache, fever, nausea, photophobia, weakness, and lethargy. This infection affects the meninges of the brain and spinal cord. The major treatment for this condition is antibiotics for infection and corticosteroids for inflammation. Prior to treatment, the client would likely have a lumbar puncture to confirm the condition. The nurse would likely administer an analgesic for the client's headache after the condition is confirmed through diagnostic testing. Physical therapy is not appropriate in the acute stage of infection. Surgery is not a treatment for meningitis. Because this infection causes fever and affects the central nervous system, the nurse would evaluate the effectiveness of client care by monitoring body temperature and neurologic status. The client does not have any respiratory distress so respiratory status and SpO$_2$ would not demonstrate care effectiveness. The client's blood pressure is also not affected by the disease process.

STAND-ALONE ITEM 8.3

Answer:

Establish peripheral venous access for fluids		Lochia amount
	Hypovolemia	
Monitor vital signs every 30–60 minutes		Blood pressure

Rationale: This postpartum client has excessive vaginal bleeding after delivering a baby causing the client to have tachycardia, lowered blood pressure, lightheadedness, and thirst. These findings suggest the client has hypovolemia from blood loss. There are no findings consistent with fluid overload or preeclampsia, and the client does not meet the criteria for clinical depression. Management of hypovolemia is focused on fluid replacement and frequently assessing vital signs to monitor fluid status. A diuretic would cause more body fluid loss which would be contraindicated. The client should not sit completely upright because blood pressure tends to decrease in a sitting position compared to when the head of the bed is lower. To assess whether the implemented plan of care was effective, the nurse would monitor blood pressure and the quantity of lochia or number of pads saturated in a period of time. Respiratory rate and SpO_2 would not be as useful. Urinary output would be expected to increase when fluids are replaced but would not be the best indicator of fluid status.

STAND-ALONE ITEM 8.4

Answer:

The nurse determines that the client is experiencing **coma** as evidenced by a **low GCS score**.

Rationale: The client had an overdose of fentanyl but is breathing independently on high-flow oxygen. The Glasgow Coma Scale (GCS) is used to assess a client's level of consciousness (LOC). A score of 15 is the highest score and indicates the client is alert and responsive. This client's score was an 8 which has decreased over several hours to a 7. A GCS score of 8 or less indicates the client is in a coma. The lower the score below 8, the deeper the coma. Although the client's heart rate decreased from 70 to 62 beats per minute, the client is not bradycardic. The client's SpO_2 on high-flow oxygen ranges between 94% and 97%, which does not reflect hypoxia.

STAND-ALONE ITEM 8.5

Answer:

The nurse analyzes laboratory findings to determine that the client is most likely experiencing **chronic kidney disease**.

Rationale: The current laboratory test results are consistent with chronic kidney disease (CKD). These findings include an elevated BUN, creatinine, potassium, and sodium. Although the blood glucose is also elevated, it is not high enough to result in diabetic ketoacidosis, which can occur in clients with type 1 diabetes mellitus (DM). Hyperglycemic hyperosmolar syndrome only occurs in clients who have type 2 DM.

REFERENCES

Betts, J., Muntean, W., Kim, D., Jorion, N., & Dickison, P. (2019). Building a method for writing clinical judgment items for entry-level nursing exams. *Journal of Applied Technology, 20*(S2), 21–36.

Burdeu, G., Lowe, G., Rasmussen, B., & Consedine, J. (2021). Clinical cues used by nurses to recognize changes in patients' clinical states: A systematic review. *Nursing and Health Sciences, 23*(1), 9–28.

Kavanaugh, J. M., & Sharpnack, P. A. (2021). A crisis in competency: A defining moment in nursing education. *Online Journal of Issues in Nursing, 26*(1). https://doi.org/10.3912/OJIN.Vol26No01Man02

National Council of State Boards of Nursing (NCSBN). (2023). *Next-Generation NCLEX®. NCLEX-RN® test plan.* NCSBN.

*Padilla, R. M., & Mayo, A. M. (2018). Clinical deterioration: A concept analysis. *Journal of Clinical Nursing, 27*, 1360–1368.

*Denotes classic reference

Note: Page numbers followed by *f* indicate figures and *t* indicate tables and *b* indicate boxes